AIDS:
Effective Health Communication for the 90s

AIDS:
Effective Health
Communication
for the 90s

Edited by

Scott C. Ratzan
Emerson College
Boston, Massachusetts

TAYLOR & FRANCIS

USA	Publishing Office:	Taylor & Francis
		1101 Vermont Avenue, N.W., Suite 200
		Washington, DC 20005-3521
		Tel: (202) 289-2174
		Fax: (202) 289-3665
	Distribution Center:	Taylor & Francis
		1900 Frost Road, Suite 101
		Bristol, PA 19007-1598
		Tel: (215) 785-5800
		Fax: (215) 785-5515
UK		Taylor & Francis Ltd.
		4 John St.
		London WC1N 2ET
		Tel: 071 405 2237
		Fax: 071 831 2035

AIDS: Effective Health Communication for the 90s

1 2 3 4 5 6 7 8 9 0   B R B R   9 8 7 6 5 4 3 2 1

This book was set in Times Roman by Taylor & Francis. The editors were Debbie Klenotic and Deena Williams Newman; the production supervisor was Peggy M. Rote; and the typesetter was Shirley J. McNett. Cover design by Michelle Fleitz.
Printing and binding by Braun-Brumfield, Inc.

A CIP catalog record for this book is available from the British Library.

∞ The paper in this publication meets the requirements of the ANSI Standard Z39.48-1984 (Permanence of Paper)

Library of Congress Cataloging-in-Publication Data

AIDS: effective health communication for the 90s / edited by Scott
   C. Ratzan.
      p. cm.
   Includes bibliographical references and index.

      1. AIDS (Disease)—United States—Prevention. 2. AIDS (Disease)—
   Prevention. 3. Communication in medicine. I. Ratzan, Scott C.
   RA644.A25A3594   1993
   362.1′969792—dc20   92-17933
                                                                  CIP

ISBN 1-56032-273-X

To Dr. John Marlier—

a colleague, teacher, and friend
      who motivates all of us to persevere, to strive,
                  and to settle for nothing but our very best.

Contents

Contributors   xiii
Foreword   xxi
Acknowledgments   xxv

INTRODUCTION   Health Communication and AIDS: Setting the
                Agenda   1
                Scott C. Ratzan
                References   11

PART 1: AIDS: EFFECTIVE HEALTH COMMUNICATION

CHAPTER 1   Developing Strategic Communication Campaigns for
                HIV/AIDS Prevention   15
                Edward W. Maibach, Gary L. Kreps,
                    and Ellen W. Bonaguro

                Principles for Strategic Communication Campaigns   18

Recommendations   30
Conclusions   31
References   32

CHAPTER 2   Health Communication as Negotiation: The COAST
               Model and AIDS   37
               Scott C. Ratzan

               The COAST Model of Negotiation   41
               The COAST Model of Negotiation Applied to a Patient
                    with Acquired Immune Deficiency Syndrome   47
               Conclusion   50
               References   51

CHAPTER 3   The Role of Care Partners in Managing AIDS
               Patients' Illness: Toward a Triadic Model of Health
               Care Delivery   55
               Eric G. Zook and Katherine I. Miller

               Health Care Provision for AIDS Patients   57
               The Role and Nature of the Care Partner's Involvement   63
               Possible Outcomes Associated with Care Partner Inclusion   67
               Conclusion   68
               References   69

CHAPTER 4   The Paradox of Accurate Information Increasing the
               Fear of AIDS   71
               Louis R. Franzini

               The Symptom Versus Syndrome Controversy   71
               The Paradox   75
               Manifestations of FRAIDS   79
               Negative Consequences of the Fear of AIDS   81
               Treatment Suggestions for the Young   83
               References   85

CHAPTER 5   Responses From the Street: ACT UP and Community
               Organizing Against AIDS   91
               Valeria Fabj and Matthew J. Sobnosky

               Overview   93
               Treatment and Support   97
               Safer Sex and Drug Use   98
               The Broader Agenda   103
               References   108

PART 2: AIDS: COMMUNICATION, EDUCATION, AND THE MEDIA

CHAPTER 6   Perceived Control in the Age of AIDS: A Review of
             Prevention Information in Academic, Popular, and
             Medical Accounts   113
             David A. Brenders and Lisaanne Garrett

             Perceived Control and Health Threat   115
             Perceived AIDS Risk Among Adolescents and College
                 Students   120
             Helplessness and Popular Accounts About AIDS   121
             Perceived Control and AIDS: How Well Do Popular
                 Accounts Activate Health Protection Motivation?   132
             References   136

CHAPTER 7   AIDS in the Media: Entertainment or Infotainment   141
             Nina Biddle, Lisa Conte, and Edwin Diamond

             Rock Hudson: Star Treatment   142
             Kimberly Bergalis: Feature Fodder   145
             Magic Johnson: "America Finds a Hero"   147
             Summing Up: AIDS News and "People" News   149
             References   150

CHAPTER 8   Crisis in Communication: Coverage of Magic
             Johnson's AIDS Disclosure   151
             J. Gregory Payne and Kevin A. Mercuri

             Purpose   152
             Method   153
             Results   154
             Discussion   163
             Summary   165
             References   165

PART 3: AIDS: THE CUTTING EDGE OF AWARENESS, ACTION, AND POLICY

CHAPTER 9   Freedom of the Press to Cover HIV/AIDS: A Clear
             and Present Danger?   175
             John Marlier

             The Problem   175
             What the Public Needs to Know About HIV/AIDS   177

Effects of Media Coverage of HIV/AIDS to Date   179
Development of an Effective Public Information Policy on
    HIV/AIDS   183
The Fourth Estate as Servant of the Public Interest   185
References   187

CHAPTER 10   Communication Disorders in Adults with AIDS   189
              Cynthia L. Bartlett

              Understanding Others' Messages   190
              Conveying Messages to Others   194
              Conclusion   200
              References   200

CHAPTER 11   Neurosurgical Professionalism and Care in the
              Treatment of Patients with Symptomatic AIDS   203
              Michael L. Levy, Joseph P. Van Der Meulen,
                  and Michael L. J. Apuzzo

              Historical Substrate   204
              Perceptions of AIDS in the Medical Community   205
              Laws Relating to Human Immunodeficiency Virus 206
              Responsibilities of Physicians   206
              The Concept of Trust   207
              Responsibilities of Physicians to Patients with Regard to
                  Information   209
              HIV Testing   209
              Neurological Manifestations of AIDS   209
              Conclusion   213
              References   213

CHAPTER 12   Adolescents and HIV: Two Decades of Denial   215
              Karen K. Hein, Jill F. Blair, Scott C. Ratzan,
                  and Denise E. Dyson

              Stereotypes, Fear, and Denial   216
              Fuel for the Future: The Adolescent AIDS Program 217
              Optimism and Activism in New York City   222
              Conclusion   227
              References   227
              Appendix 1: Straight to the Source   229
              Appendix 2: Who's Who Among American High School
                  Students: AIDS Survey of High Achievers, 1992 232

CHAPTER 13   Thinking Globally, Acting Locally: AIDS Action 2000
                 Plan   233
                 Scott C. Ratzan and J. Gregory Payne

                 The COAST Model—Health Communication as
                       Negotiation   235
                 AIDS Action 2000 Plan   237
                 Conclusion   248
                 References   248
                 Appendix   250

AFTERWORD   Communication and Prevention—They Are All We
                 Have   255
                 Scott C. Ratzan

                 Index   259

Contributors

Michael L. J. Apuzzo (M.D., Boston University) is an Edwin M. Todd/Trent H. Wells junior professor of neurological surgery at the University of Southern California School of Medicine. He is director of neurosurgery at the Kenneth R. Norris, Jr. Cancer Hospital and Research Institute and director of the Center for Stereotactic Neurosurgery and Associated Research. He has given over 60 invited professorships nationally and internationally, and has authored more than 200 scientific publications and eight volumes on topics related to stereotaxy, micro-operative techniques, brain neoplasia, and the future of neurosurgery. He has served on the editorial board of nine scientific journals and is currently editor-in-chief of *Neurosurgery*.

Cynthia L. Bartlett (Ph.D., University of Pittsburgh; M.A., Indiana University) is an assistant professor in the division of Communication Disorders at Emerson College. Prior to this, she held medical center-based clinical speech-language pathology positions. Her specialty is the acquired neuropathologies of communication in adults. She has lectured and presented workshops in her field around the United States, in Europe, and in the Soviet Union. She coauthored a chapter in *The Aging Brain,* and has published articles in *Brain and Language,* and in the *Proceedings of the Clinical Aphasiology Conference.*

Nina Biddle (M.A., New York University) is associate to the director at The Mercantile Library. She also writes for *New York Newsday,* WBAI Radio, and the *West Sider/Clinton Chelsea News* in New York City.

Jill F. Blair is special assistant to the deputy chancellor, New York City Public Schools, where she has worked with Chancellor Joseph A. Fernandez on the development of New York City Public Schools HIV/AIDS Education Program, including condom availability.

Ellen W. Bonaguro (Ph.D., Ohio University; M.A., University of Oregon) teaches organizational communication and health communication at Northern Illinois University. She has worked in the health care field as a director for a community health education center. She has written several articles focusing on various health behaviors, and has presented professional papers on both communication and health. Currently, she is a national trainer for the Association for the Advancement of Health Education for the HIV/AIDS Prevention Education Project. She has worked on the development and implementation of HIV/AIDS material for elementary, secondary, and college levels, and has designed a national training program that has been presented throughout the United States.

David A. Brenders (Ph.D., Purdue University; M.A., Ohio University) is an associate professor of communication studies at Emerson College. His research and teaching interests include health communication, interpersonal and relational communication, communication theory, research methods, and language philosophy. His publications have appeared in *The Quarterly Journal of Speech, Health Communication, Communication Yearbook 10, The Journal of Thought,* and *Mass Communication Review.* His article, "Fallacies in the Coordinated Management of Meaning," published in *The Quarterly Journal of Speech,* received the 1988 Golden Anniversary Monograph Award for outstanding scholarship from the Speech Communication Association.

Lisa Conte (M.A., New York University) is a financial editor and the assistant manager of publications for the Wall Street firm of Kidder, Peabody & Company.

Edwin Diamond (M.A., University of Chicago) is a professor of journalism at New York University, and writes the "Media" column for *New York Magazine.* He is the author of ten books, most of them focusing on the press in the political and social process. His most recent book is *The Media Show: The Changing Face of the News, 1985–1990* (MIT Press, 1991).

Denise E. Dyson (M.A., Emerson College) works in publishing and is a freelance writer in London, England. While completing her degree, she worked in the Public Relations department of Emerson College and as a contributing writer to Emerson's official publication, the *Beacon*. She has been an editor for *The Pacific Rim Business Journal* and has had articles published by Westcoast Publishing Ltd., both located in Vancouver, Canada.

Valeria Fabj (Ph.D., M.A., Northwestern University) is an assistant professor of communication studies at Emerson College, where she coordinates the division's "Teaching Scholar" program. While completing her dissertation at Northwestern University, entitled "Forgiveness and Tolerance in the Nuclear Age: The Rhetoric of the Nuclear-Weapon-Free Zone Movement in the United States," she taught courses in interpersonal communication and public speaking at the Kellogg Graduate School of Management at Northwestern University, at Loyola University of Chicago, and at Emerson College. She has delivered papers at the Speech Communication Association Convention, the Communication Theory and Methodology Mini-Conference, the Central States Speech Association Convention, the International Communication Association Convention, and the International Argumentation Conference.

Louis R. Franzini (Ph.D., University of Pittsburgh; M.A., University of Toledo) is a clinical psychologist, public speaker, and consultant on humor, psychology, and business, and professor of the psychology of humor at San Diego State University, where he has taught for 3 years. He has conducted research, published, and presented at national and international conferences and seminars on effective managerial strategies and the use of business to government agencies, school administrators, social organizations, and large corporations. He is the past president of Laughmasters, the Toastmasters International Club which specializes in humor. He has published more than 50 professional articles, ranging from children's learning to AIDS prevention strategies to identifying transsexuals. He currently is under contract with John Wiley & Sons, New York for a book on exotic syndromes called *Beyond The Bizarre*.

Lisaanne Garrett (M.A., Emerson College) has served as a mediator for small claims court in Quincy, Massachusetts, and is currently providing resolution consultation to various businesses and organizations. Her field of interest is mediation, negotiation, and conflict management.

Karen K. Hein (M.D., Columbia University's College of Physicians and Surgeons) is a professor of pediatrics and an associate professor of epidemiology and social medicine at Albert Einstein College of Medicine in New York City. In July 1987, she founded the Adolescent AIDS Program at Montefiore Medical Center in the Bronx. She currently works as director of the program. She was director of the division of Adolescent Medicine at Columbia P & S Babies Hospital from 1980–1984. She also has been on the faculty of the Albert Einstein College of Medicine. She currently is president of the Society for Adolescent Medicine. She has been the principal investigator of 20 grants; 16 of the most recent awards from foundations and federal agencies were related to HIV/ AIDS in adolescents. She serves as a consultant to many federal and health organizations, including the New York City Department of Health, Board of Education, Girls Club, and the American Medical Association. She is a manu- script and abstract reviewer for many medical journals and medical societies. She coauthored the book, *AIDS: Trading Fears For Facts,* a guide for young people, published by *Consumer Reports* Books in 1989. Through her activities in advocacy for youth, she has appeared on many television and radio shows, including special programs on AIDS in adolescence by *Nightline, MacNeil/ Lehrer News Hour,* Dr. Ruth, the *AIDS Quarterly, NBC Nightly News, The Today Show,* and National Public Radio. She has participated in a dozen AIDS educational videos for youth, and is a recipient of a 1989 U.S. federal govern- ment Assistant Secretary for Health Award for leadership in HIV service. She has written more than 100 articles, chapters and abstracts related to adolescent health, particularly focusing on high risk youth.

Gary L. Kreps (Ph.D., University of Southern California; M.A., University of Colorado) is a professor of communication studies at Northern Illinois Uni- versity. He has written many books and articles about the applications of com- munication research and theory in health care and organizational life. Recently, he coauthored the book *Health Communication Theory & Practice.* He chairs the International Communication Association's Health Communication Division and was the founding chairperson of the Speech Communication Association's Commission on Health Communication. He served as a senior research fellow with the National Cancer Institute (1985–1986), helping conduct a large-scale formative evaluation of the Physician Data Query cancer treatment information system and frame national policy for health information dissemination.

Michael L. Levy (M.D., University of California, San Francisco) is a clinical instructor in the Department of Neurological Surgery at the University of Southern California School of Medicine. He currently is completing his doctor- ate in psychology and biophysics.

Edward W. Maibach (Ph.D., M.P.H., Stanford University) is an assistant professor of behavioral science at Emory University School of Public Health. In 1991, he received the National Institute of Mental Health grant (1001MH49062-01) and grant 91061703 from the Association of Schools of Public Health and the Centers for Disease Control. He has been involved in HIV prevention research since 1987, conducting both experimental and evalua- tion research studies on effective communication strategies. He has written a number of articles and book chapters on the topic, including an examination of the implications of social cognitive theory for HIV prevention campaigns.

John Marlier (Ph.D., Michigan State University; M.A., West Virginia Univer- sity) is the divisional graduate coordinator, as well as an associate professor, in the Division of Communication Studies at Emerson College. Dr. Marlier is a communication theorist with an abiding concern for using theory in the real world. A coauthor of the GALILEO computer programs for metric multidimensional scaling, his scholarly work has appeared in such prestigious publications as the *Communication Yearbook* and *American Behavioral Scientist*. He is a founder of the Codman Square Community Development Corporation, and has served as a consultant to and/or director of numerous nonprofit organizations and government agencies.

Kevin A. Mercuri is a masters candidate in political communication in the Division of Communication Studies at Emerson College where he is a graduate member of the Emerson College Political News Study Group.

Katherine I. Miller (Ph.D., Annenberg School of Communication, University of Southern California; M.A., Michigan State University) is an associate professor of communication at Arizona State University. Her research concentrates on stress and burnout within caregiving occupations, the process of social support provision within these occupations, and empathic communication. Her work has appeared in a number of journals, including *Communication Monographs, Human Communication Research, Health Communication, Communication Research,* and the *Academy of Management Quarterly.*

J. Gregory Payne (Ph.D., M.A., University of Illinois at Urbana Champaign; M.P.A., John F. Kennedy School of Government, Harvard University) is chair and associate professor of the Division of Communication Studies at Emerson College. He is director of the Political News Study Group at Emerson and has written numerous articles and lectured extensively on political communication, docudrama, ethics, and public policy. He is the author of *Mayday: Kent State,* and the play *Kent State: A Requiem.* His most recent articles have appeared in *Political Communication and Persuasion, Journal of Ethnic Studies,* and *Health Communication.* He is the guest editor and a contributor to the *American Behavioral Scientist,* 1989 edition, entitled *Mediated Reality in the 1988 Campaign.* As a past NEH fellow, he is author of a theory of negation in American politics, provides critical commentary for the national press on campaigns, and has presented scholarly papers at conferences and symposiums throughout America and Great Britain.

Scott C. Ratzan (M.D., University of Southern California; M.P.A., John F. Kennedy School of Government, Harvard University; M.A., Emerson College) is an assistant professor of communication studies at Emerson College. He has lectured and chaired panels in health communication, negotiation, ethics, mediation, management, public relations, international dispute resolution, forensics, conflict management, health promotion, public policy, and political communication. He coauthored *Tom Bradley: The Impossible Dream,* the authorized biography of the mayor of Los Angeles, and has been published in *American*

Behavioral Scientist, Health Communication, and *The Journal of Ethnic Studies.* He coauthored legislation, the Massachusetts Drug-Free Workplace Act, for the Massachusetts Legislature and also has drafted legislation for an "AIDS Educated Workforce." Dr. Ratzan received the R.F.K. award for community service for directing the 1991 national conference, *Effective Health Communication in the 90s: The AIDS Crisis.* He has served as Medical Advisory Board chairman for *Vitality,* a leading national corporate health and wellness publication, and currently is an associate editor for the *Massachusetts Journal of Communication.* He is a consultant for business and governmental agencies, including the program design modeled after his wellness theory of POISE—Physical, Occupational, Intellectual, Social, and Emotional Balance—for *Cunard* and *the Queen Elizabeth 2.*

Matthew J. Sobnosky (Ph.D., M.A., University of Nebraska) is an assistant professor of communication studies at Emerson College. His area of expertise is the role of extremism in American politics and society. He has studied white supremacist groups on the far right, including the Ku Klux Klan and the Aryan Nations, as well as the use of extremist rhetoric by mainstream political groups and major party candidates. He also is interested in the role of religion in American politics, and has presented research at Speech Communication Association conventions and the Central States Communication Association Conventions. Dr. Sobnosky is actively involved in the forensics community and directed Emerson's nationally recognized forensics program to three national championships.

Joseph P. Van Der Meulen (M.D., Boston University) is vice president for Health Affairs and director of Allied Health Sciences at the University of Southern California. He is president of the Kenneth T. Norris Cancer Hospital and Research Institute and chairman of the Interim Governing Board of the USC University Hospital. He currently serves as chairman of the Association of Academic Health Centers and on the board of USC affiliated hospitals. He also is a board member of the Scott Newman Center, the Good Hope Medical Foundation, and Thomas Aquinas College, as well as a diplomat of the National Boards in Medicine and of the American Board of Psychiatry and Neurology. Best known for his research in the evaluation of patients with movement disorders, tremors, and loss of muscle control associated with Parkinson's disease and stroke, Dr. Van Der Meulen is a noted leader in the field of neurology who has held positions as chief physician of neurology at the Los Angeles County and USC Medical Center, as director of neurology residency training at Rancho Los Amigos Hospital and Children's Hospital of Los Angeles, as dean of the USC School of Medicine, and as associate professor of neurology and biomedical engineering at Case Western Reserve University. He is the author of many research articles published in scientific journals and medical textbooks. Dr. Van Der Meulen also has been actively involved in community service, having served on the State of California Governor's Task Force on Toxic Waste, and is the recipient of numerous awards.

Eric G. Zook (Ph.D., M.A., Michigan State University) is an assistant professor of speech communication at Pennsylvania State University. His research concentrates on the construction of illness meanings and responses via communication, the illness management systems of chronic/terminal illness, and the philosophy of communication. His work has appeared in a number of journals, including the *Management Communication Quarterly* and *Communication Research.*

Foreword

It was in Los Angeles in 1981 that the first warning signs appeared. Five cases of a rare pneumonia, previously seen only in individuals with severely depressed immune systems, were diagnosed at the UCLA Medical Center.

It was years later that the full scope of the disaster became known. An insidious virus, able to hide out in the body for years without producing symptoms, already had spread silently to hundreds of thousands of people by the time it gave that first hint of coming devastation.

As of 1990, 112,000 people in the county of Los Angeles alone had been infected with the HIV virus that causes AIDS. Sixty thousand of those people reside in the city of Los Angeles. To date, more than 5,000 city residents have developed AIDS, and well over 3,000 have died. We know that without treatment, the majority of those with the virus will develop symptomatic disease within a few short years. And we know that new cases of infection continue to occur each day.

In the city of Los Angeles, nearly half of all persons with AIDS are persons of color (African-American, Latino, Asian, and Native-American). A rapidly increasing percentage are women. The virus has gained a stronghold among intravenous drug users, high-risk youth, and adolescents in general.

But today we have ways to fight back. We know how the virus is spread. We know that infection can be prevented completely by the implementation of simple precautions. We know how to treat those who are infected in order to slow the progression of the disease and prevent some of the more serious complications. And we know that of primary importance are efforts to house and care for the sick in the most compassionate and effective ways possible.

We are no longer caught unaware. Today we have the tools to turn the corner on the greatest public health disaster of modern times. This book addresses the challenges we face as we plan our attack against HIV disease. An organized, honest, and urgent response at all levels of government throughout the 1990s must be marshaled if we are to combat the negative impact of the disease. We are thus required to review existing internal policies in a variety of areas, including confidentiality, workplace safety, discrimination, and education of employees and the community. And we must continue to update, expand, and apply our resources to govern and to create effective policies as the epidemic grows and changes.

The city of Los Angeles began this process in the 1980s, and has continued to search for creative ways to provide leadership in the battle against AIDS. In 1985, we created the City/County AIDS Task Force, which was the first local government organization to begin developing a coordinated response to AIDS. In June of that same year, the city held a series of hearings on the issue of AIDS discrimination—an issue that squarely pitted civil rights and medical facts against irrational fear and prejudice.

In August 1985, Los Angeles became the first jurisdiction in the nation to enact laws to prevent AIDS discrimination. Many cities and counties followed suit in the ensuing years. The atmosphere of safety and compassion created by this first concrete policy statement helped to improve the quality of life for thousands of people with the HIV virus and became even more important as HIV testing, and later treatment, became available.

By 1988, the AIDS crisis had grown so rapidly and significantly that every level of government came under pressure to respond in the areas of prevention, treatment, and care. Los Angeles became the first city in the country to hire a full-time AIDS coordinator to develop a city AIDS policy, a governing document which addressed a number of issues, including AIDS discrimination and the education of city employees as well as the community at large.

Since 1989, the city has committed more than $2.25 million in grant funding to AIDS-related facilities. In 1992, the city eliminated the red tape previously associated with gaining approval for facilities that serve persons with AIDS and the HIV virus.

Los Angeles has thus far been a leader in protecting the rights of persons with AIDS and the HIV virus. By leading with compassion, we can guarantee that each person with AIDS is treated with the dignity and respect he or she deserves. Every elected official and every community leader in this country must place a priority on this objective as we move into the 21st century. Our work must continue until a cure is found for the disease that inflicts thousands of our neighbors every day.

In this book, the editor and authors present appropriate ethical and effective communication strategies to prevent the spread of HIV. Readers from a variety of areas—medicine, communication, public health, and government—will find it helpful in elucidating the importance of necessary communication measures to explain the harms, risks, and preventive measures of HIV.

By integrating theory and practice through exploring the complexity of HIV prevention, *AIDS: Effective Health Communication for the 90s* promises to make an important contribution to our plight of combating this pandemic by offering innovative approaches to health communication that could benefit the overall health of our society for the 21st century.

Tom Bradley
Mayor, Los Angeles
August 1992

Acknowledgments

As of this writing, the fact that one in every 100 adult men and one in every 600 women in the United States are infected with the human immunodeficiency virus (HIV) or have acquired immune deficiency syndrome (AIDS) presents a challenge of greater importance for America than any event since World War II. Predictions by the National Commission on AIDS that three million years of life will be lost to AIDS by 1993, passing cancer, heart disease, and stroke victims with more than 200,000 individual deaths, clearly presents a communication challenge, considering at present there is no cure or vaccine on the horizon. Despite current educational efforts, the majority of Americans are still under the misconception that they are not at risk, while the federal government spends only 2% of the total designated federal AIDS funding on prevention.

This book is broad in scope, yet presents detailed analysis and actions necessary to confront the AIDS pandemic on every level of the communication realm. Hence, the list of distinguished authors represents researchers, educators, government officials, and physicians. The common theme of health communication clearly requires contribution from those schooled in a variety of fields. The contributors in this book approach this challenge from many areas, including communication, adolescent medicine, public administration, psychology, journalism, audiology, speech and language pathology, neurological surgery, preventive medicine, and public health, among others.

The idea for this book came to me as I was preparing a national conference entitled "Effective Health Communication in the 90s: The AIDS Crisis" held at Emerson College in September 1991. The impetus for the conference was the screening of the PBS/ABC Afterschool Special "In the Shadow of Love: A Teen AIDS Story," which was filmed during the summer of 1991 at Emerson's Boston campus. In the development of the conference schedule, it became increasingly clear that comprehensive information on AIDS and health communication was nonexistent. Suffice it to say, the intent of this book is to serve educators, prospective health care providers, communication scholars and students, practicing physicians and health care workers, and all those interested in the theory and practice of health communication to communicate effectively about the AIDS crisis by employing appropriate ethical studies, strategies, and instruments and thereby help combat the disease during this decade.

Many people contributed extensively to the ideals espoused in my development and conception of this book. My colleagues at Emerson College, the only college in the country devoted solely to the study of communication arts and sciences, encouraged this project from its inception. J. Gregory Payne, chair of the Division of Communication Studies, was extremely helpful in developing concepts and assimilating the ideals of education within the communication education continuum. Other colleagues in communication throughout the world also were helpful in contributing to the goal of the book, some with formal contributions. They include Philip Amato, Ina Ames, John Anderson, Cindy Bartlett, Lloyd Bitzer, David Brenders, Katherine Buckland, Larry Conner, Javier Curtis, Morton Dean, Edwin Diamond, William Elwood, Valeria Fabj, Donald Gidden, James Golden, Karen Hein, Nancy Hoar, Gary Kreps, Fred Kroger, Michael Levy, Jacqueline Liebergott, Walter Littlefield, Ed Maibach, John Marlier, Holly Massett, Ellen McDonough, Robert Norton, Helen Rose, Vito Silvestri, Matthew Sobnosky, Michael Jay Solomon, Teresa Thompson, Michael Weiler, and Chris Weir.

In the quest for cutting-edge material in the AIDS epidemic, my gratitude is expressed to Norman Stearns, dean of undergraduate medical education at Tufts University Medical School, who donated for my perusal his published and unpublished materials—reports of policy implications and educational paradigms, and formal correspondence with the government. His materials, along with the research associated with this book, will be donated to Emerson College for future use for students interested in health communication.

Personally, I could not have developed the COAST model of health communication as negotiation without the pioneering work by Roger Fisher in the field of negotiation. His mentoring in the field of negotiation since my initial coursework with him in 1987 at the Harvard Negotiation Project helped serve as the cornerstone in the win–win approach now applied to the field of health communication with COAST.

In addition, I would like to thank all of my students who applied the COAST model to their daily lives and final projects, further fine-tuning its presentation and parsimony. Jane Borrowman and Sara Burns, expert designers and graduate scholars in public relations, were phenomenal in their ability to accurately represent and help develop the COAST model visually.

Of course, I would like to thank all those who read chapter(s) at various stages of development: Brandon Arakelian, Karen Asuro, Christie Botelho, Philip Carson, Clare Ehling, Laura Goldin, Karen Levy, Laura McKeon, Caitlin Meehan, Jeremy Milner, Rebecca Miss, Janice Payne, Annabelle Rivero, and Diego Salazar. A special thanks also to department members David Calusdian and Ellen Gale, who helped coordinate and juggle the many events of a dynamic department while I worked on the book. In addition, graduate assistant Denise Dyson's continued patience in editing where appropriate and sharing of honest beliefs on the applicability of the submitted material are appreciated.

Finally, without friends and the ideals instilled in me by my parents, the labor of writing and the goals of the publication would not be worthwhile.

Scott C. Ratzan, MD

Health Communication and AIDS: Setting the Agenda

Scott C. Ratzan

The potential number of human lives—the creativity, compassion, and humanistic spirit that throughout history have prodded civilization forward—lost to acquired immune deficiency syndrome (AIDS) represents perhaps the greatest challenge to our future as we enter the 21st century. As communication technology webs humankind together as never before, we face an ever-growing pandemic reported in more than 152 countries worldwide, a pandemic with epicenters in the United States and Africa, with 204 and 150 cases per million respectively, which purportedly will cause more than 200,000 deaths in the United States alone. In an era celebrated by the promise of disappearing differences and a world opting for democracy, our shared nightmare is no longer nuclear destruction, but fear of a death more heinous than any humankind has witnessed since the advent of modern medicine. An age marked by international communication, negotiation, and cooperation must put such percepts to the test in a unified global effort to arrest the spread of the disease and to meet the ubiquitous challenges of the AIDS crisis.

When I first entered medical school in the early 1980s, AIDS was an evolving anomaly lacking a precise nomenclature and definition, with explana-

1

tions and descriptions limited to the identification of those affected, its dreaded AIDS-related complex (ARC), symptoms, sequelae and the resolution of its various related fatal diseases. Initially dubbed the "gay disease," AIDS was widely reported to be linked to Haitians. Such stereotypical constructs fanned out in the public in the effort to make sense of the growing new threat to humankind. Some concise explanations were supported by careful analysis of the target groups and research, and in 1983 the agent was identified. However, another succinct answer to what this strange disease amounted to was the erroneous yet widely held belief that specific target groups were victims of God's wrath.

As the popular media explored AIDS in slick soundbite commentary, the health community's research went beyond the headline mentality. After arriving at a widely agreed on definition of AIDS and discovering the etiological agent, researchers turned their focus on a cure for the afflicted as well as development of a vaccine. The past decade has been marked by further deductive and inductive inquiry and refinement of definitions of particular risk behaviors that promote the spread of AIDS, as well as the targeting of particular groups with specific, albeit controversial, information designed to limit their exposure to the deadly virus. Yet, despite having the technology for instantaneous communication in the 1990s, the global force of which has swept away totalitarian coups, outworn dogmas, and borders of the past, we truly suffer from a failure to communicate effectively the message of the AIDS menace. Today, we lack a coherent and effective communication campaign with specific and serious media strategies to meet this challenge and to help get the message out on how to limit the spread of AIDS. Perhaps we can term this an "acquired deficiency" of those in various sectors responsible for preventative messages.

What we have learned in the first decade of AIDS, human immunodeficiency virus (HIV), human T-cell lymphotropic virus Type III (HTLV-III), and ARC is that the answers we seek are not limited to experts in health and medicine. Insight and leadership by government and politicians have resulted in little pioneering policymaking. The AIDS crisis, like none before it, demands a strong working relationship among experts in effective health and political communication and education.

The chapters in this book, written by experts throughout the United States, are an attempt to provide timely insight on the political, educational, and health communication issues of AIDS. Common health communication themes are structured within the chapters—problems that are inherent in the status quo's inept attempt to deal with the AIDS crisis, the successes and failures of past media campaigns targeted to halt the spread of the virus, and the ethical and moral implications of our past and future efforts to quell the disease's deadly march throughout the global population.

In an era marked by economic recession and cutbacks at all levels of government, we face the task of educating the public on this national health security risk with fewer and fewer resources at our disposal. Presently, sporadic campaigns on AIDS are often obscured by the media frenzy over objections to the candid and precise language and visual representations used by other groups. Condom campaigns are criticized for promoting sexual promiscuity and identifying high-risk behaviors rather than supported as a vital role in preventing the spread of HIV. Our nation's leaders have opted to preach the findings of polling pundits, using the age-old appeal to "just say no" and to adopt abstinence, rather than spearhead a realistic effort to develop strategies that will educate the public on how to lessen their risk of contracting AIDS. The federal government allocated $247.7 million for AIDS prevention in 1990; however, only 15% of the funding went toward prevention, while $117.6 million was used for patient counseling, testing, and partner notification, despite the fact that such an approach has historically failed to decrease the spread of other sexually transmitted diseases, such as syphilis and gonorrhea (Kong, October 2, 1991).

The common denominator of the chapters in this book is effective health communication and the development of promising strategies to help educate the individual, and thereby all members of the public, about AIDS. We hope our insights will be useful to the present generation, as it attempts to cope with the onslaught of AIDS cases and the disease's tremendous financial and human costs. One of our goals is to provide constructive criticism of past efforts to meet the challenge of AIDS. Alternative strategies are presented, along with a synopsis of blueprints for the future.

Because of it reliance on strong, trusting, co-active relationships, the field of health communication is poised to play a key role in the strategizing of message content, selection of appropriate media, audience analysis, and the timing of messages on AIDS to the public. Grounded in the strong relationship that is demanded between the health communication and medical communities, future efforts should examine in detail what is implicitly explored in this book, a balance of POISE—*p*hysical, *o*ccupational, *i*ntellectual, *s*ocial/*s*piritual and *e*motional approaches to the AIDS crisis. At a time when the medical community's attention is focused on cures, treatment, and vaccines, experts in health communication must take the lead to ensure that educational information is communicated efficiently, ethically, and efficaciously to the public.

Effective health communication, focused on disease prevention and health promotion, is a mixture of art and science. However, the traditional provider, the physician, is generally trained and educated in the hard sciences with only limited or no exposure to the humanities and arts (Ling, 1989). Nichols (1964) aptly warned of the product of such a science-oriented educational process in her pioneering work in rhetorical theory: "The humanities without science are blind, but science without the humanities may be vicious" (p. 18). It is clear that the AIDS pandemic demands that a devoted scientific community work closely in concert with humanistic and ethical experts in the communication arts in crafting effective rhetorical messages and campaigns.

Western medicine's perspective and infatuation with reporting health by "ruling out" particular disease, disorder, or illness in the quest to make accurate diagnosis has traditionally contributed to the difficulty in defining health communication. Although many humans have a definition of illness—whether it be "sickness of body or mind" (*American Heritage Dictionary*, 1982), the "night side of life" (Sontag, 1978), or another—few have a clear definition of health. Health communication—promotion, prevention, policy, price, public health, population, education, etc.—often is viewed as a multidimensional discipline in its infancy in higher education and therefore faces a similar dilemma. Definitions and scope are subjects of discussion and debate.

The synergistic nature of health and communication is rooted in the writings of ancient Greece. The Homeric ideal outlined the virtues of being a speaker of words and doer of deeds, as well as the need to be of sound body and mind. Plato and Aristotle devoted large sections of their writings to outlining regimens not only for rhetoric's role in society, but also for the achievement of balance between the mind, body, and spirit. Plato's philosopher-king was a special rhetorician—a physician of the soul.

On the contemporary scene, reflective of interpersonal communication's interest in health communication is evident in Costello's (1977) study of how patients process health- and medical-related information into a meaningful context. Costello identified four areas as strategic to effective communication: diagnosis, cooperation, counseling, and treatment. Thompson's (1984) research confirmed the importance of effective communication in the health area: "Evidence indicates that communication can have a *direct* impact on patient pain and recovery" (p. 4).

Definitions of health also reflect widespread interest and expanding areas of influence for health communication. Northouse and Northouse (1985) and Friedman and DiMatteo (1979) noted the infancy of the health communication area and its spillover into health psychology, medical sociology, biomedical communication, behavioral medicine, behavioral health, and medical communication.

Kreps and Thornton's (1984) definition of health communication is "human interaction in the health care process" (p. 2). Cassata (1980) described health communication as "the study of communication parameters (levels, functions, and methodologies) applied in health situations and contexts" (p. 2). Northouse and Northouse (1985) defined health communication as "health-related transactions between individuals who are attempting to maintain health and avoid illness. . . . Health communication is a subset of human communication that is concerned with how individuals in a society seek to maintain health and deal with health related issues" (pp. 4–6). In 1988, Kreps described health communication as "pervasive, ubiquitous, and equivocal" (p. 239).

Noting its popularity as a field of study, Ling (1989) commented that "while health communication is now an established subject in a growing number of schools of communication, it has yet to become a regular course in training institutions for health personnel'' (p. 259). Furthermore, Ling identified the typical home for such research, ''in institutions in which health communication is taught, it deals with interpersonal and group communication'' (p. 259).

A purpose of this book is to expand the realm of health communication to include communication that traditionally has been associated with advocacy, deliberation, and the political arena due to the impact of such areas in the emerging field of health communication. Given the importance and crucial role of the communication process and mass media in packaging information and disseminating it to various publics, it is paramount that health communication is viewed as concerned not only with the health of individual members of society, but also with the well-being of the community, nation, and humankind. Such an approach to policymaking in the health area can focus on elimination of the bureaucratic maze and scientific jargon that research demonstrates tends to dominate health communication from a more interpersonal perspective.

Health communication for the 1990s and for the 21st century should be viewed as ''the process and effect of employing ethical persuasive means in human health care decision-making.'' In contrast to earlier definitions, this construct is not based solely on health promotion or the avoidance of illness. It is a broader, neo-Aristotelean approach that views health communication strategies as dependent on publics, contexts, timing, and the traditional elements of the rhetorical act. This approach values scientific facts as its data, but places at its apex the effective and ethical employment of Aristotle's artistic proofs and audience analysis in promoting the public good through effective communication.

This view of health communication has value on both the individual and mass public level. On a provider–patient level, it prods the physician to expand beyond the favored scientific model, beyond the use of hypothesis and evidence in the American medicine model, to a more humanistic and personal approach. Ethically based, it promotes education and understanding built on quantitative and qualitative support. This view is consistent with that offered by Edgar, Hammond, and Freimuth (1989), who outlined the following pertinent areas of concern in the formation of an effective campaign against AIDS: ''Identifying target audiences, using credible sources, using effective repetition, focusing on simple skills, balancing logic and emotion, and judiciously using fear and humor'' (p. 9).

This expanded definition of health communication carries increased ethical responsibility of all of those agents involved in the health communication process: physician/health care providers and patient, family, and group communication; media sources and publics; leaders (political, occupational, intellectual, spiritual, social, athletic, emotional, and arts and entertainment figures) and their respective followers—all are co-active participants in the synergistic communication process. The effectiveness of health communication has intrinsic as well as extrinsic benefits. The reception of persuasive and relevant health information is the primary social process that can empower individuals to take charge of their own health; hence, health communication is a crucial element to the preventative approach to public health (Reardon, 1988).

Furthermore, this active approach is a necessity given an aging population and the danger of fatal transmissible diseases such as AIDS. Key components of this new perspective include awareness, diagnosis, counseling, cooperative decision making, education, prevention, life-style adjustments, pain relief, rehabilitation, and relationship building. It is clear that traditional perspectives must give way to new approaches as we begin a new century with our quest to treat and cure new diseases like AIDS, as well as to seek answers to those illnesses and infirmities that have plagued humankind since our beginning. Pepper (1989) highlighted the paradox we now face in a world of technological advancement, where there is so little hope for those with a disease that threatens life as we know it: "Certainly, epidemics were not considered a possibility in a civilized world—AIDS has changed this way of thinking. Modern medicine was caught off guard, and so far has been unable to solve the problem" (p. 264).

During this epidemic we must seek not only a cure and treatment but a new way of communicating effective and ethical health policy and prevention to our neighbors who share the global village.

The exploration by the different authors in this book of the role of the media, interpersonal relationships, advertising, popular/academic/scientific articles, public service announcements and brochures, computer-based interactions, and government in the AIDS crisis clearly demonstrates the complex interaction of the different systems at work in reaching the intended audience on health issues.

Part I presents the framework for effective health communication. In the first chapter, following a description of the challenges inherent in a health communication campaign, Maibach, Kreps, and Bonaguro present ideas for implementation of a wide range of different prevention messages and campaign strategies targeted at several audiences to curtail the spread of AIDS. Their proposed Strategic Health Communication Campaign model, with five major stages and 12 key steps, incorporates the many facets of the health communication agenda. Following the description of the important preplanning of goals and objectives of HIV/AIDS education, the authors lay the theoretical foundation of health communication in exchange and behavioral theory, identifying the vast application and background necessary for an efficient HIV/AIDS campaign. Their analysis of communication, in which they draw on their own extensive individual and collaborative research, identifies audience analysis and segmentation, formative research, and channel analysis as necessary prerequisites to implementation of a communication strategy. The marketing mix, process evaluation, macrosocial considerations, long-term involvement, and institutionalization all contribute to the goal of long-lived change, which constantly should be evaluated and reoriented.

Maibach et al.'s final 12 recommendations provide excellent examples for the design and implementation of strategic HIV/AIDS campaigns. The first recommendation attests to the extensive exploration of proposed ideas in subsequent chapters: "No one campaign or general campaign strategy is likely to achieve the diverse demands of HIV/AIDS prevention. A wide range of different campaigns, using different communication strategies and messages targeted at different audiences, will have to be employed to help curtail the spread of HIV/AIDS."

In Chapter 2, I offer a new approach for individual health providers to effectively communicate health issues to the appropriate public. The ethical and effective co-active communication process between the patient and the provider serves as the foundation for the COAST model for health communication as negotiation. In summary, COAST mandates that during the health communication encounter, both parties in the dyad *communicate* a particular medical exigence and brainstorm all available *options*. This procedure is followed by a focus on identifying *alternatives* that could/should be employed to reach a common goal based on application and analysis of specific *standards*. An essential element that should be pervasive throughout the various phases of the dyadic encounter is *trust*, helping to build relationships that are a positive prediction of the degree of compliance and overall satisfaction. Following paradigmatic, descriptive, and schematic representations of COAST, the model is applied to an AIDS patient's case in which the communication techniques of two physicians are compared.

The intrinsic value of the relationship between patient and physician is further highlighted by Zook and Miller, who explore care partners as an important addition to the treatment context in Chapter 3. The physician–patient relationship, concepts of illness, and the locus of care are appropriately discussed with both theoretical and case study analysis. The authors contend that "the traditional physician–patient model of health care delivery has served society well; however, it is dysfunctional for the social situations that are associated with the greater chronicity of illness." They argue that with regard to the AIDS crisis, this premise necessitates care partners as a part of a health communication/delivery triad. "The need for care partners to negotiate legitimate forms of involvement with both the patient and the physician is evident from the centrality of the patient–physician relationship in health care delivery." Zook and Miller further identify the appropriate application of a negotiation model to the COAST health communication context: "It is likely that if such relationships are to succeed, a contract model of health care provision is necessary."

Communicating accurate information on AIDS in the 1990s is the subject of Franzini's exploration of the fear of AIDS in Chapter 4. Franzini aptly describes the fear of AIDS (FRAIDS) as perpetuated by all areas of American society, from the individual health professional to the legal system. This FRAIDS manifestation suppresses improvements in health care quality, which in turn hinders HIV treatment. As a psychologist, Franzini suggests the use of appropriate "standard methods of psychotherapy and behavior therapy in treating FRAIDS." He posits the shared responsibility of journalists, the government, and the health care community to prevent AIDS disinformation. Various potential modalities to reach the public are presented, from television dramas to rock music. This chapter elucidates many studies, including a recent study in which Franzini described sexual and social behavioral changes of university students.

In the last chapter in Part I, rhetorical scholars Fabj and Sobnosky address the communication efforts of the AIDS Coalition to Unleash Power (ACT UP) with various audiences. Fabj and Sobnosky's analysis sheds light on the goals of an effective health communication campaign's efforts to halt the spread of AIDS through safer sex and drug use. In addition, an expanded agenda for social reform is presented as an ultimate solution to the AIDS epidemic. The description of the ACT UP's actions, from displaying messages at major league baseball games ("No glove, no love. . . . AIDS is no ball game") to confronting the mainstream American media (producing a video in response to an erroneous *Cosmopolitan* article on women and AIDS) enlightens the reader to the challenges of activist groups. This examination highlights ACT UP's rhetoric as representing "those who cannot speak, whose words are insignificant in today's society because they are people of color, intravenous drug users, prostitutes, or prisoners." Finally, they conclude with heuristic applicability that ACT UP and AIDS activism "will continue to change the nature of medical care (including cancer, Alzheimer's disease, and other diseases) in profound ways."

Part II focuses on the magazine coverage of AIDS during the first decade of discovery. In Chapter 6, Brenders and Garrett explore health communication control theories to examine the control-relevant premises embedded in popular accounts of AIDS prevention from 1987 to 1991. Their analysis suggests that early popular accounts of AIDS risk and prevention strategies emphasized a high degree of helplessness and loss of personal freedom. As the AIDS epidemic grew, press coverage became more balanced, but many accounts are still ambivalent about the efficacy of prevention approaches. Nonetheless, Brenders and Garrett conclude that despite an infatuation with the sensationalizing of AIDS in which many popular accounts of AIDS have been presented, the public is still significantly uneducated: "There is still enough doubt and confusion to incite the fears of the 'worried well' yet encourage the complacency of those wishing to depersonalize their risk."

In Chapter 7, Biddle, Conte, and Diamond describe media coverage of AIDS cases in celebrities such as Rock Hudson and Magic Johnson as medical "infotainment sometimes and uninformed hysteria at others." Their analysis reveals the euphemisms and evasions of modern-day journalism, and evolves into a discourse of biographical star treatment and the turning of the Kimberly Bergalis case into feature fodder. Finally, in an analysis of the Magic Johnson case, Biddle et al. identify three stages of media coverage of celebrity AIDS cases: surprise, then heroic treatment, followed by second thoughts of the media. The success of such sensationalism, the authors conclude, make it easy for "the media to avoid learning the lessons they might have learned after 10 years of the AIDS experience."

A content analysis of press coverage of the Magic Johnson incident is presented by Payne and Mercuri in Chapter 8. In their study, Payne and Mercuri analyzed the press coverage in different regions of the country for 4 weeks after Johnson disclosed he has AIDS. They found that Johnson, looked on by millions as a superstar, experienced a debunking of his ethos in the wake of the news coverage of his frequent sexual encounters. The authors conclude that even with such media scrutiny, Johnson's credibility persevered as he took the initiative to become a spokesperson against the AIDS epidemic. The authors suggest that given the pervasive global impact of AIDS, serious questions on journalistic ethics in reporting those diagnosed demand careful study and further investigation. This is especially significant given *USA Today's* threat in April 1992 to disclose his HIV status that ultimately forced Arthur Ashe to publicly announce he has AIDS.

The final part of the book describes the cutting edge of AIDS awareness and preventative action. In Chapter 9, Marlier suggests that many public policy issues remain unresolved and undebated after a decade of media coverage. He suggests that this "represents a threat to the economic as well as the medical security of the nation and the world." The arguments in this chapter on the discrimination and the omission of those with HIV from the American policy-making agenda calls for a public information policy that the author believes "offers great hope of stimulating effective individual and collective responses to the threat of HIV/AIDS than that which has occurred to date." Marlier's support for the public interest dates back to Oliver Wendell Holmes with a conclusion of a need for a consistent HIV policy to promote media coverage with agenda-setting and ethical omission and insertion.

In Chapter 10, speech–language pathologist Bartlett presents an important analysis of communication with individuals with impaired communication ability. Clearly, medical decision making and patient comprehension, insight, and judgment are often impaired in people with AIDS as HIV crosses the blood–brain barrier. Bartlett offers specific recommendations for the health care provider to maximize their effectiveness in communicating with people with AIDS. In addition, language disorders (aphasic and nonaphasic), as well as dementia are discussed in the chapter, with suggestions for dealing with a constellation of symptoms. "Attending to the communicative needs of these individuals has the potential to assist in ensuring quality health care," Bartlett concludes, "and is central to the preservation of dignity."

Complementing specific actions by the health care provider in people with AIDS is Levy and Apuzzo's description of neurosurgical professionalism and care in symptomatic AIDS patients in Chapter 11. These authors present a number of examples of diagnosis, surgical management, and treatment of HIV-positive patients. The examples of their work at the Los Angeles County/ University of Southern California Medical Center—the largest teaching hospital in the United States—suggest professional perceptions of AIDS in the medical community as well as of HIV transmission and confidentiality. Levy and Apuzzo caution that "education of the physician and general population is essential to return AIDS to its categorization as an infectious disease and return patient care to the level of the patient–physician relationship." In addition to emphasizing the necessity of education, this chapter describes hospital-based policies that do not adequately address the epidemic. In fact, the authors conclude, "The fear of both the disease and its political ramifications has compromised physicians' ability to provide care."

Hein, Blair, Ratzan, and Dyson focus on the adolescent AIDS population in Chapter 12, describing the scope and magnitude of lessons learned during the first decade of the HIV/AIDS pandemic. The information provided can be applied by educators, counselors, physicians, and public health professionals when designing programs to reach the fastest growing population of HIV incidence. By examining the research of the New York City Adolescent AIDS Program, the authors provide more comprehensive understanding of the needs and conflicts of the adolescent that will aid efforts to develop appropriate strategies for addressing these issues. The newly implemented New York City school system plan is explored as a potentially replicable program. The structure and procedures defined by the plan combine to offer "a powerful weapon, fighting the epidemic on three levels, through the insistence of factual awareness, the development of necessary communication skills, and the expansion of available services." A survey that highlights the attitudes and behaviors of the adolescent community concerning HIV/AIDS is included, along with a case study of a sexual education/HIV/AIDS prevention course conducted in a Connecticut high school.

In the final chapter, the idea of thinking globally and acting locally is presented from a perspective incorporating many of the ideals of effective health communication presented in previous chapters. Along with my colleague Payne, I assimilate ideals of communication, medicine, and public administration into a working model to help providers and patients, government and media, as well as infected and uninfected citizens understand the virus and potentiate the effectiveness of their health and well-being. Furthermore, an AIDS Action 2000 Plan is presented to assist in controlling the spread of HIV. It is rooted in proactive communication, more specifically that detailed in the health communication as negotiation (COAST) model outlined in Chapter 2. Beginning the campaign from the level of the healthy individual through the various spheres of family, group, media, government, and health polity, the AIDS Action 2000 plan comes full circle back to the individual level, the AIDS patient.

The shared goal of the authors as well as the editor of this book is to nourish a humane understanding of an epidemic that challenges the scientific know-how as we enter the next millennium.

REFERENCES

American Heritage Dictionary. (1982). Boston, MA: Houghton Mifflin.

Cassata, D. M. (1980). Health communication theory and research: A definitional overview. In D. Nimmo (Ed.), *Communication yearbook 4* (pp. 583–589). New Brunswick, NJ: Transaction Books.

Costello, D. E. (1977). Health communication theory and research: An overview. In B. Ruben (Ed.), *Communication yearbook 1* (pp. 557–567). New Brunswick, NJ: Transaction Books–International Communication Association.

Edgar, T., Hammond, S. L., & Freimuth, V. S. (1989). The role of the mass media and interpersonal communication in promoting AIDS-related behavioral change. *AIDS and Public Policy Journal, 4*(1), 3–9.

Friedman, H. S., & DiMatteo, M. R. (1979). Health care as an interpersonal process. *Journal of Social Issues, 35,* 1–11.

Ling, J. C. (1989). New communicable diseases: A communication challenge. *Health Communication, 1,* 253–260.

Kreps, G. L., & Thornton, B. C. (1984). *Health communication: Theory and practice.* New York: Longman.

Kreps, G. (1988). The pervasive role of information in health and health care: Implications for health communication policy. In J. Anderson (Ed.), *Communication yearbook 11* (pp. 238–276). Newbury Park, CA: Sage.

Kong, D. (1991, October 2). AIDS group faults CDC in effort to halt disease. *Boston Globe.*

Nichols, M. H. (1963). *Rhetoric and criticism.* Baton Rouge, LA: Louisiana State University Press.

Northouse, P. G., & Northouse, L. L. (1985). *Health communication: A handbook for health professionals.* Englewood Cliffs, NJ: Prentice-Hall.

Pepper, G. L. (1989). AIDS and its metaphors. *Health Communication, 1,* 261–264.

Reardon, K. K. (1988). The role of persuasion in health promotion and disease prevention: Review and commentary. In J. Anderson (Ed.), *Communication yearbook 11* (pp. 277–297). Newbury Park, CA: Sage.

Sontag, S. (1978). *Illness as metaphor.* New York: Farrar, Straus & Giroux.

Thompson, T. L. (1984). The invisible helping hand: The role of communication in the health and social service professions. *Communication Quarterly, 32*(2), 148–163.

Part One

AIDS: Effective Health Communication

Chapter One

Developing Strategic Communication Campaigns for HIV/AIDS Prevention

Edward W. Maibach
Gary L. Kreps
Ellen W. Bonaguro

Strategic health communication campaigns are currently the best available public health strategy for curtailing the spread of human immunodeficiency virus (HIV)/acquired immune deficiency syndrome (AIDS), considering that there are no effective techniques for vaccinating the public against the disease (Brown, 1991; Edgar, Hammond, & Freimuth, 1989; Nussbaum, 1989; Reardon, 1990). Strategic campaigns must be designed to help targeted audiences recognize their HIV risk, convey appropriate strategies for minimizing risk, and motivate audiences to implement these strategies (Atkin, 1981; Kreps & Maibach, 1991; Rubinson & Alles, 1984; Tones, 1986). Health communication is a crucial element in disease prevention and health promotion campaigns because the provision of relevant and persuasive health information is the primary social process that can empower individuals to take charge of their own health (Kreps, 1988; Reardon, 1988).

Effective health communication campaigns are deceivingly complex (Portnoy, Anderson, & Eriksen, 1989). Health communication planners cannot assume that mere exposure to relevant health information will lead directly to desired behavior change (Edgar et al., 1989; Tones, 1986). The tenuous and multifaceted relationship between communication and long-term behavior change must be addressed (Flay, DiTecco, & Schlegel, 1980). A well-designed communication campaign can play an instrumental role in facilitating behavior change, but the behavior change process takes considerable time. Therefore, to be highly effective, communication campaigns must consider a long-term perspective. Campaign planners must take into consideration the nature of the health risk, the specific audience targeted, and the behavioral changes they wish to encourage audience members to adopt when making difficult decisions about the best message strategies and communication channels for reaching and influencing targeted audiences (Flay & Burton, 1990; Rogers & Storey, 1987). Effective campaigns use a variety of appropriate channels of communication to provide relevant publics with persuasive information that will facilitate recognition and evaluation of health risks and encourage the adoption of prescribed health behaviors to reduce these risks (Kreps, 1988).

HIV/AIDS campaigns, in particular, are complicated by several factors. First, because the individuals who are at greatest risk for HIV/AIDS contagion are diverse, both culturally and behaviorally, it is unlikely that campaign planners can develop a general set of effective campaign messages that will work equally well with all audiences. There are three primary audiences at highest risk for infection that are currently targeted by most HIV/AIDS prevention campaigns: (a) homosexual and bisexual men, (b) drug users who share needles and syringes (and their sex partners), and (c) high-risk groups who are particularly hard to reach through the usual health care and educational channels (such as runaway youths, men who have sex with other men but do not consider themselves to be homosexual, individuals who exchange sex for drugs or money, prisoners, and men and women who do not know they are at risk because of their partner's risky behaviors; Rugg, O'Reilly, & Galovotti, 1990). To further complicate prevention efforts, these groups are not mutually exclusive; individuals often move from one category to another as their behaviors or other factors change. Effective HIV/AIDS prevention campaigns targeted to these different audiences must set different objectives, use different communication strategies, and have different measures of success (Rugg et al., 1990).

In addition to targeting populations who currently engage in high-risk behavior, HIV/AIDS communication campaigns should be designed to discourage others who do not currently engage in risky behavior from adopting behaviors that would put them at risk. For example, HIV/AIDS prevention campaigns need to target adolescents to prevent the initiation of high-risk behavior. These efforts need to be continued with reminder campaigns that build on previous campaigns as members of the target groups move through their teen and adult years.

We contend that a wide range of different prevention messages and campaign strategies targeted at several audiences have to be employed to help curtail the spread of HIV/AIDS. This perspective on HIV/AIDS campaigns is supported by Gilchrist (1990), who suggested that at least three different types of intervention approaches are necessary for the prevention of HIV/AIDS with youths, depending on the target population's potential risk of transmitting or acquiring the virus: The first is a *universal* approach that is broad in scope and entails dissemination of general information about AIDS and decision making to a wide audience, primarily through the schools. The second is a *selective* approach that is more intensive and emphasizes self-esteem and communication skill building by employing peer-led stress management programs to be used with youth whose risk for AIDS is high, such as those in areas where the rates of drug use, teenage pregnancy, or sexually transmitted disease are high. The third is a sustained and highly personalized *indicated* behavior change approach for adolescents who are already engaging in high-risk behaviors, to be delivered through programs with access to high-risk youth (such as shelters, social service agencies, support groups, and detention centers).

Because HIV/AIDS campaigns invariably concern personal, habitual, and often taboo topics such as sexual practices and illegal drug use, communicating about these topics can be difficult. Certain messages about sexual practices and illegal drug use are likely to be perceived as inappropriate and in bad taste by many publics, suggesting that campaign planners will have to carefully craft prevention messages to avoid censorship and unanticipated and unwanted consequences among other audiences. Particular messages regarding safe sex behavior or the use of clean needles and syringes may be perceived as condoning or encouraging sexual practices and drug use. Campaign planners need to take into consideration that certain campaign messages targeted at a specific group may create effects in groups that are not targeted, which may result in positive and/or negative outcomes. These potential influences of HIV/AIDS campaign messages can often be constructively addressed by involving representatives of many different community groups in the early stages of the message planning process. Because it is very difficult to persuade people to change personal and entrenched behaviors such as sexual practices and drug abuse, campaign planners have to develop powerful and personally meaningful communication strategies for motivating targeted audiences to change habitual behaviors.

To target at-risk populations with information meant to educate, motivate, and enable risk reduction behavior, effective health communication campaigns often employ a wide range of message strategies and communication channels, such as interpersonal counseling, support groups, lectures, workshops, newspaper and magazine articles, self-help approaches, computer-based information systems, school- and primary care-based educational programs, billboards, pamphlets, posters, radio/television programs, and public service announcements. Modern campaigns have become increasingly dependent on integrating interpersonal, group, organizational, and mediated communication to effectively disseminate health information to specific at-risk populations (Atkin & Wallack, 1990; Reardon & Rogers, 1988).

To help address several of the critical issues in strategic HIV/AIDS campaign design, we offer a Strategic Health Communication Campaign model that includes five major stages and 12 key issues for consideration in guiding campaign development and implementation. Our model is informed by the Stages in Health Communication model developed by the National Cancer Institute (Office of Cancer Communications, 1989), and by discussions of social marketing by Lefebvre and Flora (1988) and Maibach (1991). The first stage is *planning*, in which two issues are addressed: campaign objectives and consumer orientation. The second stage is *use of theory*, in which a variety of theoretical perspectives useful in guiding campaign design are described, including exchange theory and various behavioral theories. The third stage, *communication analysis*, includes three components for consideration in developing communication strategies: audience analysis and segmentation, formative research, and channel analysis and selection. In the fourth stage, *implementation*, we describe four issues for consideration in conducting campaigns: marketing mix, process evaluation, macrosocial conditions, and long-term involvement and campaign institutionalization. The fifth stage is *evaluation and reorientation*, which includes the use of outcome evaluation and its implications for ongoing conduct of the campaign and development of future campaigns. Outcome evaluations provide campaign planners with information about the relative success of campaigns and identify areas for further intervention, which leads campaign planners back to the first stage of the model (see Figure 1). In this chapter, we describe the model in the context of designing effective HIV/AIDS health communication campaigns.

PRINCIPLES FOR STRATEGIC COMMUNICATION CAMPAIGNS

Stage 1: Planning

Before a health communication campaign can be initiated, a great deal of planning must occur. There are many questions that need to be answered before an effective campaign can be designed and implemented. Who is at risk? Is a health information campaign an appropriate vehicle for addressing this risk? What campaign objectives are most realistic and cost-effective for this health issue and target audience? What are the target audience's needs and cultural orientations? The planning stage of strategic health communication campaigns provides the campaign planner with answers to these important questions.

Campaign Objectives Individuals planning strategic HIV/AIDS campaigns must set realistic goals for influencing public health behaviors. Current

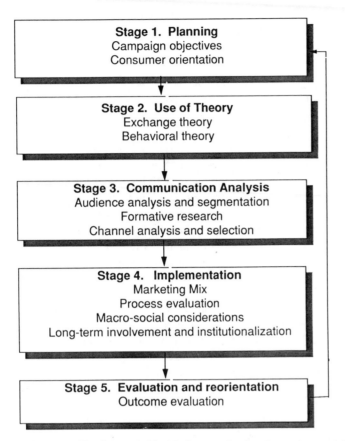

Stage 1. Planning
Campaign objectives
Consumer orientation

Stage 2. Use of Theory
Exchange theory
Behavioral theory

Stage 3. Communication Analysis
Audience analysis and segmentation
Formative research
Channel analysis and selection

Stage 4. Implementation
Marketing Mix
Process evaluation
Macro-social considerations
Long-term involvement and institutionalization

Stage 5. Evaluation and reorientation
Outcome evaluation

Figure 1-1   The Strategic Health Communication Campaign model.

research suggests that most campaigns have only moderate and intermediate effects on the health behaviors of target audience members (Flora, Maccoby, & Farquhar, 1989; McCombs & Shaw, 1972; Rogers & Storey, 1987). Rather than expecting campaigns to result in dramatic and permanent changes in health behavior, campaign planners should view their goals as a hierarchy of effects ranging from becoming aware of the health issue, to becoming knowledgeable about the issue, to adopting behavior changes, and finally to maintaining the changes (McGuire, 1989).

Because HIV/AIDS campaigns have the potential to influence a wide variety of outcomes at several different levels of analysis, objectives should be both specific and realistic. The outcomes achieved will be determined by the nature of the campaign, the campaign design, and the way the campaign is conducted. A certain level of effort is generally required to achieve even the most basic campaign objectives. Campaign planners should evaluate their resources to ensure that their efforts will produce at least the minimum acceptable set of objectives. Aggressive campaign objectives should be given careful scrutiny because of the amount of resources they will require.

Consumer Orientation Effective HIV/AIDS health communication campaigns must be designed to reflect the target audiences' specific concerns and cultural orientations; in other words, the campaign must be a reflection of the "consumer's" orientation (Kotler, 1975). Effective campaigns appeal to the interests and orientations of target audience members to gain their attention, increase the likelihood they will comprehend and be moved by campaign messages, encourage their participation in campaign activities, and ultimately to enable them to adopt the campaign's strategies and recommendations (Andraesen, undated; Maibach, 1991). The goals of such campaigns are developed in response to the perceived needs of the audience. Campaign efforts must identify and satisfy audience needs. Campaign planners must also monitor the audience to ensure that communication efforts continue to meet those needs and to identify any new or changing needs to which future messages can be targeted (Lefebvre & Flora, 1988).

A consumer orientation is predicated on identification of the most appropriate target audiences. Campaign planners must identify specific target audiences before they can gather the audience information that guides campaign design and message strategy. Audiences should be identified who either are at high risk for HIV/AIDS or are potentially part of the problem's resolution. These broad categories of people should be the highest priority targets for HIV/AIDS awareness and behavior change campaigns.

Consumer orientation is an expression of the audiences' interests in, and sensibilities regarding, the campaign topic and goals. This includes their involvement with the topic, recognition of the problem, knowledge about the topic, past experience with the topic, expectations about the topic, social norms regarding the topic, time available to spend on the topic, language use regarding the topic, and values or mores concerning the topic (Bandura, 1986; Grunig, 1989; Maibach, 1991). Effective campaigns require the participation of target audiences with program planners (Childers, 1991). Members of the target audience must be involved in developing message strategies, at least in terms of providing formative input (see Formative Research). True participatory planning is complicated in strategic HIV/AIDS campaigns by geographically diverse target audiences, large social distances between campaign planners and target audiences, and bureaucratic factors that inhibit the involvement of audience members. To avoid alienating target audiences, planners must address these organizational constraints before planning and delivering an HIV/AIDS campaign.

Stage 2: Use of Theory

Effective health communication campaigns are carefully designed and guided by established theory. Theory provides campaign planners with a clear direction and rationale for using specific communication strategies with target audiences. Theory also helps campaign planners predict a campaign's influence on the target audience's health beliefs and health behaviors. Both the social marketing literature and the broader literature of the behavioral sciences lend important theoretical perspectives to campaign design. We shall discuss these perspectives under the respective headings Exchange Theory and Behavioral Theory.

Exchange Theory Exchange theory suggests that health communication campaigns involve a voluntary exchange of resources (Lefebvre & Flora, 1988). Effective HIV/AIDS campaigns disseminate prevention messages that can be seen as products or services that are bought and sold for the mutual benefit of, and at costs acceptable to, both campaign planners (the sellers) and target audiences (the buyers). For audience members to respond to campaign messages, HIV/AIDS campaigns must show that the benefits of adopting preventive behaviors outweigh the costs of "purchase" (adoption), because the perceived costs and benefits of embracing campaign recommendations are critical to the adoption decisions made by audience members.

Costs Campaign planners must be aware of the potential costs to target audience members in adopting prevention behaviors. Health behavior changes may cost the consumer money, time, convenience, physical and/or mental ease, social standing, and comfort (Lefebvre & Flora, 1988). These costs can often be identified by conducting focus group discussions with members of the target audience. Although most people demonstrate concern for their health and are willing to make some sacrifices (incur some costs) to maximize their health, it is difficult to predict which costs they are willing to incur and which they are not. For example, the costs of insisting that clients wear condoms may or may not be acceptable to sex workers. Similarly, individuals who use intravenous (IV) drugs can experience economic, psychological, and social costs as a result of resolving to use only clean needles and syringes. Information on the audience's perception of costs is absolutely vital in efforts to develop a campaign that successfully proposes certain costs in exchange for certain benefits. By understanding the various costs of preventive actions, campaign designers can make efforts at reducing these costs (through "product design" or implementation strategies) thereby encouraging the adoption of the recommended practices (Kreps & Maibach, 1991).

Benefits There are many different benefits associated with adopting most preventive health behaviors. Such benefits can include:

- improving physical and/or psychological health,
- minimizing health risks,
- decreasing mortality,
- improving self-esteem,
- contributing to the common good,
- enhancing personal satisfaction, and
- promoting self-empowerment.

The target audience's perception of the costs and benefits directly influences their willingness to adopt campaign recommendations. For example, individuals who use IV drugs may desire the disease prevention benefits of needle cleaning but be unwilling to adopt the practice if there are likely to be significant social costs. Campaign planners must work with these individuals to design an approach to needle cleaning that minimizes the costs incurred. Commercial advertisers often suggest that health messages should focus on benefits that are not necessarily health related. HIV/AIDS campaign planners should consider their target audience's desires for love, security, status, and acceptance in creating campaign messages and should clearly communicate these benefits. For example, campaign messages directed to adolescents might focus on adolescent identity, the desire to be autonomous, and the importance of the peer group (McLeRoy, Bibeau, Steckler, & Glanz, 1988).

Incentives are benefits that campaign planners can offer to members of target audiences to encourage adoption of health behavior innovations (Bandura, 1986). Material inducements may be effective in helping consumers minimize the financial costs of adopting a health innovation, particularly among low-income target audiences. For example, health departments can offer free child immunizations to mothers who attend an HIV education session. Status incentives (such as public recognition of successful behavior changes) can be used as an inexpensive yet potentially effective motivating factor. The Centers for Disease Control's innovative AIDS Community Demonstration Projects use status incentives by creating educational media that feature the "role model stories" of people in the target audience. Self-evaluative incentives (i.e., feeling better about oneself as a result of adopting the recommended practice) also represent a powerful set of benefits that HIV/AIDS campaign planners can use to promote goal accomplishment among high-risk target audiences (Bandura, 1992; Schnell, Galovotti, & O'Reilly, 1991).

Exchange theory encourages explicit acknowledgment of the costs and benefits of actions to be promoted in a campaign and, moreover, efforts to minimize the costs and maximize the benefits. The actual processes of identification of the costs and benefits perceived by a target audience and the subsequent development of appropriate campaign materials are described later in our planning model (see Formative Research and Marketing Mix).

Behavioral Theory Theories of human behavior (e.g., Bandura, 1986, 1991) and communication processes (e.g., Bandura, in press; Rogers, 1983) enable campaign planners to predict, explain, and prescribe strategies for influencing risky health behaviors. Behavioral theories provide insights into health behaviors at the individual, dyadic, social network, organizational, and societal levels of analysis (Flora, Maibach, & Maccoby, 1989). Different HIV/AIDS health communication campaigns can be targeted at each of these levels using behavioral theories to interpret and predict behavior.

Individual-level theories include social learning (Bandura, 1986), expectancy (Ajzen & Fishbein, 1980), information processing (McGuire, 1989), risk perception (Slovik & Lichtenstein, 1971), and decision making (Kahneman & Tversky, 1972). For example, Bandura's (1986) social cognitive theory can be used to explain and predict the internal and external influences on risky behavior and the cognitive mechanisms (such as self-efficacy, outcome expectations, personal standards, and self-evaluations) that specify how to construct communication campaigns to facilitate behavioral changes. Network-level theories, such as diffusion of innovations (Rogers, 1983; Rogers & Kincaid, 1981), explain how to facilitate adaptation of health innovations within a social system, enhancing campaign planners' ability to promote health innovations. Organizational-level theories describe the diffusion of innovations through networks of organizations (Hage & Aiken, 1970; Zaltman & Duncan, 1977). Societal-level theories, such as agenda setting (McCombs & Shaw, 1972), spiral of silence (Noelle-Neumann, 1974), theories about public opinion (Price & Roberts, 1987), and theories about the effects of the information environment (Weick, 1979), explain societal influences on health behaviors. The theory of agenda setting, for example, explains how the mass media influence what people think about (McCombs & Shaw, 1972), demonstrating how media coverage of the health risks of HIV/AIDS has helped to publicly legitimize HIV/AIDS campaigns by directing public attention to the issue and placing HIV/AIDS prevention on the public policy agenda (Brown, Wazak, & Childers, 1989; Price & Roberts, 1987).

Stage 3: Communication Analysis

Although planning and theoretical considerations are important steps in setting up a strategic campaign, communication analysis is at the core of the planning process. Communication analysis begins with target audience analysis and emphasizes the need to segment the larger at-risk audience into a number of smaller more homogeneous target audiences. Formative research is the process through which campaign planners work with members of the target audiences to better understand their orientation(s) and enable appropriate exchanges. Formative research can also be thought of as giving the target audience a voice in the development of the campaign. Careful specification of target audiences as well as activities that give these audiences a voice facilitates the final element of communication analysis: channel selection.

Audience Analysis and Segmentation   HIV/AIDS campaigns are more likely to be effective if they target relatively homogeneous audiences. Audience segmentation, subdividing large heterogeneous populations into smaller and more homogeneous target audiences, enables campaign planners to target audiences for whom the campaign's goals are most relevant and to design messages that meet those audiences' specific needs. Doing so increases the likelihood that audience members will pay attention to the message, be persuaded by the message, and adopt the health action suggested by the message (Kotler & Roberto, 1989). There are many strategies for segmenting target audiences; these can be described as geographic, demographic, psychographic, behavioral, or combinational strategies (Maibach, 1991). To guide audience segmentation efforts, campaign planners must gather data from target populations concerning these segmentation variables and/or use secondary data compiled by existing health agencies or other organizations.

Geographic segmentation identifies audiences on the basis of location, examining physical size, location, density, and climate of the region. For example, in HIV/AIDS campaigns, urban areas are likely to be more critical target areas than rural locations. Geographic variables can be extremely useful in segmentation because of the pervasive cultural influence on attitudes and behaviors and the fact that culture develops differentially by location.

Demographic segmentation examines audience variables such as age, sex, ethnicity, religion, family size and structure, education, occupation, and income. The utility of demographic segmentation is intuitive (i.e., men are likely to respond differently to campaign messages than women, and adolescents are likely to respond differently to campaign messages than adults). HIV/AIDS campaigns must be particularly sensitive to the ways in which culture influences target audience members' perceptions of sexuality, sexual behavior, and gender roles (Bonaguro, 1991a).

Psychographic segmentation examines consumer conditions, attitudes, personalities, and life-styles to identify target audiences. Psychographic segmentation enables campaign planners to locate individuals within geographic or demographic target populations who share similar perspectives on reality. For example, the Stages of Change model is a psychographic segmentation strategy that has been used in HIV/AIDS and other health campaigns to divide a potential target audience into subaudiences on the basis of readiness to change health-risk behavior (Prochaska, Velicer, DiClemente, & Fava, 1988; Schnell et al., 1991).

Behavioral criteria, such as how often and under what conditions members of the target audience engage in a high-risk behavior, can productively be used to segment target audiences (Kotler & Roberto, 1989). In HIV/AIDS campaigns, important behavioral segmentation variables include type of sexual partners, numbers of sexual partners, use of condoms, and the sharing of needles and syringes for IV drug use.

Campaign planners often use a combination of complementary segmentation strategies. For example, a campaign seeking to promote the use of clean works among individuals who use IV drugs might first behaviorally segment users on the basis of frequency of use (occasional users vs. regular or addicted users) and current needle hygiene practices (use only clean works vs. do not always use clean works). Next, at-risk IV drug users (i.e., those who do not always use clean works) might be geographically segmented according to where group members live, congregate, or seek health care to determine which individuals can be reached with campaign messages and to design strategies for channel use and message delivery. Finally, psychographic segmentation strategies might be used to further segment the target audience by identifying the individuals who are most inclined to adopt the recommended practice of using sterile needles and syringes.

Once target audiences are segmented, campaign planners must carefully analyze each audience still under consideration. Original formative research is typically the main vehicle for this analysis, although secondary data analyses and the published literature also offer invaluable information. Formative research allows campaign planners to design messages that are most likely to reach the target audience with an acceptable and potentially effective health-promoting message.

Formative Research Formative research is the mechanism through which consumer orientation is established. Formative research guides the conceptualization and development of campaign messages before and during the course of the campaign (Lefebvre & Flora, 1988; National Research Council, 1991; Palmer, 1981). In concept development, the first stage of formative research, campaign planners use focus groups, interviews, surveys, observations, etc. to identify the general message concepts that are most likely to achieve campaign objectives. The focus of concept development activities is to evaluate the audience members' understanding of, and predispositions toward, the actions to be promoted in the campaign. Concept development helps HIV/AIDS campaign planners develop culturally specific and developmentally appropriate messages to effect changes in risk-related behaviors (Bonaguro, 1991b).

In addition to concept development, formative research is used to develop specific messages most likely to be effective. Analysis of formative data can suggest the most relevant prevention messages, productive strategies for presentation of those messages, appropriate terminology, and credible spokespersons to deliver the messages. Finally, formative research is used to test campaign messages on members of the target audience, evaluating how well the message captures audience members' attention, is comprehended, is perceived as being relevant, achieves campaign objectives (e.g., to impart HIV/AIDS-resisting skills or enhance self-efficacy to resist HIV/AIDS), as well as to assess the likelihood that the messages will result in unintended consequences.

Channel Analysis and Selection   Strategic campaign planning involves the selection of communication channels on the basis of the target audience's channel use characteristics and preferences. Channels that have been used in HIV/AIDS campaigns include television (broadcast and video), film, radio, print media (e.g., newspapers, magazines, books, pamphlets, and posters), interpersonal communication, folk media, and computerized information systems. In analyzing the channels available for use, it is important to assess their

- reach (how many people access the information via this channel),
- specificity (which groups of people use this channel), and
- rate of influence (what impact messages received via this channel will have on those it reaches; Chaffee & Mutz, 1988).

Interpersonal channels are generally described as having low reach, high specificity, and a high potential rate of influence, whereas mediated channels are generally characterized by high reach, low specificity, and a low potential rate of influence.

Because different channels have different strengths and weaknesses (in terms of reach, specificity, influence, credibility, and ability to convey different types of information), it is preferable for campaign planners to use multiple channels of communication to maximize an individual channel's strengths and overcome its weakness by using it in tandem with a complementary channel (Flay & Burton, 1990; Rogers & Storey, 1987). Interpersonal channels have been found to be an effective complement to mediated channels (Hall, 1977; Rogers & Storey, 1987; Worden et al., 1988), and printed media an effective complement to electronic media (Bettinghaus, 1988; Flay, 1987). Edgar et al. (1988) recommended synergistic integration of mediated and interpersonal channels in HIV/AIDS prevention campaigns.

Entertainment media, such as popular music, music videos, popular television programming, and movies, can be used as powerful communication channels for conveying relevant HIV/AIDS information to the public and promoting behavior change. These media are pervasive, sought out by target audiences, involving, and persuasive (Rimon, 1990). Posters, cartoons, theatrical productions, and films are examples of popular media that have been used successfully to disseminate information about HIV/AIDS to groups at risk (Brown, 1991; Brown et al., 1989; Keaveney, 1989).

Health communication campaigns have typically relied on (free) public service time to air campaign messages on television and radio. Restricted financial resources often prevent planners from purchasing premium air time. Some strategies that might be used to address this financial problem include encouraging local television and radio stations to offer reduced rates for premium air time, negotiating a set ratio of free to paid time, seeking corporate sponsorship to purchase air time, incorporating health messages into corporately purchased commercials, and involving broadcasters in campaign planning.

Stage 4: Implementation

There are a number of important issues to be considered in campaign implementation. The information developed during Stages 1 through 3 must at this point be integrated into the development and delivery of a set of complementary campaign messages or behavior change strategies. The actual delivery of the campaign must be monitored closely so that midcourse corrections can be made, if needed. There are bound to be important macrosocial conditions that negatively influence the target audience's HIV/AIDS risk behaviors. Campaign planners must consider these conditions and decide if campaign strategies are an appropriate means to counteract some of these cultural, environmental, and organizational influences. Finally, campaign planners must consider the length of time required to create lasting changes in the targeted risk behaviors.

Marketing Mix   Marketing mix (i.e., the 4 Ps: product, price, placement, and promotion) is a key element of the social marketing process that suggests that health communication goals should be pursued in a fashion similar to the marketing of consumer products (Kotler, 1975). Campaigns should create a product or product line (such as media programs, advertisements, public service announcements, pamphlets, posters, training programs, or information systems) designed to meet the target audience's needs (Kotler & Roberto, 1989). A product line can be assessed in terms of

- width (the number of different target behaviors addressed),
- depth (the number of target audiences addressed), and
- diversity (the variety of products offered; Lefebvre & Flora, 1988).

Behavior changes advocated in social marketing products always have a price (or cost). Such costs may be economic but can also be psychological and social, influenced heavily by subjective perceptions and self-evaluations. Campaign planners must minimize price by designing approaches to health behavior change in a fashion that facilitates their relative ease of adoption. The place dimension of the marketing mix refers to channels of distribution for the social marketing products. Campaign products must be placed in a fashion that reaches members of the target audience in a manner capable of influencing their behavior. Placement decisions for mass-mediated products typically involve consideration of competing mass media channels and the timing of delivery within the channel, which depends on the target audience's life paths (Lefebvre & Flora, 1988; Worden et al., 1988). Product promotion lets the target audience know when and where they can obtain the social product, depending on their needs and habits.

Process Evaluation   In process evaluations, campaign planners monitor the progress of campaign messages and products to determine the extent to which campaign objectives are being achieved. Process evaluations provide data that answer such questions as what proportion of the target audience was exposed to the campaign messages, how many times the average audience member was exposed to the messages, and how audience members who were exposed reacted. Measures of audience reach are an important check on campaign process, as are the reactions of the target audience to campaign programs and messages. Process evaluations are an essential part of campaign implementation because they enable campaign planners to identify potential problems with campaign strategies and programs so these problems can be rectified and the campaign refined while it is in progress. The campaign's success should be determined by data collected prior to, during, and after the campaign.

Macrosocial Conditions   Campaign planners must be aware of the many macrosocial conditions that influence health risks, such as societal norms, information environments, the structure and culture of relevant organizations, and public policies. These macrosocial contributions can be either direct, such as laws influencing the availability of sterile needles, or indirect, such as cultural influences on sexual practices or IV drug use. The influence of macrosocial conditions on the target audience's risk practices must be analyzed and placed in perspective to the individual determinants of risk behavior.

There are three basic campaign strategies available should planners decide that one or more macrosocial conditions must be altered to facilitate risk reduction:

1   Persuade government officials to change public health policies.
2   Influence organizational/corporate officials to discontinue problematic practices/policies and support solutions.
3   Mobilize support among the general public to influence macrosocial conditions through legislation and changes in public policy.

HIV/AIDS campaigns can target government officials with information to help achieve several goals: to establish a clear agenda for HIV/AIDS education and prevention, to expand government officials' knowledge base about HIV/AIDS to enable them to make better policy decisions, and to propose politically acceptable HIV/AIDS prevention strategies for government agencies. ACT UP (the AIDS Coalition to Unleash Power) is undoubtedly the organization that has most visibly embraced this strategy. Similarly, campaigns can target nongovernmental organizations, corporations, and employers to discourage conditions that contribute to risk and mobilize organizational support for HIV/AIDS prevention. For example, a number of mainstream campaigns (including the Centers for Disease Control's America Responds to AIDS) have attempted to reduce the stigma of AIDS in the workplace. Perhaps most important, campaigns can also encourage the general public to exert pressure on political and corporate systems (Hornik, 1980; Price & Roberts, 1987). For example, in San Francisco and New York, gay community groups instigated government action to formally affirm the rights of people with AIDS to receive health care by sending letters to elected officials, signing petitions, responding to public opinion polls, and creating media events to convey their messages to elected officials (Shilts, 1987). Strong public pressure on elected officials provides them with powerful motivation to enact, or at least support, legislation to satisfy their constituencies. Another example of a community-based effort to mobilize public attention and action is the "Names Project," which has used public showings of a huge quilt composed of a shockingly large number of cloth panels representing individuals who died from AIDS to increase public awareness of the magnitude of the AIDS health risk and to spur legislation concerning HIV/AIDS (Biemiller, 1991).

Long-Term Involvement and Institutionalization Campaign planners must determine the amount of time needed to achieve their health communication goals, because time is a crucial element in the campaign process. Entrenched health behaviors are generally resistant to change, and campaign programs and messages must be long-lived, providing continued educational outreach to influence these behaviors (Rogers & Storey, 1987). The more time invested by campaign planners and campaign participants, the more the campaign is likely to achieve. By empowering consumers to get personally involved with campaign programs, strategies for accomplishing campaign goals can be institutionalized into the target communities. Grieser (1991) has proposed the following indicators of campaign success: (a) grass roots participation in campaign activities, (b) beneficial effects on policy in the public and private sectors, (c) transformation of a project (or campaign) into a program, and (d) sustainability of the program over time. HIV/AIDS campaigns that intend to promote local empowerment and institutionalization as campaign objectives must plan to maintain the campaign for a number of years to be successful (Lefebvre, 1990).

Stage 5: Evaluation and Reorientation

After health communication campaigns are implemented, campaign planners must evaluate the influences of the campaign (both positive and negative) on the target audience. Evaluations of campaign outcomes almost always identify health risks that have not been minimized, suggesting new directions for developing health communication campaigns and leading the campaign planner back to the first stage of the Strategic Health Communication Campaign model.

Outcome Evaluation   Outcome evaluations in which data are gathered about the overall effects of the campaign on target audiences and on the public's health are a critical part of health communication campaigns. Such evaluations are conducted to assess the strengths and weaknesses of the campaign at a variety of levels (Flay & Cook, 1989). *Effectiveness evaluation* determines how individuals exposed to the campaign changed as a result. *Impact evaluation* determines the range of effects a campaign had on the aggregate of individuals, organizations, or communities to which it was targeted. *Causal evaluation* examines why campaigns did or did not have the intended effects on target audiences, often indicating directions for revising campaign strategies. *Cost-effectiveness evaluation* determines whether a campaign achieved its objectives at a reasonable cost, by examining the amount of resources required (in terms of money, time, personnel, and physical resources) to achieve some specified unit of change in the outcome measure.

Outcome evaluations assess not only the success of health communication campaigns, but also the inevitable weaknesses, problems, and shortfalls in achieving campaign objectives. Data are gathered on the different health risks and health communication needs of target audiences that were not fully addressed by the campaign. Outcome evaluations help identify additional strategies for segmenting target audiences, as well as new audiences to address with future health communication efforts. They also help identify new strategies for more effectively designing and implementing campaigns. Such information is critical for planning future prevention efforts, leading the campaign planner full circle back to initiating and planning new health communication efforts in the Strategic Health Communication Campaign process.

RECOMMENDATIONS

Our analysis has led us to several recommendations for the design and implementation of strategic HIV/AIDS campaigns:

1   No one campaign or general campaign strategy is likely to achieve the diverse demands of HIV/AIDS prevention. A wide range of different campaigns, using different communication strategies and messages targeted at different audiences, will have to be employed to help curtail the spread of HIV/AIDS.

2   Campaigns must be designed to reflect the specific concerns and cultural orientations of the target audiences.

3 Campaigns require extensive involvement of target audiences in all stages of planning.

4 Campaigns should address target audiences who are as homogeneous as possible through careful audience segmentation.

5 Campaigns must set specific and realistic objectives for influencing public health behaviors.

6 Campaign planners should attempt to use multiple complementary channels of communication to maximize an individual channel's strengths and overcome its weaknesses.

7 Campaigns must persuasively demonstrate that the benefits of adopting preventive behaviors outweigh the costs of adoption.

8 Campaign strategies should be informed by theories of human behavior and communication process at the individual, dyadic, social network, organizational, and societal levels.

9 Campaign planners must consider macrosocial conditions that influence health risks when designing and implementing campaigns. Moreover, campaigns can be used to influence macrosocial conditions in three ways: to educate and influence government officials, to educate and influence nongovernmental officials and organizations, and to mobilize the general public to exert pressure on political and corporate systems.

10 Campaigns should create a message or product line designed to meet the target audience's needs.

11 Campaign efforts should be appropriately long-lived and should be institutionalized into target communities by empowering consumers to get personally involved with campaign programs.

12 Campaigns should be evaluated throughout their life span through formative, process, and outcome evaluation.

CONCLUSIONS

The importance of strategic campaigns in curtailing the spread of HIV/AIDS is clear. Yet prevention is a complex, multifaceted process that blends both art and science. To overcome the complexities of prevention in developing effective HIV/AIDS campaigns, we suggest careful examination of the implications and applications of the Strategic Health Communication Campaign model.

Effective HIV/AIDS prevention campaigns must begin with careful campaign planning in which campaign goals are determined, the target audience's specific needs and orientations are examined, and the target audience is segmented into homogeneous groups. The communication strategy should be carefully analyzed to identify accessible and effective communication channels, design campaign messages, and test these messages for use with target audiences. Relevant communication, persuasion, and behavioral theories should be used to guide campaign strategies. Campaigns should be implemented with awareness of macrosocial and cultural constraints; be designed to influence an audience's motivation to engage in behavior change; be evaluated to refine campaign process, products, and strategies; and be sustained for a sufficient amount of time to promote long-term behavior change. Finally, campaign outcomes must be carefully evaluated so that the influences of the campaign on health behaviors and directions of future risk prevention and health communication efforts can be identified.

REFERENCES

Ajzen, I., & Fishbein, M. (1980). *Understanding attitudes and predicting social behavior.* Englewood Cliffs, NJ: Prentice-Hall.

Andraesen, A. (Undated). *Social marketing: Its potential application to child survival.* Washington, DC: Academy for Educational Development.

Atkin, C. (1981). Mass media information campaign effectiveness. In R. Rice & W. Paisley (Eds.), *Public communication campaigns* (pp. 265–280). Beverly Hills, CA: Sage.

Atkin, C., & Wallack, L. (Eds.). (1990). *Mass communication and public health.* Newbury Park, CA: Sage.

Bandura, A. (1986). *Social foundations of thought and action: A social cognitive approach.* Englewood Cliffs, NJ: Prentice-Hall.

Bandura, A. (1991). Self-efficacy mechanism in physiological activation and health-promoting behavior. In J. Madden (ed.), *Neurobiology of learning, emotion, and affect* (pp. 229–269). New York: Raven Press.

Bandura, A. (1992). A social cognitive approach to the exercise of control over AIDS infection. In R. D. Clemente (Ed.), *Adolescents and AIDS: A generation in jeopardy* (pp. 89–116). Newbury Park, CA: Sage.

Bandura, A. (in press). Social cognitive theory of mass communication. In J. Bryant & D. Zillman (Eds.), *Media effects advances in theory and research.* Hillsdale, NJ: Erlbaum.

Bettinghaus, E. P. (1988). Using the mass media in smoking prevention and cessation programs: An introduction to five studies. *Preventive Medicine, 17,* 503–509.

Biemiller, L. (1991, May 29). For three days at Dartmouth. *Chronicle of Higher Education,* 37:A28.

Bonaguro, E. (1991a, August). *HIV prevention education for teachers of elementary and middle school grades.* Training program presented at the National Training of Trainers for HIV Prevention Education Meeting of the Association for the Advancement of Health Education, Washington, DC.

Bonaguro, E. (1991b, September). *K–12 preservice guidelines for the development of HIV/AIDS prevention education programs.* Paper presented at the Western College Health 2000 Conference, San Diego.

Brown, J. D., Wazak, C. S., & Childers, K. W. (1989). Family planning, abortion and AIDS: Sexuality and communication campaigns. In C. Salmon (Ed.), *Information campaigns balancing social values and social change* (pp. 85–112). Newbury Park, CA: Sage.

Brown, W. J. (1991). An AIDS prevention campaign: Effects on attitudes, beliefs, and communication behavior. *American Behavioral Scientist, 34,* 666–678.

Chaffee, S., & Mutz, D. (1988). Comparing mediated and interpersonal communication data. In R. Hawkins, J. Wiemann, & S. Pingree (Eds.), *Advancing communication science: Merging mass and interpersonal processes* (pp. 19–43). Newbury Park, CA: Sage.

Childers, E. (1991). *Communication in popular participation: Empowering people for their own development* (Working document). New York: United Nations.

Edgar, T., Hammond, S. L., & Freimuth, V. S. (1989). The role of the mass media and interpersonal communication in promoting AIDS-related behavioral change. *AIDS and Public Policy Journal, 4,* 3–9.

Flay, B. (1987). Mass media and smoking cessation: A critical review. *American Journal of Public Health, 77,* 153–160.

Flay, B., & Burton, D. (1990). Effective mass communication strategies for health campaigns. In C. Atkin & L. Wallack (Eds.), *Mass communication and public health* (pp. 129–148). Newbury Park, CA: Sage.

Flay, B., and Cook, T. (1989). Three models for summative evaluation of prevention campaigns with a mass media component. In R. Rice & C. Atkins (Eds.), *Public communication campaigns* (2nd ed., 175–195). Newbury Park, CA: Sage.

Flay, B., DiTecco, D., & Schlegel, R. (1980). Mass media and health promotion: An analysis using an extended information-processing model. *Health Education Quarterly, 7,* 127–147.

Flora, J., Maccoby, N., & Farquhar, J. (1989). Communication campaigns to prevent cardiovascular disease: The Stanford community studies. In R. Rice & C. Atkin (Eds.), *Public communication campaigns* (2nd ed., pp. 233–252). Newbury Park, CA: Sage.

Flora, J., Maibach, E., & Maccoby, N. (1989). The role of mass media across four levels of health promotion intervention. *Annual Review of Public Health, 10,* 181–201.

Gilchrist, L. (1990). The role of schools in community based approaches to prevention of AIDS and intravenous drug use. In C. Leukfeld, C. Battjes, & Z. Amsel (Eds.), *AIDS and intravenous drug use: Future directions for community based prevention research: NIDA research monograph 93* (Department of Health and Human Services Publication No. ADM 89-1627). Washington, DC: U.S. Government Printing Office.

Grieser, M. (1991). *Case studies in environmental education and communication* (Position paper). Washington, DC: Office of Education, Bureau for Science and Technology, U.S. Agency for International Development.

Grunig, J. E. (1989). Public, audiences, and market segments: Segmentation principles for campaigns. In C. Salmon (Ed.), *Information campaigns: Balancing social values and social change* (pp. 189–228). Newbury Park, CA: Sage.

Hage, J., & Aiken, M. (1970). *Social change in complex organizations.* New York: Random House.

Hall, B. (1977). *Mtu ni afya: Tanzania's health campaign.* Washington, DC: Agency for International Development.

Hornik, R. (1980). Communication as a complement in development. *Journal of Communication, 30,* 10–24.

Kahneman, D., & Tversky, A. (1972). Subjective probability: A judgement of representativeness. *Cognitive Psychology, 3,* 430–454.

Keaveney, M. M. (1989, November). *A cross-cultural analysis of AIDS messages: AIDS pamphlets in Norway, France, and Japan.* Paper presented at the Speech Communication Association conference, San Francisco.

Kotler, P. (1975). *Marketing for non-profit organizations.* Englewood Cliffs, NJ: Prentice-Hall.

Kotler, P., & Roberto, E. (1989). *Social marketing: Strategies for changing public behavior.* New York: Free Press.

Kreps, G. L. (1988). The pervasive role of information in health and health care: Implications for health communication policy. In J. Anderson (Ed.), *Communication yearbook 11* (pp. 238–276). Newbury Park, CA: Sage.

Kreps, G. L., & Maibach, E. W. (1991, May). *Communicating to prevent health risks.* Paper presented at the International Communication Association conference, Chicago.

Lefebvre, C. (1990). Strategies to maintain and institutionalize successful programs: A marketing framework. In N. Bracht (Ed.), *Health promotion at the community level* (pp. 209–228). Newbury Park, CA: Sage.

Lefebvre, C., & Flora, J. (1988). Social marketing and public health intervention. *Health Education Quarterly, 15,* 299–315.

Maibach, E. (1991). *Social marketing for the environment using information campaigns to promote environmental awareness and behavior change* (Position paper). Washington, DC: Office of Education, Bureau for Science and Technology, U.S. Agency for International Development.

McCombs, M., & Shaw, D. (1972). The agenda setting function of the mass media. *Public Opinion Quarterly, 36,* 176–187.

McGuire, W. J. (1989). Theoretical foundations of campaigns. In R. Rice & C. Atkin (Eds.), *Public communication campaigns* (2nd ed., pp. 43–67). Newbury Park, CA: Sage.

McLeRoy, K., Bibeau, D., Steckler, A., & Glanz, K. (1988). An ecological perspective on health promotion programs. *Health Education Quarterly, 15,* 351–377.

National Research Council. (1991). Evaluating media campaigns. In S. Coyle, R. Baruch, & C. Turner (Eds.), *Evaluating AIDS prevention programs* (Expanded ed., pp. 50–82). Washington, DC: National Academy Press.

Noelle-Neumann, E. (1974). The spiral of silence. *Journal of Communication, 24,* 43–51.

Nussbaum, J. F. (1989). Directions for research within health communication. *Health Communication, 1,* 35–40.

Office of Cancer Communications. (1989). *Making health communication programs work: A planner's guide* (National Institutes of Health Publication No. 89-1493). Washington, DC: National Cancer Institute.

Palmer, E. (1981). Shaping persuasive messages with formative research. In R. Rice & W. Paisley (Eds.), *Public communication campaigns* (pp. 227–238). Newbury Park, CA: Sage.

Portnoy, B., Anderson, D. M., & Eriksen, M. P. (1989). Application of diffusion theory to health promotion research. *Family and Community Health, 12*(3), 63–71.

Price, V., & Roberts, D. (1987). Public opinion processes. In C. Berger & S. Chafee

(Eds.), *Handbook of communication science* (pp. 781–816). Newbury Park, CA: Sage.

Prochaska, J., Velicer, W., DiClemente, C., & Fava, J. (1988). Measuring processes of change applications to the cessation of smoking. *Journal of Consulting and Clinical Psychology, 56,* 520–528.

Reardon, K. K. (1988). The role of persuasion in health promotion and disease prevention: A review and commentary. In J. A. Anderson (Ed.), *Communication yearbook 11* (pp. 277–297). Newbury Park, CA: Sage.

Reardon, K. K. (1990). Meeting the communication/persuasion challenge of AIDS in workplaces, neighborhoods, and schools: A comment on AIDS and public policy. *Health Communication, 2,* 267–270.

Reardon, K. K., & Rogers, E. M. (1988). Interpersonal versus mass communication: A false dichotomy. *Human Communication Research, 15,* 284–303.

Rimon, J. (1990). Sing and the world sings with you. *Development Communication Report, 71,* 8–9.

Rogers, E. M. (1983). *Diffusion of innovations.* New York: Free Press.

Rogers, E. M., & Kincaid, D. (1981). *Communication networks: Toward a new paradigm for research.* New York: Free Press.

Rogers, E. M., & Storey, J. D. (1987). Communication campaigns. In C. Berger & S. Chafee (Eds.), *Handbook of communication science* (pp. 817–846). Newbury Park, CA: Sage.

Rubinson, L., & Alles, W. F. (1984). *Health education: Foundations for the future.* St. Louis: C. V. Mosby.

Rugg, L., O'Reilly, K., & Galovotti, C. (1990). AIDS prevention evaluation: Conceptual and methodological issues. *Evaluation and Program Planning, 13,* 79–89.

Schnell, D., Galovotti, C., & O'Reilly, K. (1991). *An evaluation of behavior change using statistical and cognitive models.* Unpublished manuscript, Division of STD/HIV Prevention, Center for Prevention Studies, Centers for Disease Control.

Shilts, R. (1987). *And the band played on: Politics, people, and the AIDS epidemic.* New York: St. Martin's Press.

Slovik, P., & Lichtenstein, S. (1971). Comparison of Bayesian and regression approaches to the study of information processing in judgment. *Organizational Behavior and Human Performance, 6,* 649–744.

Tones, B. K. (1986). Health education and the ideology of health promotion: A review of alternative approaches. *Health Education Research, 1,* 3–12.

Weick, K. (1979). *The social psychology of organizing* (2nd ed.). Reading, MA: Addison-Wesley.

Worden, J., Flynn, B., Geller, B., Chen, M., Shelton, L., Seckerwalker, R., Solomon, D., Solomon, L., Couchey, S., & Costanza, M. (1988). Development of a smoking prevention mass media program using diagnostic and formative research. *Preventive Medicine, 17,* 531–558.

Zaltman, G., & Duncan, R. (1977). *Strategies for planned change.* New York: Wiley.

Chapter Two

Health Communication as Negotiation: The COAST Model and AIDS

Scott C. Ratzan

Traditional studies on the doctor–patient relationship indicate that when a physician improves his or her interviewing and interpersonal skills, there is reciprocal improvement in a patient's proclivity to comply with the prescribed medical regimen (Alroy, Ber, & Kramer, 1984; Barrows, 1990; Bartlett, Grayson, & Barker, 1984; Kreps & Thornton, 1984; Roberson, Kowlowitz, Jenkins, & Hoole, 1989; Rowland-Morin & Carroll, 1990; Sivertson & Stone, 1983; Stewart & Roter, 1989; Thompson, 1986). Unfortunately, focusing on the physician–patient relationship exclusively vitiates the synergistic interpersonal dynamic so important to effective health communication. By employing the essential components of the art of negotiation to emphasize the importance of dyadic co-dependency in establishing effective health communication, researchers and health professionals alike can enhance their overall efficacy in the health communication encounter.

This chapter centers on applying shared decision making, mutually beneficial interests, and common goals and objectives—inherent traits of the negotiation process—as they relate to the patient–physician encounter. Application of principles of negotiation, which encourage "back and forth communication designed to reach an agreement" (Fisher & Ury, 1981, p. xi), to the health communication encounter provides a unique and realistic focal point. For, as one might surmise from personal experience as well as past research (Inui & Carter, 1985; Wasserman & Inui, 1983), the patient–physician equation is neither static nor independent. In the effort to meet the individual patient's health needs, there is a continual interactive dialogue among the dyad participants.

Viewing the medical encounter[1]—the health care provider–patient relationship—as a negotiation process can be beneficial to both parties. Beisecker (1990) stated that when an encounter between a physician and a patient is characterized by dialectical discussion and increased emphasis on patient responsibility in a proposed treatment plan, the patient is more realistic and self-reliant in his or her clinical expectations. Furthermore, studies have revealed that a patient's compliance with a prescribed regimen depends on his or her level of satisfaction with the overall medical experience, which is based primarily on the physician's communication skills (Street & Wiemann, 1987). In addition, research has identified the patient's overall level of satisfaction as related directly to the quality of the communication that takes place between the patient and the doctor (Ballard-Reisch, 1990; Beisecker, 1990; Lane, 1983). Researchers have warned that increased reliance on technology in the physician–patient relationship, as well as the loss of communication skills in patient–physician negotiation, further threatens the final satisfaction of the dyad (Fitzgerald, 1990; Norfolk, 1990).

Sharing responsibility for a favorable outcome between the client and the health care provider is necessary in the health communication encounter. The more active role by the patient increases his or her locus of control, thereby diminishing feelings of helplessness and passivity and increasing participation and acceptance of the optimal decision (Rowland-Morin & Carroll, 1990; Stiles & Putnam, 1989). Furthermore, the physician benefits through effective inquiry and frank discussion of treatment, costs, and other factors that reflect the patient's individualized interests and needs. In addition to enhancing satisfaction among those involved in the dyadic health encounter, increased patient participation that uses negotiation concepts also can prove beneficial for third parties, such as insurance companies and other members of the health polity. Patients involved from the start as active agents in the health encounter might

---

[1]In this chapter, negotiation (defined as "shared decision-making rooted in communication; to arrange or settle by conferring or discussing; an act or process of dealing with another to reach agreement") refers to professionals at any level of health care—physician, psychologist, nurse, third-party payer/provider, etc.—and the client/patient. Hence, the phrase *health communication encounter* is used interchangeably with *physician–patient, health care provider–patient, medical/ health encounter,* and *health communication as negotiation.* The author's background principally guides examples in this chapter to the doctor–patient encounter. It is interesting to note the term *doctor* stems from its etymology derived from the Latin verb *docere* which means "teacher." In contrast, the word *patient* is derived from the Latin verb *patior*, meaning "to suffer."

be less likely to claim malpractice (Robertson, 1985). Of course, this could be an additional benefit to government, physicians, and patients, considering that malpractice insurance premiums increased from $1 billion in 1980 to $3 billion in 1988.

Since the days of Hippocrates, there has been some form of communication, albeit principally unidirectional, in the patient–physician encounter. In fact, the Greeks and Romans both stressed the importance of *mens sana in copore sano,* a healthy mind in a healthy body. Later, the famous 19th century Canadian physician Sir William Osler espoused, "It is much more important to know what sort of patient has the disease than what sort of disease the patient has" (Norfolk, 1990, p. 4). Yet, given the expansion of the rhetorical and technological options that are involved in treatment and other aspects of health maintenance and prevention, the demands on today's health communication process necessitate going beyond what researchers have labeled the traditional "universal topoi"—the standard medical history protocol for clinical diagnosis of the physician–patient act. The message clearly demonstrates is that the quality of communication in the negotiation directly affects the overall satisfaction of the patient–physician relationship. According to Samora, Saunders, and Larson (1961),

> If the goal of medicine is the diagnosis and treatment of disease, the quality of communication between practitioner and patient makes little difference, so long as an adequate medical history can be obtained and the necessary cooperation of the patient in doing or refraining from doing certain things can be assured. But if the goal is more broadly interpreted, if the concern is with the person who is sick . . . the quality of communication assumes instrumental importance. (p. 92)

The major theme of this chapter is that the quality of communication can be enhanced significantly when the health communication encounter is approached as a negotiation.

The concept of applying negotiation to the doctor–patient relationship has support in prior research. In 1982, the President's Commission for the Study of Ethical Problems in Medicine and Biomedical and Behavioral Research stated that "'shared decisionmaking' is the appropriate ideal for patient-professional relationships" (p. 30). In its final report on health care decisions, the commission cited Katz's (1980) observation that physicians missed the opportunity to move toward "a new and unaccustomed dialogue between physicians and their patients . . . in which both, appreciative of their respective inequalities, make a genuine effort to voice and clarify their uncertainties and then to arrive at a mutually satisfactory course of action" (p. 122).

Quill (1983) argued that a physician–patient relationship is consensual and not obligatory, that each participant must willingly choose to be a part of the encounter. He further advocated that in situations characterized by difficult patient problems, a "contract" should be agreed on that clearly outlines the limitations and expectations of each party. Furthermore, Ballard-Reisch (1990) stipulated that the patient–physician encounter should be characterized by participative decision making rather than the traditional paternalistic relationship. A major factor that influenced Ballard-Reisch's recommendation is the changing legal system, which encourages patient knowledge and participation in medical decisions. Succinctly stated, today's health agenda presents an increasingly crowded context that demands a focused, dynamic, negotiation perspective.

In addition, time constraints on today's patient–physician encounter negatively affect the quality of the health communication process: Information exchange often is incomplete because of inept encoding and decoding within the time-specific context. Patients misunderstand instructions, forget key steps of a treatment plan, or fail to comply with directions (Ballard-Reisch, 1990; Robertson, 1985). Yet, prior research suggests that actual length of time of the dyadic encounter to be only one variable that affects the encounter. Beisecker (1990) found that even though a positive correlation exists between a high level of information exchange and compliance with the physician's instructions, patients are still reluctant to ask their physicians questions, regardless of the amount of time spent together.

The explanation provided for this lack of inquiry lies in the physician's perceived role in the traditional relationship. In the attempt to maintain control of the health communication encounter, physicians frequently change the topic, respond ambiguously, and ignore patient inquiries, which results in an unsatisfactory communication act for the patient. The message conveyed is to not question the doctor—the amount and quality of input will be decided on solely by the physician (Beisecker, 1990; Thompson, 1986). Such an approach is the antithesis of a negotiation-oriented communication encounter—the exchange/ sharing of information for the benefit of the recipient—and also hinders the transference phenomenon.

The use of negotiation in the health encounter optimizes a positive outcome by introducing nonquantifiable communication factors often described as transference (Strachey, 1958; Brody, 1977; Seldes, 1985). In a pejorative sense, Ben Franklin's old adage "God heals but the doctor takes the fee" and French surgeon Abroise Pure's "I treated him—God cured him" also echo the transference phenomenon. In modern days, Bok (1978) identified the unquantifiable placebo effect as a positive effect on the patient's health. Furthermore, Aristotle termed *ethos* the most important factor in communication. Sixteenth century German physician Philipius Aureolus Paracelcus, often referred to as the "Luther of Medicine," stated, "Medicine is not really a science but an art. The character of the physician may act more powerfully upon the patient than the drugs employed" (Seldes, 1985, p. 321).

THE COAST MODEL OF NEGOTIATION

A visual model illustrating the COAST model of negotiation is provided below in Figure 1. The continuous flow of the process, as represented by the arrow, demonstrates the dynamic and ongoing interaction necessary in its application to the physician–patient health communication encounter. Communication is the foundation and focal point of the model; without communication, there would not be a negotiation. The entire process begins with the initial communication act. As the negotiation develops, options are presented and discussed, along with appropriate alternatives, all within a context of mutually agreed on objective standards that imbue the process with trust, in the joint effort to reach a satisfactory and successful outcome while building an effective ongoing relationship.

Communication

Effective and ethical communication is the key ingredient of a mutually satisfying doctor–patient relationship. Several crucial outcomes of a physician–patient relationship depend on the type and quality of the health communication encounter. These include exploring/discussing the interests of each party; exercising effective listening skills; understanding personalities, cultures, backgrounds, attitudes, values, and beliefs; establishing an agreed on agenda; setting ground rules; and asking/answering pertinent questions.

More specifically, interests—needs, desires, and concerns—are the motivating forces behind the people involved in the specific negotiation (Fisher & Ury, 1981). Interests should be explored and determined without being affected by fixed or predetermined positions. The patient's interests usually stem from what Bitzer (1968) termed the "exigence," the imperfection that initiates the encounter. In the health context, the exigence could be symptoms, illness, pain, change in homeostasis, mental outlook, stressors, etc. The physician's interests generally center on alleviating the patient's existing ailments, providing answers to questions, fulfilling the necessary services in a reasonable amount of time, developing a clientele/practice, and collecting a fee for services rendered.

The common interest shared by the doctor and the patient is the patient's health and well-being. Communicating together, the physician and the patient should explore the reason(s) for the encounter and outline their shared goals and objectives during the initial "two-way" interview/meeting (and during their subsequent activities). Plato's traditional view of the dialectical encounter is an excellent model for the proper investigation and determination of such objectives. Of course, there is one major exception to the Platonic dialectical approach that must be elucidated. There are no philosopher kings conveying grand views of truth through unidirectional communication to the masses. Parties involved in the negotiation-based health communication encounter should have reciprocal respect and credibility.

The patient's ability to self-disclose, a product of the degree of trust endemic in the encounter, can provide tremendous insight into the situation, thereby enabling the health professional to select the appropriate rhetorical map beyond the predetermined medical interview when proceeding with the negotiation.

The physician, in turn, should listen actively to the patient's attitudes, emotions, fears, beliefs, and concerns and inquire with probing yet reasonable questions, atypical of the standard medical interview (Thompson, 1986). (This, in fact, has been referred to as the "art" of medicine and has received considerable criticism for being neglected in modern day medicine; "Three Possible Futures," 1990.) A major requirement is that the physician demonstrates empathy and genuine concern for the patient (Quill, 1983). If the patient is reluctant to disclose any information beyond merely outlining the problem, the physician must respond with appropriate strategic ethical and emotional rhetorical appeals that encourage and explain the crucial importance of opening up such lines of communication. Although this places a heavy burden on doctors, their fortunate position of possessing expert power and having the medical knowledge and expertise (Quill, 1983) can help induce patients to step beyond the traditional, paternalistic physician–patient model (Ballard-Reisch, 1990). Furthermore, it is incumbent that the physician abandon the traditional omnipotent power role to maximize the success of the health communication encounter.

Although the communication agenda and ground rules often are affected by time constraints, the imprecision of language, the inability of parties to communicate clearly, attitudes, beliefs, role expectations, and religious perspectives, the physician and patient must make the effort to establish an open relationship, thereby ushering in a two-way process of decision making (Quill, 1983). Without such an active agenda objective, shared by both participants, health communication as negotiation will be stymied. Beisecker (1990) echoed this communication-centered approach reemphasizing Nelson's (1981) finding that "before they can make a choice about their medical care, patients must first decide that they have a right to choose" (p. 115).

Opting to pass on such vast responsibility to the physician is a viable alternative to the patient. Yet, the important negotiation principle is that the patient actively is engaged in decision making. Addressing the shared responsibility by patients in such an encounter, Ballard-Reisch (1990) wrote that a patient should be able to choose to (a) have the ultimate say in decision making, (b) pass the responsibility on to the physician, (c) work with the physician in the decision-making process, or (d) decide the relationship would be better if terminated because of irreconcilable differences.

Following the establishment of goals and objectives through the dialectical health communication encounter, the patient and physician proceed to an action

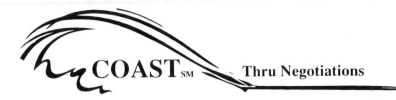

Communication

- Communicate your interests and theirs without fixing positions.
- Establish an agenda and set ground rules; ask questions to clarify.
- Listen to the other side; understand personalities, education, culture, and style.

Trust

- Establish trust and complete deal with authority.
- Be honest and open.
- Develop an agreement which is compliance-prone.
- Build relationships through communication and trust between parties.

Options

- Generate creative options by brainstorming ideas which satisfy each party's interests.
- Continue dialogue without judging.
- Strengthen your options before negotiating; know other opportunities for possible agreement.

Standards ← Alternatives

Standards
- Locate and share objective standards (i.e. comparable sales, legal precedents, other research, etc.)
- *Separate people and personalities from the problem.*

Alternatives
- Know your best alternative; it is not always prudent to agree/settle on the first attempt.
- Explore competitive, cooperative and realistic ideas which can strengthen your alternatives.
- Let each party know various alternatives.

Everyone can be satisfied - - resulting in a win-win,
a good outcome and a successful negotiation.

Dr. Scott C. Ratzan
Emerson College, Division of Communication Studies
100 Beacon Street, Boston, MA 02116

Figure 2-1 The COAST model of health communication as negotiation.

plan that benefits the patient's best interests (if the patient is incompetent or otherwise impaired, the family's best interests), maximizing the doctor's expertise (Quill, 1983).

At this juncture, it is important to emphasize that if the patient chooses autonomy or abdication, communication is a key component in the event that the type of relationship changes and future negotiations need to be conducted. Appropriate oral and written communication might be necessary to redefine the physician–patient encounter, especially if the ultimate joint decision is—in negotiation terms, an impasse. Clearly, a communication-based negotiation model centers on a multiagent approach to determine the respective parties' best interests rather than employing a "substituted judgment" decision.

Options

Exploration of options, the second component of the health communication encounter as negotiation, invites the doctor and patient to engage in brainstorming potential solutions that could satisfy each party's interests. At the outset, however, there must be an understanding that the first effort should be to create as many options as possible, without criticism or analysis (Fisher & Ury, 1981). The advantage of the brainstorming process is that it provides a wider variety of options to be considered by the patient and physician often beyond the scope of the traditional physician-centered medical interview. Furthermore, it results in a strong bond and identification with the decision, a product of a joint decision-making effort (Ballard-Reisch, 1990). It also increases satisfaction in the decision-making process and hence increases compliance (Beisecker, 1990). The ability to generate ideas through dialogue, emphasizing inductive and deductive reasoning further enhances outcome potential. Inductive empiricist Francis Bacon stated, "A wise man makes more opportunity than he finds." Furthermore, Campbell's (1987) hypotheticodeductive model of diagnosis helps the physician generate options by suggesting data from experiments and clinical simulations and studies.

Alternatives

During the decision-making process, the physician and patient should protect against hasty selection of an inappropriate course of action. Each should consider viable and workable alternatives in an effort to strengthen the satisfaction levels of both. Determining alternatives frequently includes conferring with family members, consulting other health colleagues, and obtaining second opinions. The major focus in this part of the negotiation health encounter is to continue the dynamic flow of communication among the dyad participants. Employing traditional formal and informal decision analysis (probabilities, reasoning, heuristics, etc.) with frank discussion of advantages and disadvantages regarding each alternative can aid involved parties in eliminating weak alternatives and strengthening the ultimate decision.

During the negotiation procedure, it should be reaffirmed that there is nothing permanent or obligatory in the health communication encounter. If either party views the encounter from an unsatisfactory perspective, barring a resolution of the differences, potential termination of the relationship remains, however unpleasant, an alternative, which could increase ultimate compliance with realistic/rational decisions.

Standards

Another pertinent component of the health communication encounter act is standards, the criteria by which alternatives are measured and assessed. Common standards include individual determinism, designation of the final authority in determining the outcome of the negotiation, legal precedents, designation of the parties involved if the patient is no longer able to render rational decisions, divergent perspectives on medicine (Food and Drug Administration, Western, Eastern, holistic, etc.), use of prescription drugs/life-support devices to prolong life, quantity versus quality of life, and outcomes of controlled research experimentation.

The agreement on and use of specific standards—objective criteria—in the decision-making process are a crucial component in enhancing the efficacy of the health communication encounter. Of course, given the negotiation perspective, there is room for compromise and acceptance; the key step is for mutual agreement through communication. For example, a patient might be motivated by moral standards and a physician by professional standards. According to Fisher and Ury (1981), each must realize that "one standard of legitimacy does not preclude the existence of others" (p. 89). The physician and patient must discuss, and eventually concur on, what they both consider to be appropriate standards to refer to in their health communication encounter.

Trust

Trust, one of the most important elements in the negotiation health communication encounter, is a reciprocally enhanced product of each of the aforementioned areas. As open communication is encouraged, all possible options and alternatives discussed, and objective standards agreed on, both the patient and the physician have already begun the process of establishing an abiding trust and relationship. Trust is at the communication core of an effective relationship in the dyadic encounter. Communication with disclosure of information further enhances trust and the relationship (illustrated in Figure 1 by the double arrows and handshake).

Trust is the final element in the COAST model of the health communication encounter as negotiation. The COAST paradigmatic dialectical design presents an added opportunity for disclosure by the interested parties, thereby further deepening the level of trust. If present, trust imbues the encounter with honest and open dialogue (Bromberg, 1981; Deutsch, 1958; Jabusch & Littlejohn, 1990; Kremenyuk, 1991; Linzey & Aronson, 1989). The intrinsic value of trust is also evident beyond the initial health communication encounter. Past studies have found that patients would rather be provided all available information and be made aware of the possible side effects and consequences of treatment rather than be cushioned from the stark realities of ill health (Korsch & Negrete, 1972).

Nonetheless, research on the typical traditional relationship reveals that physicians feel uncomfortable discussing unpleasant information, often opting to keep such information from the patient (Beisecker, 1990). Commenting on the interpersonal needs of the patient in such situations, Bernarde and Mayerson (1978) wrote, "It is essential that the patient be made to believe that he is an independent, worthy person entitled to the most clearly stated information possible . . . respect is demonstrated by being responsive" (p. 1413). The product of open dialogue, even discussion of troublesome issues between the patient and physician, has its benefits to the health care provider. Thompson (1986) found a positive correlation between the frequency of physicians' caring and unselfish attitudes toward patients and the development of referent power for the physicians because patients liked them, trusted them, and considered them role models.

Ultimately, the COAST model of the health communication encounter as negotiation is merely a theory that builds trust, a necessary objective for the model's practical and efficient application. Relationships are formed over time with trust built from disclosure and effective communication between parties (Silvestri, 1987). The relationship—the double arrow in Figure 1—is perhaps the unquantifiable resource employed in the COAST negotiation health communication model. With a strong relationship (communication and trust), the outcome efficacy of future health encounters is enhanced, adding positive human factors that often are the most important indicators of a treatment plan's success (Fisher & Brown, 1988; Norfolk, 1990; Northouse & Northouse, 1985; "Three Possible Futures," 1990).

As the relationship matures, options will evolve naturally based on trust. The patient and physician will no longer need to specifically negotiate these two stages because they will be understood and accepted. This will streamline the overall efficacy of the health communication encounter, allowing the participants to pay greater attention to open communication and searching for the best possible alternatives. This positive relationship within the COAST model (identified with the icon of a handshake) can be a most effective component in combating disease.

The biological/psychological response to a beneficent trusting relationship is often termed the *placebo* (meaning "feel good" in Latin) *effect* (Brody, 1987; Fish, 1973; Norfolk, 1990; Simons, 1989). The placebo effect, the benefits to a patient beyond the pharmacological effects of a certain drug, is generally measured by giving a "dummy pill" with no apparent pharmacological value to subjects. Its effect has been found in a recent study at New York's Mt. Sinai School of Medicine, cited by Norfolk (1990), to be dependent on two factors: the positive attitude of the patient to the drug (placebo) and the degree of trust the patient placed in the doctor. The latter was related to communication variables—the doctor's status, physical attractiveness, enthusiasm, warmth, empathy, and general likability. Norfolk concluded that "of the two factors, the patient's trust in the doctor proved to be three times more important than the faith they [sic] had in the dummy pill" (p. 43). These modern-day prescriptions of trust again have their roots in classical rhetoric, which the Greeks identified as *vis medicatrix nature*—the healing power of nature.

Discussion

In contrast to the Socratic style of inquiry stressed in medical schools, the COAST model of the health communication encounter as negotiation does not follow a semistatic scientific/decision-tree analysis approach. However, the open communication of alternatives offers individuals the opportunity to apply different standards, whether scientific, religious, or other beliefs deemed important to participants in the encounter. In place of the traditional communication patterns widely adopted in health settings, the negotiation model of the physician–patient encounter clearly emphasizes the importance of mutual decision making through ethical and effective communication. As stated, major ingredients and by-products of such an approach include a relationship and a sense of patient empowerment to be involved and responsible throughout the health communication encounter.

Overall, the application of COAST—Communication, Options, Alternatives, Standards, and Trust—to a physician–patient dyad can result in what negotiation scholars would term a win–win situation for both parties involved in the health communication encounter.

THE COAST MODEL OF NEGOTIATION APPLIED TO A PATIENT WITH ACQUIRED IMMUNE DEFICIENCY SYNDROME

The following case study illustrates the value of the COAST model of negotiation in the health care setting involving a 34-year-old Caucasian male patient with acquired immune deficiency syndrome (AIDS) who underwent 2 years of therapy in Chicago. The first year after learning he had the human immunodeficiency virus (HIV), the patient was under the direction of Physician 1, who did not apply any of the basic principles in COAST in the physician–patient encounter. The patient subsequently switched to the care and guidance of Physician 2 because of irreconcilable differences with Physician 1. This is explained in both narrative form and Figure 2.[2] He died of complications due to AIDS on July 4, 1991.

Physician 1

Communication, Trust, and Standards Physician 1 rarely smiled or greeted the patient in a friendly manner. She was formal and standoffish, and would open the consultation period without visual contact with the patient by examining the patient's chart and inquiring directly into the nature of his specific affliction, his chief complaint. Visits were scheduled in 5- to 10-min allotments, always at the end of the day. Physician 1 would terminate the visit by looking at her watch. She would state that she had to "find the time" to fit the patient into her busy schedule. She often would not return the patient's urgent phone calls for up to an hour, and even then she would often have her nurse perform this function. Physician 1 frequently reminded the patient that he was covered on a public aid insurance policy, implying that her treatment was a favor to the patient. Occasionally, Physician 1 would make blunt and straightforward statements, such as "No one has of yet survived this disease."

The patient found it difficult to establish a bond of trust with Physician 1 because Physician 1 displayed the minimal, if not substandard, amount of communication necessary to discover the patient's symptoms and prescribe treatment.

Alternatives and Options Physician 1 did perform a myriad of diagnostic tests/procedures without emotion, and her staff was often visibly nervous and overly cautious given the infective nature of the disease. The test results often took 1 to 2 days to be completed, with minimal explanations provided. The patient perceived that Physician 1 regarded him as only a statistic, rather than an individual human being inflicted with a disease. Although the patient kept files on information about AIDS, attended seminars on the disease, and kept updated on all the latest developments of the epidemic, Physician 1 never recognized his knowledge, information, or opinion. There was no two-way dialogue as prescribed by COAST. Ideas and alternatives were not explored together; information from the patient was discouraged. The physician used a "This is the only way" attitude in regard to the administering of zidovudine (AZT) treatment, even though the patient was skeptical and wished to avoid its use. The overall approach of Physician 1 seemed to the patient and family to be

---

[2]All patient information was provided by Holly Massett, sister of the late patient.

Coast Model		Physician #1	Physician #2
Communication	Agenda/Questions	Standard questions Standoffish, formal	Detailed, specific questions Personable, friendly, warm
	Listen and understand	Technical language, statistics	Understandable terms, detailed description
	Communicate interests	Imposing on time schedule; financial Little hope, a favor to see the patient Low level of empathy	Not time driven; interested in patient's well-being Positive outlook High level of quality
Options	Generate options	Only FDA approved drugs	FDA drugs and potential for non-approved drugs and therapy
	Continue dialogue	No psychotherapy/counseling suggested	Psychotherapy/counseling suggested
	Strengthen options	No assistance (financial/social/psychotherapy) IV-food hook-up Diet/exercise/vitamins casually mentioned	Direct involvement in diet/exercise/vitamin regimen strongly suggested Research potential Suggestion of variety of other treatment sites and plans
Alternatives	Know best alternative	End relationship if not satisfied	End relationship if not satisfied, but broadened boundaries
	Explores ideas together	Outside information discouraged	Encouraged second opinions
	Let each party know various attempts	"This is the only way" attitude "Take it or leave it"	Outside information encouraged -- it could help refine treatment plan Financial/family support and hospice services discussed
Standards	Locate objective standards	Quantity of life FDA approved drugs only Text book style of medical treatment	Quality of life FDA approval not necessary
	Establish authority	Physician initiates questions/responses; physician makes decisions	Patient's requests considered. Could deviate from standard, accepted method of treatment Open, two-way communication and decision making
	Separate people from the problem	An infected person who has a lifestyle disease	A person who has contracted HIV
Trust	Establish trust	Factors best interest over patient's	Mutual respect for good relationship
	Honest and open	Ideas that the patient is "buying time," rather than sustaining life	Patient has a role in his health; not just another statistic; shared ideas
	Develop compliance-prone agreement	Low compliance with doctor's suggestions and treatment	High compliance to a joint treatment, desire to keep fighting disease; discouragement low

Figure 2-2 Examples of ineffective (Physician 1) and effective (Physician 2) use of the COAST model of health communication as negotiation with a patient with AIDS.

to wait for the inevitable death of the patient, although lessening the pain of its consequences.

Physician 2

Communication, Trust, and Standards   Physician 2 maintained a cheerful, personable disposition, making certain that he always greeted the patient and listened to the patient while maintaining direct eye contact. Visits consisted of the amount of time necessary to answer all of the patient's questions to his satisfaction. Physician 2 often encouraged the patient with advice such as, "A cure may be found any day. Keep up the fight." He used humor to relax the patient and open channels of communication. The groundwork for a trusting relationship was evident from the first patient-physician encounter. The patient was encouraged to call the physician any time. If the physician was unavailable for the call, the call would be returned personally, generally within a half hour. Unlike Physician 1, who would schedule appointments only when the patient suffered opportunistic infections, Physician 2 treated the patient on a preventative basis.

Options and Alternatives   Physician 2 treated the patient as an individual, not as a statistic, emphasizing the fact that the patient had a role in his health. Because trust and communication had been encouraged and established, Physician 2 was able to work with the patient on his level to discover a program maximizing satisfaction of mutual interests. Test results were always ready within 3 hr. Physician 2 did not insist that the patient take AZT treatments but instead deviated from standard, accepted methods of treatment, experimenting with drugs with which the patient felt more comfortable. Because the patient disliked hospital stays, Physician 2 helped him find a nurse to administer treatment in his own home. Physician 2 researched the patient's individual case, involving the patient in the decision-making process. The relationship with Physician 2 reestablished the patient's independence and will to fight for his life and maintain hope.

CONCLUSION

The medicalization of disease, and specifically HIV/AIDS, follows the traditional dehumanizing medical model/paradigm of defining ill health located in the body, in tissues, organs, and glands replete with a "medicobabble" of lymphocytes, antibodies, and syndromes. The individual and communication process sometimes become lost in the polysyllable profundity. Unfortunately, health care providers are trained more in the immunology of the replication of the retrovirus on the microscopic level than in the communication theories and practices that can be crucial to altering attitudes and risk behavior ("Three Possible Futures," 1990). Communication of the appropriate social response by the health care team is necessary, yet grossly ineffective in its current approach.

The medical response to the AIDS epidemic contributes to the perfidy and misguided approaches of many physicians who are unable to employ traditional methods of communication in approaching the medical encounter as a negotiation. The application of the COAST model at the initial contact with the patient—the early phase of disease—presents an opportunity for a physician to build one of the most powerful components, the *sine qua non*, of effective health communication—a relationship built on trust and effective communication.

The ethical application of the COAST model of health communication as negotiation, specifically to the AIDS crisis, by health care providers/patients, institutions, and political groups can further the prospect for appropriate social responses, including individual behavior and attitude change as well as institutional and governmental policymaking to educate the American public.

REFERENCES

Alroy, G., Ber, R., & Kramer, D. (1984). An evaluation of the short-term effects of an interpersonal skills course. *Medical Education, 18,* 85–89.

Ballard-Reisch, D. S. (1990). A model of participative decision making for physician-patient interaction. *Health Communication, 2*(2), 91–104.

Barrows, H. S. (1990). The pedagogical importance of a skill central to clinical practice. *Medical Education, 24,* 3–5.

Bartlett, E. E., Grayson, M., & Barker, R. (1984). The effects of physician communication skills on patient satisfaction, recall, and adherence. *Journal of Chronic Diseases, 37,* 755–764.

Beisecker, A. E. (1990). Patient power in doctor-patient communication: What do we know? *Health Communication, 2*(2), 105–122.

Bernarde, M., & Mayerson, E. W. (1978). Patient-physician negotiation. *Journal of the American Medical Association, 239,* 1413–1415.

Bitzer, L. F. (1968). The rhetorical situation. *Philosophy and Rhetoric, 1,* 1–14.

Bok, S. (1978). *Lying.* New York: Pantheon Books.

Brody, H. (1977). *Placebos and the philosophy of medicine.* Chicago: University of Chicago Press.

Bromberg, M. D. (1981). The new medical-industrial complex. *New England Journal of Medicine, 304,* 233.

Campbell, E. J. M. (1987). The diagnosing mind. *Lancet, 1,* 849–851.

Deutsch, M. (1958). Trust and suspicion. *Journal of Conflict Resolution, 11,* 265–279.

Fish, J. M. (1973). *Placebo therapy.* San Francisco: Jossey-Bass.

Fisher, R., & Brown, S. (1988). *Getting together: Building a relationship that gets to yes.* Boston: Houghton Mifflin.

Fisher, R., & Ury, W. (1981). *Getting to yes.* New York: Penguin Group.

Fitzgerald, F. T. (1990). Physical diagnosis versus modern technology—A review. *Western Journal of Medicine, 152*, 377–382.

Inui, T. S., & Carter, W. R. (1985). Problems and prospects for health services research on provider-patient communication. *Medical Care, 3*, 521–538.

Jabusch, D. M., & Littlejohn, S. W. (1990). *Elements of speech communication.* San Diego: Collegiate Press.

Katz, J. (1980). Disclosure and consent: In search of their roots. In A. Milunsky & G. J. Annas (Eds.), *Genetics and the law II.* New York: Plenum Press.

Korsch, B. M., & Negrete, V. F. (1972). Doctor-patient communication. *Scientific American, 227*(2), 66–74.

Kremenyuk, V. A. (Ed.). (1991). *International negotiation: Analysis, approaches, issues.* San Francisco: Jossey-Bass.

Kreps, G. L., & Thornton, B. C. (1984). *Health communication: Theory and practice.* New York: Longman.

Lane, S. D. (1983). Compliance, satisfaction, and physician-patient communication. In *Communication yearbook 8* (pp. 772–799).

Linzey, G., & Aronson, E. (1989). *The handbook of social psychology: Volume 5* (2nd ed.). Reading, MA: Addison-Wesley.

Nelson, M. K. (1981). Client responses to a discrepancy between the care they want and the care they receive. *Women and Health, 6*, 135–152.

Norfolk, D. (1990). *Think well, feel great.* London: Michael Joseph.

Northouse, P. G., & Northouse, L. L. (1985). *Health communication: A handbook for health professionals.* Englewood Cliffs, NJ: Prentice-Hall.

President's Commission for the Study of Ethical Problems in Medicine and Biomedical and Behavioral Research. (1982). *Making health care decisions, Volume I,* Washington, DC: U.S. Government Printing Office.

Quill, T. W. (1983). Partnerships in patient care: A contractual approach. *Annals of Internal Medicine, 98*, 228–234.

Roberson, D. W., Kowlowitz, V., Jenkins, P. C., & Hoole, A. J. (1989). The development of medical students' interviewing skills: An observational study. *Medical Encounter, 6*(1), 3–5.

Robertson, W. O. (1985). *Medical malpractice: A preventive approach.* Seattle: University of Washington Press.

Rowland-Morin, P. A., & Carroll, J. G. (1990). Verbal communication skills and patient satisfaction: A study of doctor-patient interviews. *Evaluation and the Health Professions, 13*(2), 168–185.

Samora, J. L., Saunders, L., & Larson, R. F. (1961). Medical vocabulary knowledge among hospital patients. *Journal of Health and Human Behaviors, 2*, 92.

Seldes, G. (1985). *The great thoughts.* New York: Ballantine Books.

Sharf, B. F. (1990). Physician-patient communication as interpersonal rhetoric: A narrative approach. *Health Communication, 2*(4), 217–231.

Silvestri, V. N. (1987). *Interpersonal communication: Perspectives and interfaces* (2nd ed.). Boston: American Press.

Simons, H. W. (1989). *Rhetoric in the human sciences.* Newbury Park, CA: Sage.

Sivertson, S. E., & Stone, H. L. (1983). Efficiency in examining adult patients on preceptorship. *Journal of Medical Education, 58*, 657–659.

National Underwriter Company. (1990). *Statistical abstract of the United States 1990* (Chart 857). Cincinnati, OH: Author.

Stewart, M., & Roter, D. (Eds.). (1989). *Communicating with medical patients.* Newbury Park, CA: Sage.

Stiles, W. B., & Putnam, S. M. (1989). Analysis of verbal and nonverbal behavior in doctor-patient encounters. In M. Stewart & D. Roter (Eds.), *Communicating with medical patients* (pp. 211–222). Newbury Park, CA: Sage.

Strachey, J. (Ed.). (1958). *The standard edition of the complete psychological works of Sigmund Freud* (Vol. 12). London: Hogarth Press.

Street, R. L., Jr., & Wiemann, J. M. (1987). Patient satisfaction with physician's interpersonal involvement, expressiveness, and dominance. In M. L. McLaughlin (Ed.), *Communication yearbook 10* (pp. 591–612). Newbury Park, CA: Sage.

Thompson, T. L. (1986). *Communication for health professionals.* New York: Harper & Row.

Three possible futures for medicine (Editorial). (1990). *Western Journal of Medicine, 152*(4), 114.

Wasserman, R. C., & Inui, T. S. (1983). Systematic analysis of clinician-patient interactions: A critique of recent approaches with suggestions for future research. *Medical Care, 21,* 279–293.

Chapter Three

The Role of Care Partners in Managing AIDS Patients' Illness: Toward a Triadic Model of Health Care Delivery

Eric G. Zook
Katherine I. Miller

In the years since acquired immune deficiency syndrome (AIDS) was first recognized and then developed into a national health "crisis," there has been an
explosion in the number of persons afflicted and an accompanying expansion in
the range of services and treatments available (Clement, 1989; Schofferman,
1988). However, the response of our health care system has been variously
criticized as too slow, overly political, and inefficient (Perrow & Guillen,
1990). Although critiques of today's health care system range from discussions
of inadequate funding for research and service development to insufficient preventive public education, we are concerned in this chapter with examining the
failure to adequately account for the role of care partners (CPs) in managing the
illness of persons with AIDS.

We use Grieco and Kowalski's (1987) term "care partner" in place of the
more traditional referent "caregiver" for two reasons. First, "caregiver" is a
broad term that requires a qualifying adjective to make its referent explicit and
useful, such as "professional caregiver" or "family caregiver." Second, and
more important, "caregiver" carries connotations of "doing for." Recognizing
the strain created by nonreciprocity in relationships (Pearlin, Semple, & Turner,

1988) and the significant problem of informal carers' stress and burnout, we prefer to emphasize the positive interaction and participation the care dyad can establish. The term "care partner," then, is not simply a designation, but establishes a normative standard wherein an illness is shared by the patient and some informal third party; it takes the onus off the CP and acknowledges the dignity and limited, but nonetheless real, independence of the patient.

The lack of specific information regarding the number of CPs working with AIDS patients parallels the lack of knowledge concerning those who assist the millions of people incapacitated by accidents and a variety of chronic diseases, such as arthritis, Alzheimer's disease, Lou Gehrig's disease, cancer, cerebral palsy, childhood disorders, chronic lung disease, chronic mental illness, Huntington's disease, Parkinson's disease, premature birth, and stroke. What is clear, however, is that an increasing amount of care is being provided at home and family members are heavily involved in this process.

Bishop and Karon (1989) reported that total Medicare spending on home health services more than doubled between 1980 and 1985, totaling approximately $1.8 billion. Between 1980 and 1983, the annual rate of growth for home health services expenditures was 28.3%; between 1983 and 1985, the growth slowed to 12.6% but continued its upward trend. Combined with the tripling of Medicaid payments for such services between 1980 and 1985, "total public spending on home health shows a steady increase in the amount of public resources flowing into the home health market" (Bishop & Karon, 1989, p. 142). These authors also reported that the number of agencies providing home health services expanded at the rate of 15.8% per year between 1980 and 1984, resulting in an overall increase from 2,858 agencies in 1980 to 5,964 by 1985. Such growth supports Halmandaris's (1985) and Goodhue's (1984) claims that home health care is the wave of the future in health care delivery.

Although Goodhue (1984) and Halmandaris (1985) extolled the economic growth potential of the home care market, the fact is that much of the burden of care falls on the family. Estimates of family involvement range from 75% to 90% (Brody, 1985; Brody, Poulshock, & Masiocchi, 1978). Such figures, combined with the growth in professional home health care, have led Strauss and Corbin (1988) to argue that "the home should [now] be at the very center of care. All other facilities and services should be oriented toward supplementing and facilitating work done at home" (p. 150).

With the number of diagnosed AIDS cases recently topping 200,000, and given the significant late-stage deterioration of individuals with AIDS, it seems clear that many CPs' are aiding in the management of patient illness. Many agencies (e.g., the Gay Men's Health Crisis in New York City and the Shanti Project in San Francisco) have developed support groups for CPs, and books such as Eidson's (1988) *The AIDS Caregiver's Handbook* have been published to facilitate CPs' work with individuals who have AIDS. These resources are valuable for the emotional and informational support they provide, but they have little to say about CP relations with medical personnel. This lack is critical, considering that Greif and Porembski (1988) found that medical personnel's treatment of the AIDS patient and difficulty in accessing adequate information about the patient's health are significant concerns of CPs. Similar concerns were common in a study we recently conducted (Zook, 1991; Zook & Miller, 1992).

To fully understand the importance of a CP's relations with both the patient and the physician, it is necessary to establish the context in which health care is delivered. In the following section, we discuss important contextual factors and note areas where human immunodeficiency virus (HIV)/AIDS care departs from that of other illness situations. In particular, we consider three aspects of health care delivery: the primacy of the patient–physician relationship, Strauss and Corbin's (1988) concept of illness trajectories, and locus of care. Our discussion of these issues draws on both extant theory and research and our own intensive study of 23 CPs of AIDS patients.[1]

HEALTH CARE PROVISION FOR AIDS PATIENTS

The Primacy of the Patient–Physician Relationship

Medical care has traditionally been delivered primarily through patient–physician interaction (Engel, 1977). To be sure, both participants operate in accordance with roles within a wider system: The patient comes from and returns to his or her family, who have their own concerns and conceptions about the patient's health status; the physician carries out his or her diagnosis and treatment only with the assistance of a wide array of allied health professionals. However, so long as the patient is of sound mind and retains confidence in the

---

[1]Our research on relationships between CPs and medical professionals in the context of HIV/ AIDS is based on the experiences of 23 CPs. Participants were drawn from the client population of a government-funded case management agency servicing the needs of patients with HIV infection in a large Midwestern city. The sample consisted of patient mothers (45%), lovers (23%), siblings (18%), an aunt, an ex-wife, and a friend. Half the sample was or had been involved in caring for a patient with full-blown AIDS (55% of these patients were deceased at the time of the interview); 39%, with asymptomatic HIV; and 4%, with AIDS-related complex. Fifty-nine percent of the patients were Black compared with 41% White, and patients were predominantly male (91%). The primary route of transmission was intravenous drug use (32%), followed closely by sexual transmission through homosexual relations (30%). Other forms included unknown (14%), heterosexual sex (8%), and multiple risks (8%).

Data were collected by the first author via semistructured interviews that assessed the degree and nature of CP involvement with the patient, CP burden, professionals involved in patient care, and communication patterns between CPs and medical personnel. Initially, CPs were asked to provide a brief history of their patient's experience, particularly noting the crisis periods of illness and medical contacts. Participants were then asked about their interactions with each individual who provided medical care to the patient, focusing on those who participated regularly in the care, including community nurses and social workers who assisted the CPs with home care planning and management.

physician's expertise, the majority of information exchange occurs within the patient–physician relationship. The patient thereby retains control over the amount and nature of information shared with his or her social network, as well as over treatment decisions.

The primacy of the physician–patient relationship is typically justified on the basis of expertise and confidentiality. That is, the physician is seen as the expert with regard to diagnosing and treating physical dysfunctions, and the patient is viewed as the expert concerning the impact of the underlying disease on his or her physical and social being (Quill, 1983). Moreover, there is a continued belief that illness is related to personal failing, whether insufficient moral virtue or lack of rational prevention behaviors. Thus, the attending social stigma and discrimination that may occur increase concerns about maintaining patients' confidentiality (Sontag, 1978). A concern for confidentiality has been significantly justified throughout the brief history of AIDS (Brandt, 1987; Sontag, 1989). Because grave repercussions can arise from the revelation of diagnoses such as AIDS, patient control over whom is informed about medical diagnoses has long been supported and even codified into law.

The traditional patient–physician model of health care delivery has generally served society well; however, it is dysfunctional for the demands that are typically associated with the chronic nature of illnesses such as AIDS. Increasingly, a person's functional independence is undermined long before death, necessitating the sharing of illness. In such situations, it is useful, and perhaps even necessary, for CPs to have direct interaction with the primary care physician. Several arguments can be made for such interaction.

First, a CP may well have different concerns than the patient. As a result, the CP could be inadequately informed even if the patient gives him or her a full account of each medical encounter. Second, even such "full" accounts are subject to substantial distortion and filtering by the patient, both intentional and unintentional. That is, the patient may actively withhold information from the CP to maintain denial or in an effort to protect the CP from further worry. Patient recountings also represent a consolidation and interpretation of the full information exchanged during the encounter—an inherently selective picture.

To the extent that CPs are increasingly asked to assume ever larger and more technical roles within patient illness management systems, these concerns with information flow are significant. Assumption of care responsibilities requires adequate preparation and ample opportunity for clarification regarding care regimens. We cannot expect CPs to provide basic forms of nursing care if they do not have adequate access to general medical and patient-specific information (Nichols, 1987, 1984).

Patients' ability to gatekeep information also applies to information flowing from the patient to the physician. Patients in denial or those who fear their health is worsening may underreport symptoms; others may simply forget or be unaware of behavioral details that are noticed by the CP. Inclusion of the CP in a triadic relationship reduces the patient's ability to gatekeep in either direction, improving the efficiency and completeness of communication and, ideally, the overall efficacy of treatment. Such outcomes raise significant ethical issues, but these may be mitigated by respecting patient autonomy. The key is not to force involvement if not desired, but rather not to hinder it when it is desired.

In general, however, CPs are excluded from the patient–physician relationship. Of course, CPs do find opportunities to talk directly with the physician, but these opportunities are subject to numerous restrictions. If communication occurs during routine medical appointments, it is typically after the patient examination. Because the patient examination usually consumes most of the allotted time, little time is left for the CP's questions. At the hospital, pressing demands from other patients limit the amount of time for CP–physician interaction, not to mention the fact that physician rounds often occur during early morning hours when the CP is not present. This leaves the telephone. Phone contact suffices for specific issues, but hardly replaces ongoing, open-ended interactions that might increase the CP's understanding of critical care issues. Finally, although CPs often seek out printed information on HIV and AIDS, such information can be made more real and useful through discussions with appropriate medical personnel.

Ironically, the greatest limitation on CP–physician interaction may be the CP's own belief that he or she does not have the right to impose on the physician. That is, CPs themselves question the legitimacy of their desire to communicate more fully and directly with the physician about issues relating to patients' health and care. In our research (Zook, 1991; Zook & Miller, 1992), CPs frequently mentioned the patient's adult status as automatically excluding them from more direct interaction with health care professionals. Patient desires for independence also promoted this hesitance on the part of CPs.

Negotiation of the Care Partner's Involvement in Health Care

The need for CPs to negotiate legitimate forms of involvement with both the patient and the physician is evident from the centrality of the patient–physician relationship in health care delivery. Support for increased CP involvement can be extrapolated from calls for greater negotiation (Quill, 1983) and accommodation (Siegler, 1981) between physicians and patients in the wake of a more consumerist notion of medical care. Although little specific research has been done on the process through which CPs negotiate involvement, we identified several important issues in our research on CPs of people with AIDS.

In general, the illness situations we examined began with acceptance of the traditional model of health care delivery. Patients wanted to maintain this model as a form of normalization, which is to say they wished to continue functioning as a normal adult for as long as possible (Pearlin et al., 1988). The departure from the norm of health care delivery represented by CP inclusion could be interpreted as an indication that the patient can no longer successfully manage his or her own illness independently. The issue of normalization is even more important to persons with HIV/AIDS because most of them are young and thus heavily invested in living. Many of the CPs we interviewed never deviated from the traditional patient–physician model of health care. For many, this was simply the way that health care has to be done. Thus, they never questioned their exclusion from this model.

For those CPs who did achieve greater inclusion, the primary impetus for inclusion was declining patient health. As the patient's ability to function independently decreased, the CPs assumed a greater role in illness management (Pearlin et al., 1988). Declining health typically provided CPs with greater opportunity for direct interaction with the physician and also prompted many CPs to insist on inclusion in health care discussions that had previously been restricted to the patient–physician dyad. One CP we interviewed described the discussion he had with his partner when the latter could no longer drive himself to medical appointments:

> I told him at that point that I wanted to start going in with him to the appointment. Because I told him quite frankly that, "I don't want to wait until you're in the hospital to form some kind of relationship with this person. I want to be visible."

In the main, our research indicated that physicians' acceptance of increased participation by CPs was important. However, it was clear that patient wishes predominated. Thus, agreement between the CP and patient regarding the CP's inclusion formed the basis for presenting a unified desire for greater CP involvement to the attending physician. In all but 1 of the 23 situations we investigated, the attending physician willingly accommodated such requests.

For most CPs, however, acquiring the motivation and ability to talk with the physician and other medical staff regarding the patient was only the first step. The aim of most CPs was to establish a sense of partnership with the health care team and with the patient. To this end, the CPs we talked with stressed the importance of being strong, competent, clearly open to truthful information about the patient's status, and flexibly insistent on issues of patient care. Social status and education can also be influential, as indicated by one CP. Her relationship with her daughter's physician became tense fairly early when she was critical of a treatment decision. The CP, an insistent, direct person, felt that some of the physician's continuing resistance to her was due to her poverty and lack of formal schooling. The CP believed the physician considered demographic characteristics and ignored her sound knowledge of AIDS and awareness of her daughter's health.

Because physicians were not included in our sample, we were unable to assess the actual influence of these characteristics on the strength and valence of the CP–physician relationship. However, some related support is available on physician evaluations of various patient characteristics. Harris, Rich, and Crowson (1985) presented four groups of characteristics that were negatively viewed (60% or more of the physicians indicated willingness to treat only occasionally or rarely) by a sample of internal medicine residents and staff physicians. These included characteristics that (a) might hinder effective doctor–patient communication (e.g., not speaking English or being uncooperative), (b) reflect general societal rejection of certain qualities (e.g., unpleasant odor), (c) are associated with self-destructive tendencies (e.g., drug addiction or intoxication), and (d) reflect psychological problems or aspects of illness (e.g., organic brain disease or personal life difficulties). Positively viewed (90% or more of the physicians were willing to treat regularly or mostly) characteristics included cardiac disease; controllable, chronic disease; compliance; middle age; multiple current diseases; age over 65; and good grooming.

It is interesting to note that residents reported preferences for intelligent, middle-income patients with acute, curable diseases. By contrast, staff physicians ranked the following patient characteristics as positive: having a low income, being a veteran, and belonging to a different racial or ethnic group. This finding is important because it shows that whereas staff physicians appear to be the best candidates for delivering service to low-income minorities living in the inner cities, it is usually residents who work in the publicly funded hospitals where many such patients are treated. Coupled with the high prevalence of drug addiction in these patients, this suggests that both the patient and the CP may find it difficult to establish a partnership with the physician. This is further complicated by the transient nature of residents' hospital assignments, which creates ruptures in the continuity of care. Intravenous-drug-using HIV-positive patients being treated at public hospitals often reported seeing a different physician at each appointment.

Factors That Affect Care Partner Involvement

In sum, the successful inclusion of CPs in health care contexts traditionally dominated by the patient–physician dyad can be difficult to achieve. It is likely that if such relationships are to succeed, a contract model of health care provision will be most appropriate. Quill (1983) provided an overview of basic assumptions that underlie doctor–patient contracts that can be extended to cover doctor–patient–CP contracts. These are:

1 Each party has unique responsibilities,
2 The relationship is consensual rather than obligatory,
3 Each party must be willing to negotiate, and
4 Each must gain something from the transaction.

Quill (1983) and Siegler (1981) pointed out that such negotiated relationships must be dynamic to accommodate contextual changes. The primary cause of flux in such contracts will be the patient's movement along an illness trajectory, its attendant influence on the locus of care, and the health care professionals included in the patient's illness management system.

Illness Trajectories   Corbin and Strauss (1988) conceptualized illness trajectories through the use of two central ideas. First, illness trajectories vary in form, duration, and requisite tasks. Such variability "is determined by a combination of (1) the nature of the illness and the person's physiological and emotional response to it, and (2) management schemes instituted by health professionals and the ill (Corbin & Strauss, 1988, p. 45). Second, trajectories consist of at least five different phases: acute, comeback, stable, unstable, and downward. On average, AIDS patients experience a slow downward trajectory following full-blown diagnosis, with two or three comebacks and stable phases prior to death. The ability of health care professionals and CPs to adapt the illness management system in response to changes in the patient's health is vital to successful management.

Locus of Care   Health care is most often delivered in one or more of three basic contexts: hospital, clinic, and home. The appropriate care context depends on the patient's place on the illness trajectory (Martin, 1988). For the AIDS patient, severe acute ailments such as pneumocystis pneumonia require hospital care; less immediately threatening ailments such as Kaposi's sarcoma and those of a chronically recurrent nature are treated through outpatient services, where, increasingly, even sophisticated forms of treatment such as chemotherapy are being applied. Typically, outpatient treatment requires some form of home care as well, ranging from patient self-medication and symptom monitoring to mobility assistance that requires CP involvement.

Ideally, the three contexts interlock—home and hospital provide the two options for patient residence, and the clinic serves as an interface between these two loci. Each context has attendant advantages for meeting the patient's needs: Hospitals have the constant presence of trained medical personnel to monitor health and provide treatment, as well as important diagnostic equipment to track and manage the plethora of complications common to persons with AIDS. Clinics provide a forum for intermediary consultation with a variety of specialists, as well as prescriptions and other forms of simple treatment. The home provides the emotional support of family, friends, and routine surroundings and lessens the financial burden of health care. Each context also carries its own implications for the nature of CP involvement.

Medical Professionals Involved   A variety of medical professionals are employed as a patient with AIDS moves along the illness trajectory. Foremost among these, at least in terms of directing the formal medical treatment, are the various physicians: the patient's primary care physician; an internal medicine physician whose task it is to track manifestations and developments in the patient's underlying infection; and allied specialists to cover problems with the respiratory, circulatory, and digestive systems. Nurses provide the majority of the actual care required during hospitalization, and are supported, along with the physicians, by a host of allied health professionals including laboratory and x-ray technicians, orderlies and aides, dietary consultants, and physical therapists. The work in hospitals and clinics also relies on receptionists and business managers; hospitals also provide discharge counseling and chaplain services, the latter serving to meet patients' desire for spiritual as well as physical guidance. Social workers also play an important role in health care, integrating patient and family needs with a variety of hospital and community services that provide assistance for psychosocial, financial, and care management difficulties.

All of these personnel contribute more or less directly to the patient's well-being. And in interacting with the patient, they are likely to interact, to some degree at least, with the CP. Although the CP's most important relationship outside the patient is with the patient's physician, CPs may also need to negotiate an "involvement contract" with each of the different persons who regularly interact with the patient (Zook & Miller, 1992). This is particularly true of the nursing staff that is charged with day-to-day patient care.

Given these various contextual factors that shape the nature of CP involvement in the management of persons with AIDS, it is important for us to go beyond Grieco and Kowalski's (1987) presentation of the CP as someone whose primary involvement takes place in the home. Rather, significant amounts of participation take place during hospitalizations and, to some degree, during and around medical appointments as well. In short, it is important to incorporate the CP more fully into the illness management system rather than limiting him or her to simply one phase or locus of care (Greif & Porembski, 1988). We turn next to the various tasks that CPs can negotiate into their roles as the patient passes along an illness trajectory. Our consideration of involvement options is based on our interviews with 23 CPs of AIDS patients (Zook, 1991; Zook & Miller, 1992; for additional information, see Tiblier, Walker, & Rolland, 1989).

THE ROLE AND NATURE OF THE CARE PARTNER'S INVOLVEMENT

In investigating care partner participation in illness management systems, we found various forms of context-appropriate functions, as well as factors that promote or impede CPs' decision to become involved. The first form of involvement for many care partners is likely to be *emotive sharing* with the patient following a diagnosis of HIV or AIDS. The patient is usually beset with an immediate sense of loss and grieving; the sudden trauma that accompanies such a diagnosis and so often produces denial requires acceptance and support. The CP may face traumatic feelings of loss and grief as well, and it is important that patient and CP work together to cope with the disease and its implications.

The next form of involvement usually takes the form of participation in an *information search*. The CP assists the patient in locating information on, for example, how HIV is transmitted, how it works to deplete the immune system, what diseases are commonly associated with it, and what treatments exist. Participation in the information search can range from passive involvement (e.g., scanning mass media sources but not seeking out information) to full involvement (e.g., active individual search of media sources, questioning of interpersonal contacts, and participation in HIV/AIDS information networks).

In the early stages of cases in which the patient is only HIV positive (i.e., asymptomatic), there is not a pressing need for the CP to attend *medical appointments*, and few do. CPs may help the patient with transportation to and from the appointments but typically remain in the waiting room. However, we must distinguish between direct involvement at this time, of which there is little, and indirect involvement, which varies greatly from CP to CP. Indirect involvement concerns the extent to which the CP seeks full disclosure from the patient regarding each appointment. Of course, the CP's reliance on the patient for this information permits patient gatekeeping and the accompanying danger that information will be presented selectively. Nonetheless, discussing appointments thoroughly keeps the CP up to date on health developments, yet enables the patient to maintain a sense of independence and control over his or her life.

So long as the patient's health remains fairly stable, the CP's involvement is likely to be maintained along the preceding three lines: emotional involvement accompanied by varying levels of information search and indirect medical involvement. However, the breadth and depth of the CP's involvement increase following an acute illness crisis that necessitates patient hospitalization. At a minimal level, CPs provide *companionship* and *emotional support* through visitation when the locus of care moves to the hospital. We found that the amount of time spent at the hospital is contingent on such variables as the CP's work requirements, the seriousness of the patient's condition, the strength of the CP–patient relationship, and staff willingness to disregard standard visiting hours (see also Pearlin et al., 1988).

Many CPs also perform small *comfort tasks* for the patient. At minimum, the CP serve as the patient's mobility—getting drinks, helping the patient to the bathroom, and calling nurses. Other CPs seek to perform more complex tasks that require greater interaction with staff and the use of hospital supplies, such as bathing the patient or cleaning incontinence.

Probably the most important role for CPs in the hospital context, however, is *monitoring patient care* and serving as an *advocate* when necessary. This level of CP involvement includes watching for oversights (e.g., spiking fevers and missed medication) and outright errors (e.g., mixing incompatible medications and ignorance of the patient's allergies to particular medicines). One element unique to monitoring the care of HIV/AIDS patients is the CPs' concern with the attitudes of hospital personnel during patient interaction. The CP often seeks to protect the patient from slights from hospital staff that might imply that the patient is unclean, unwhole, or less than a person. In our study of CPs of AIDS patients, however, we found medical personnel to be on the whole quite supportive; the only reported refusals to enter the patient's room or insistence on being fully gowned from head to toe were practiced by housekeeping or dietary personnel.

Even the best hospitals make mistakes, and because of the complexity of AIDS, the presence of a knowledgeable CP who has shared the patient's illness from the outset can be invaluable. We found that although few CPs believe at the outset that monitoring of patient care will be necessary, monitoring activities usually intensify following the first incident in which the patient's comfort or health is significantly jeopardized.

Following simple monitoring, CPs often move on to become patient advocates. Whether a CP simply calls a problem to the attention of the staff or informs staff superiors in the hope of preventing recurrence, it is sometimes deemed necessary for the patient's well-being to seek redress of the situation. One CP in our study even went so far as to insist on a permanent staffing change following continued inept behavior by a nurse who had inadequate knowledge of AIDS treatment.

The typical AIDS patient is hospitalized two or three times prior to death. To the extent that health stabilizes following an acute episode, establishing the necessary care requirements for the patient's return home becomes important. At this point, CPs often interact with discharge personnel to fashion a home care plan. The most critical issue at this juncture is the identification of a case manager who will serve as the responsible contact for the patient and/or CP. The case manager ensures adequate service delivery during the patient's home stay. Case managers may be drawn from either free-standing community case management agencies or the hospital. Given the relatively new status of this occupational position, there is a great deal of variability in the professionals who perform case management services. Physicians, nurses, and social workers have all been seen as likely candidates, although social workers have tended to predominate, largely because of their greater knowledge of and practice in assisting with the integration of the vast array of community services patients may require. Physicians and nurses typically possess more technical and specialized health knowledge.

Social workers are far from being assured the primary role in case management (Philbin & Altman, 1990), however. The specific needs of individual patients could well dictate whether medical specialty is of greater importance than what might be termed "social needs" specialty. It is important to note that case management is more conceptually than operationally effective. Because of professional disputes over who should serve case management functions and the untenable case loads currently carried by case managers, many responsibilities often fall into the domain of the CP, who must become a *de facto* case management expert.

Whoever assumes case management responsibilities, the important outcome to achieve is the provision of adequate care at home. This usually takes the form of a needs assessment in which the patient's health status is examined at the time of discharge. Among the possible services required are the provision of:

- technical equipment necessary to sustain patient health (e.g., intravenous drips, feeding pumps, and equipment for administering aerosol pentamidine),
- products that facilitate ease of patient care (e.g., hospital beds, walkers, and portable commodes),
- visits of home health providers to monitor patient health, and
- chore assistance if necessary to give CPs a break from overly burdensome care requirements.

It is also important to assess the CP's understanding of the patient's health status and skills in managing the technical aspects of patient home care (Nichols, 1984). Once home, the CP again can become involved to a greater or lesser degree in the management of the patient's illness.

To the extent that the patient's health is sufficiently poor that technical equipment is required for medication and sustenance, the CP is likely to assume more complete responsibility for the administration of all medications. Typically, patients retain control of these issues until they are clearly unable to handle the responsibility. CPs in our study mentioned medication as an area in which most patients clearly wanted to maintain autonomy as long as possible.

Thus, CP involvement can include emotional support, information searches, case management, patient advocacy, administration of medication, and comfort tasks such as cleaning incontinence. From this smorgasbord of options, CPs interviewed in our study (Zook, 1991; Zook & Miller, 1992) created widely varied packages of involvement. Six CPs practiced full involvement in all areas: full information search, strong participation in medical appointments, intensive interactions with medical staff characterized by information exchange and patient advocacy, and heavy involvement in both home and hospital contexts. Such CPs appeared to bond with the patient to such a degree that the medical staff came to view and interact with them as one and the same in many regards. In short, these CPs did whatever they, the patient, or medical care providers saw as necessary for the good of the patient.

Other CPs limited themselves to intensive participation in one or a few categories. Ten CPs focused their efforts primarily on either the home or hospital context, providing emotional and instrumental support to the patient. Five CPs devoted large blocks of time to dealing with government agencies on items such as filing for disability, securing Medicaid, and applying for chore grants. Another CP directed most of his assistance to intensive information search, decision making about treatments, and emotional support of the patient.

What appears significant in these admittedly limited findings is that no single model of CP involvement is likely to be identified. Although further research might provide helpful suggestions on effective versus ineffective participation, the appropriateness and efficacy of CP actions will likely depend on the personal characteristics of the patient, CP, and physician, as well as the various contextual factors discussed earlier.

POSSIBLE OUTCOMES ASSOCIATED WITH CARE PARTNER INCLUSION

When considering outcomes of CP involvement, we look first and foremost at the patient. Being HIV positive or having the diagnosis of AIDS is very real and very frightening. A person who receives such a diagnosis must grapple not only with the loss of hope (ideally only temporary), but also with the fear of social ostracization and discrimination (Tiblier et al., 1989). Even in the asymptomatic stages, the identification of a CP who will agree to stand by the individual through the illness can offset many concerns. The importance of identifying someone who cares underlies buddy programs that have been used extensively by AIDS-related service agencies around the country. These services are especially beneficial if the person with AIDS lacks a relational partner or family member who can and will assume CP duties. However, a buddy system can rarely surpass the care, time, knowledge, effort, and support devoted by most of the CPs we talked with in our research (Pearlin et al., 1988; although see Shelp, DuBose, & Sunderland, 1990, for discussion of intensive church-based support programs).

In a triadic relationship that includes the patient, physician, and CP, patients are able to access a knowledgeable partner for assistance in making treatment decisions and altering illness management as the disease progresses. The CP can also provide the physician with information the patient might forget or be unaware of and can help the patient remember what was said during medical appointments. In short, the person with AIDS who has a CP can often establish a mutually agreed on sharing of the illness that protects the patient's wishes for autonomy. With the help of a CP, the patient benefits by being able to devote him- or herself more fully to all aspects of managing the illness.

For physicians, the additional information and input provided by CPs can aid in designing and altering treatment regimens. Early interaction between the CP and physician enables the development of the relationship over time, such that potentially difficult milestones in the patient's illness trajectory (e.g., negotiating the moment of death with regard to life-support wishes and Do Not Resuscitate orders), will be more easily reached. Long-term partnerships form a more solid basis for interaction than waiting for the patient to become incapacitated before moving beyond a basic acquaintanceship with the CP.

Finally, the CP stands to benefit greatly from formal inclusion in the care triad. CPs are already heavily involved, informally, in the tasks and concerns regarding the patient's health. We contend that increased sharing of information with the CP and freer access between CPs and medical professionals will enable CPs to share the very real burdens of care involvement with individuals who have AIDS. Support groups for medical professionals working with AIDS patients were established early in recognition of the emotional toll exacted in such work. Although similar groups have also been developed for CPs, it would seem more effective and efficient to encourage a natural ongoing "support group" in the form of a health care team that includes the CP. The interaction stemming from formal recognition of a patient–physician–CP triad may well be a more functional form of support in the long run, one that will keep both CPs and medical professionals functioning with minimal strain and burnout while benefiting patients through higher quality care in both the home and hospital.

CONCLUSION

It is important to note that the triadic model of health care we have advocated herein is an ideal case. In particular, it presumes a stable financial and social base from which patients and loved ones may build a time-consuming, albeit rewarding, partnership. The sad truth with respect to AIDS, however, is that it strikes many who are homeless or who lack the requisite income and social network to provide extensive care partnering assistance (Schietinger, 1988). Though there are publicly funded residences for the homeless with AIDS, demand far exceeds availability. The largest group home, New York City's Bailey House, has only 44 rooms; overall, there are fewer than 500 rooms available in the city for a homeless population of individuals with AIDS estimated to be as high as 13,000 (Brown, 1992).

The structural inadequacies present in our society today are many: poverty, limited opportunity, violent crime, drug use, inadequate food and housing, and racial tension, to name a few. The fact that these limit the availability and/or adequate involvement of care partners for individuals with AIDS, particularly in our inner cities, does not invalidate our central thesis about the need for greater sharing of illness and its attendant burdens; it simply underscores that individuals cannot conquer the ills of our health care system alone. In addition to caring partners, illnesses such as AIDS require caring communities.

REFERENCES

Bishop, C. E., & Karon, S. L. (1989). The composition of home health care expenditure growth. *Home Health Care Services Quarterly, 10* (1/2), 139–175.

Brandt, A. M. (1987). *No magic bullet: A social history of venereal disease in the United States since 1880.* New York: Oxford University Press.

Brody, E. M. (1985). Parent care as normative family stress. *The Gerontologist, 25,* 19–29.

Brody, E. M., Poulshock, S. W., & Massiocchi, C. F. (1978). The family caring unit: A major consideration in the long-term support system. *The Gerontologist, 18,* 556–561.

Brown, C. (1992). A last good place to live: Inside a residence for the homeless with AIDS. *Harper's, 284*(1701), 48–55.

Clement, M. (1989). Opportunistic infections, AIDS-associated malignancies, and their management. In N. Rapoza (Ed.), *HIV/AIDS: Infection and disease* (pp. 145–162). Chicago: American Medical Association.

Corbin, J. M., & Strauss, A. (1988). *Unending work and care.* San Francisco: Jossey-Bass.

Eidson, T. (1988). *The AIDS caregiver's handbook.* New York: St. Martin's Press.

Engel, G. L. (1977). The need for a new medical model: A challenge for biomedicine. *Science, 196*(4286), 129–136.

Goodhue, S. V. R. (1984, August). Home care: The answer to tomorrow's health care needs. *Caring,* pp. 5–7.

Greif, G. L., & Porembski, E. (1988). AIDS and significant others: Findings from a preliminary study. *Health and Social Work, 13*(4), 259–265.

Grieco, A. J., & Kowalski, W. (1987). The "care partner." In L. Bernstein, A. Grieco, & M. Dete (Eds.), *Primary care in the home* (pp. 71–82). Philadelphia: J. B. Lippincott.

Halamandaris, V. I. (1985, October). The future of homecare. *Caring,* pp. 4–11.

Harris, I. B., Rich, E. C., & Crowson, T. W. (1985). Attitudes of internal medicine residents and staff physicians toward various patient characteristics. *Journal of Medical Education, 60,* 192–195.

Martin, J. P. (1988). Hospice and home care for persons with AIDS/ARC: Meeting the challenges and ensuring quality. *Death Studies, 12,* 463–480.

Nichols, K. A. (1984). *Psychological care in physical illness.* Philadelphia: Charles Press.

Nichols, K. A. (1987). Chronic physical disorder in adults. In J. Orford (Ed.), *Treating the disorder, treating the family* (pp. 62–85). Baltimore, MD: Johns Hopkins University Press.

Pearlin, L. I., Semple, S., & Turner, H. (1988). Stress of AIDS caregiving: A preliminary overview of the issues. *Death Studies, 12,* 501–517.

Perrow, C., & Guillen, M. F. (1990). *The AIDS disaster.* New Haven, CT: Yale University Press.

Philbin, P., & Altman, D. (1990, August). HIV/AIDS home care: An HMO experience. *Caring,* pp. 42–45.

Quill, T. E. (1983). Partnerships in patient care: A contractual approach. *Annals of Internal Medicine, 98,* 228–234.

Schietinger, H. (1988). Housing for people with AIDS. *Death Studies, 12,* 481–499.

Schofferman, J. (1988). Care of the AIDS patient. *Death Studies, 12,* 433–449.

Shelp, E. E., DuBose, E. R., & Sunderland, R. H. (1990). The infrastructure of religious communities: A neglected resource for the care of people with AIDS. *American Journal of Public Health, 80,* 970–972.

Siegler, M. (1981). Searching for moral certainty in medicine: A proposal for a new model of the doctor-patient encounter. *Bulletin of the New York Academy of Medicine, 57,* 56–69.

Sontag, S. (1978). *Illness as metaphor.* New York: Farrar, Strauss, and Giroux.

Sontag, S. (1989). *AIDS and its metaphors.* New York: Farrar, Strauss, and Giroux.

Strauss, A., & Corbin, J. M. (1988). *Shaping a new health care system.* San Francisco: Jossey-Bass Publishers.

Tiblier, K. B., Walker, G., & Rolland, J. S. (1989). Therapeutic issues when working with families of persons with AIDS. In E. B. Macklin (Ed.), *AIDS and families* (pp. 81–128). New York: Haworth Press.

Zook, E. G. (1991). *Toward a theory of care partnering: The role of third-party carers in the illness management systems of AIDS patients.* Unpublished doctoral dissertation, Michigan State University, East Lansing, MI.

Zook, E. G., & Miller, K. I. (1992, May). *Care partner involvement and communication in the illness management systems of AIDS patients.* Paper presented at the annual convention of the International Communication Association, Miami, FL.

Chapter Four

The Paradox of Accurate Information Increasing the Fear of AIDS

Louis R. Franzini

The fear of acquired immune deficiency syndrome (AIDS) is easier to transmit than the disease itself. Evelyn Fisher in 1986 may have been the first to use the term "FRAIDS" to refer to the second epidemic—the fear of AIDS. FRAIDS indeed can reach phobic proportions and produce serious negative consequences for individuals whose reactions can become irrational and debilitating.

On the surface it does not seem inappropriate to fear AIDS or any other serious illness, such as cancer, or even death. The abnormality of this fear is defined by its consequences and effects on individuals' daily lives and psychological well-being.

This chapter discusses the symptom versus syndrome controversy, the paradoxical effect of accurate information on FRAIDS, the presently known facts about AIDS that contribute to FRAIDS, the manifestations of FRAIDS, the negative consequences of FRAIDS, and some suggestions for treatment and action.

THE SYMPTOM VERSUS SYNDROME CONTROVERSY

Excessive reactions to the fear of AIDS are now being described in the literature. A potpourri of case reports and attempts at creating a new nosology have

included "pseudo-AIDS" (Miller, Green, Farmer, & Carroll, 1985), "facti-
tious AIDS" (Evans & Gill, 1988; Miller, Weiden, Sacks, & Wozniak, 1986;
Robinson & Latham, 1987), "AIDS-induced psychogenic state" (O'Brien &
Hassanyeh, 1985), "AIDS panic" (Windgassen & Soni, 1987), "AIDS phobia" (Jacob, John, Verghese, & John, 1987; Jager, 1988a; Winslow, Rumbaut,
& Hwang, 1990), "fear of AIDS" (Chodof, 1987; Kamlana & Gray, 1988),
"delusional AIDS" (Altamura, Mauri, Coppola, & Cazzullo, 1988; Lawlor &
Stewart, 1987; Rapaport & Braff, 1985), "FRAIDS" (Fisher, 1986; Franzini,
1987; Winslow, Rumbaut, & Hwang, 1989), "excessive concern about AIDS"
(Lippert, 1986), "intractable AIDS worry" (Salt, Miller, Perry, & Bor, 1989),
and even "fraudulent AIDS" (Tyson & Fortenberry, 1987).

Controversy has arisen as to whether all these labels and case descriptions
represent a new psychiatric syndrome or merely a delusional symptom with
contemporary content that indicates a standard underlying psychiatric distur-
bance (cf. Bor & Miller, 1989; Jacob, John, Verghese, & John, 1989; Lipkin,
1988; Mahorney & Cavenar, 1988; O'Brien, 1987; Riccio & Thompson,
1987; Segal, 1988). Those who suggest that the fear of AIDS reflects an
underlying psychiatric disorder (e.g., Fenton, 1987) have suggested a variety
of core diagnoses: depression, anxiety state, panic, paranoia, obsessive–
compulsive disorder, hypochondriasis, alcoholism, simple phobia, mania, and
even nonspecific psychopathology. Complicating the diagnostic picture is the
possibility of Munchausen syndrome masquerading as AIDS-induced depression, as suggested by McDonald and Wafer (1989), and simple misdiagnosis
of AIDS (factitious or misinterpreted false-positive human immunodeficiency
virus [HIV] tests), which can generate excessive fear of the disease in the
unfortunate individuals (Vernon, Hoagland, & Perlman, 1987; Wu, Kennedy,
& Paradise, 1988).

Jager (1988b) provided a list of "indications for AIDS phobia" for patients
who wrongly believe that they have AIDS and cannot be dissuaded otherwise.
His signs include: telephone contacts often from afar, no membership in the
principal risk groups, negative HIV test results, mistrust of those results, an
unconscious or conscious conviction of having AIDS, guilt-laden past sexual
contacts, previous efforts at counseling, belief that the problem will be solved
by medical research, and disrupted social relationships.

As Mahorney and Cavenar (1988) reminded us, "the content of delusions
varies tremendously and often represents an external focus for the patients'
internal wishes and fears. It is common clinical experience that delusions tend
to incorporate material which is of popular interest at the moment" (p. 1130).
Rapaport and Braff (1985) described two cases of AIDS delusion accompanied
by homosexual panic, a topic they noted has conspicuously diminished in the
literature in recent years.

It is important to distinguish three aspects of the fear of AIDS that have
been blended in past reports. Some patients are disturbed psychologically, and

part of their clinical presentation includes the unsubstantiated fear that they actually have AIDS (or are HIV infected) at this time. Other patients, the "worried well" (see Bor, Perry, Jackson, & Miller, 1989), engage in a variety of unnecessary and perhaps irrational behaviors to avoid being infected, but are otherwise psychologically healthy. These behaviors can be considered irrational because there is no evidence and no likelihood that these individuals are exposed to possible modes of infection or transmission. Finally, there are those patients who have been correctly diagnosed as HIV infected and whose consequent symptoms include fear of AIDS, depression, anxiety, paranoia, hopelessness, etc. This latter group are not addressed in this chapter because their reactions are somatopsychic and realistic.

Similarly, it is not the purpose of the present discussion to resolve the diagnostic debate of whether the fear of AIDS is merely a symptom of another disorder or a new syndrome that deserves its own etiology, typical symptom pattern, and treatment. The intricacies of this problem have been captured well by Bruhn (1989): "The fear of AIDS is not solely a private fear of the client seeking help; its etiology is societal, and it is reinforced daily by the media and the many uncertainties about the disease" (p. 455).

The fear of AIDS is very much present and increasing in our society. For example, it is reflected in the popular literature (e.g., Thomas, 1985; Wein, 1987) as well as the professional literature, which documents its effects on university students (e.g., Adame, Taylor-Nicholson, Wang, & Abbas, 1991) and health care professionals (e.g., Gerbert, Maguire, Badner, Altman, & Stone, 1988). In a survey of the general public taken as long ago as mid-1987 ($N = 1,540$ adults in the six-county Chicago metropolitan area), only 3.2% of the sample "had never heard of AIDS" (Albrecht, Levy, Sugrue, Prohaska, & Ostrow, 1989).

Print and electronic lay media (Thomas, 1985), plus the professional literature (cf. Weiss & Thier, 1988), daily discuss concerns over the safety of the nation's blood supply (e.g., Callero, Baker, Carpenter, & Magangal, 1986); the advisability of mandatory HIV antibody testing; the ethics of disclosure of patients' HIV status by physicians, dentists, and the patients themselves (Kantrowitz et al., 1991); budgetary debates on the proportion of available funding that should be devoted to AIDS research; and the priorities of research in terms of possible treatments, prevention, education, aftercare, and so on. Even the conservative corporate culture is considering AIDS education programs in the workplace to reduce employees' fears, to assist employees who seroconvert, and to reduce the likelihood of summary dismissal of such a person (cf. Puckett & Emery, 1989). Clearly, this high degree of public attention in so many arenas is partially fueled by the fear of AIDS (cf. Muir, 1991).

Adame et al. (1991) surveyed 226 freshman college students at a university in the southeastern United States, 72.4% of whom were "afraid of getting AIDS." More than half indicated they would rather get any other disease than AIDS. In their survey of 1,793 high school students, Skurnick, Johnson,

Quinones, Foster, and Louria (1991) found that 83% feared getting AIDS and commonly exaggerated the risk of social contacts with infected persons. Skurnick et al. stated that students' "fear was associated with misperceptions" and "was not always dispelled by knowledge" (p. 21). Negy and Webber (1991) found no differences in the fear of AIDS among White, Black, and Hispanic college students in southern California, but their female students expressed less fear than did males. Skurnick et al. also found males to be more fearful. At this time, the AIDS epidemic apparently threatens males more because most of the cases thus far have been male.

Although college students are currently underrepresented in AIDS statistics, it is generally assumed that many students are presently being infected because "too few students understand how HIV is transmitted" (Stevenson & Stevenson, 1990) and because of the frequently obtained finding that adolescents and college students are not changing their behaviors that put them at risk for HIV infection (Becker & Joseph, 1988; Booth, 1988; Goodman & Cohall, 1989; Hingson, Strunin, & Berlin, 1990; Kegeles, Adler, & Irwin, 1988; McKusick, Conant, & Coates, 1985).

The best available data on HIV seroprevalence among college students comes from Gayle et al.'s (1990) blinded survey of 16,863 blood specimens obtained from 19 U.S. universities. Seroprevalence was 0.5% for men and 0.02% for women. Although these rates are lower than those of known high-risk populations, the authors reiterated the clear potential for spreading the infection in the college student population, especially in view of students' continuing engagement in high-risk behaviors.

Bruhn (1989) suggested that some individuals may be especially prone to developing an excessive fear of AIDS because of prior hypochondriacal or anxious features in their personalities. Of course, those in high-risk groups such as promiscuous gay men or needle-sharing intravenous drug users may also be very susceptible. The presence of FRAIDS in the general public and even in technically educated health care professionals indicates that life-style variables do not sufficiently account for this "fear of contagion." Bruhn, citing Brandt (1988), added, "The public historically has had a considerable fear of sexually transmitted diseases and of death, especially when it is debilitating and painful, as is the case with AIDS" (p. 455).

Muir (1991) discussed the "general public" as one of the major "environmental contexts" of AIDS. She suggests that AIDS by implication involves four kinds of deviance in American society: immorality, illegality, infidelity, and illness. Furthermore, it involves the "fear of contagion," which in U.S. society is heightened by negative associations of bodily fluids. Many people are suspicious that the general public is not receiving complete or correct information from the authorities about the virus or the course of the disease. She argued that each of these psychologically sensitive factors serves to heighten the public's irrational response (fear) to AIDS.

Muir added:

> To compound the problems of credibility, a variance of opinions, aired almost daily in the media by persons who may be speaking outside their sphere of expertise or knowledge, contributes to an environment of uncertainty and fear. Everyone who holds an important post or who speaks convincingly (but particularly physicians and scientists) has access to the media, who then edit the information for the public. Despite the best intentions of all those involved in the chain of information, skirmishes to report will inevitably result in headlines and news stories that present not only clear and credible but also confused and conflicting information. (1991, p. 73)

When the risk of infection of a fatal disease is not zero, there necessarily will be fear of infection. That fear can become excessive and disproportionate to the actual risk. One of the intriguing aspects of FRAIDS is that it can be heightened not only by misinformation and rumors, but also by scientifically accurate information and known gaps in our factual knowledge.

THE PARADOX

Unlike other unrealistic fears, such as the fear of flying, the fear of AIDS is not necessarily reduced by accurate information about the disease and its modes of transmission. The paradox is that the facts about AIDS, as they are presently known, can actually enhance FRAIDS.

U.S. Air airline offers a 21-hr series of classes for its potential customers who have aviaphobia. The coinstructor of the course is a U.S. Air pilot who educates the phobic customers about the safety features of commercial aircraft, navigational procedures in inclement weather, and the tight control of air traffic. The clinical social worker who is the other instructor teaches relaxation techniques and discusses possible related fears such as claustrophobia and fear of dying. Their reported success rate of 97% (Walker, 1992) is impressive and undoubtedly is at least partially attributable to the accurate information on safety and instrument redundancy that the authoritative source, the uniformed captain, provides.

New knowledge about AIDS-related research emerges daily. The following is a randomly ordered, nonexhaustive list of facts about the transmission and risk of HIV infection that actually exacerbate many people's fear of AIDS.

  1 Although there are some relatively long-term survivors of the disease, AIDS appears to have a 100% mortality rate.
  2 No cure for AIDS or vaccine against HIV infection is available or imminent. (These two dramatic facts and their implications are also not lost upon physicians with concerns for their own personal safety; see Fribourg, 1989.)
  3 The research reports present widely varying estimates of the incuba-

tion period of HIV (e.g., Falkner von Sonnenburg & Eichenlaub, 1988; National Academy of Sciences, 1988; Petit, 1988). Therefore, even a negative antibody test result cannot completely alleviate fear. One can never really be sure that enough time has elapsed after an incident of possible exposure that one can feel secure that one is infection free.

4 Newspapers, magazines, and television daily document the continual increase of AIDS and HIV infection with frightening headlines, for example, "AIDS Danger Stalks Millions Worldwide" in the Palm Springs, California, *The Desert Sun* ("Aids Danger Stalks," 1991). The grim statistics that followed stated that up to 10 million people are infected thus far, with an additional 5,000 more each day. In the United States more than 123,000 of the 200,000 infected have died. Estimates are that by the year 2000, between 30 and 40 million people will be infected worldwide. In 8 years the first 100,000 individuals were infected in the U.S. It has taken just 26 months for the second 100,000 to be infected. As of June 30, 1992, 230,179 people in the U.S. have been diagnosed with AIDS; 152,153 have died.

5 Heterosexually acquired AIDS continues to increase in the United States, especially among women, Blacks, and Hispanics in inner-city populations (Holmes, Karon, & Kreiss, 1990). The most recent data from the Centers for Disease Control (CDC) through November 1991 confirm no change in these trends (Knight-Ridder, 1992). The disease is not just that of gay men and drug abusers. Computer model predictions for the proliferation of the virus in Asia, Latin America, and Africa are "very frightening" even to the epidemiologists (Palca, 1991).

6 In April 1992, the CDC began enforcing a new definition of who has AIDS in the United States. If the patient's blood shows fewer than 200 CD4 T cells per cubic millimeter, that person can be classified as having AIDS even though he or she is otherwise without symptoms. The estimates are that the new definition will qualify three times as many people for the diagnosis in San Diego County, California (Clark, 1991). When these new data are reported, the tripling of the AIDS caseload will surely alarm many citizens.

7 The most widely recommended HIV infection prevention measure, other than abstinence, is the use of condoms. However, condoms sometimes fail, even when used correctly. Falkner von Sonnenburg and Eichenlaub (1988), citing research on partners of HIV-infected patients who subsequently seroconverted, concluded that the use of condoms over 18 months "reduced the transmission rate to about one-fifth." *Consumer Reports* evaluated 40 varieties of condoms for defects and strength ("Can You Rely on Condoms?" 1989). Among the readers surveyed by the magazine, one in four had experienced a condom breaking in the past year. One in eight reported two instances of breakage. The magazine calculated differential breakage rates depending on the sexual activity: one condom in 105 for anal sex and one in 165 for vaginal sex. Widely publicized condom failure rates can only add to one's uncertainty about their ability to protect from HIV infection.

8 State laws on required reporting of infections are quite variable and of little assurance to the average citizen. HIV seropositivity is reportable in only

15 states and the District of Columbia, whereas AIDS is reportable in all 50 states (Lamboi & Sy, 1989).

9 Underreporting of AIDS cases by physicians in practice because of insufficient training and occasional political differences has been a problem for public health officials from the beginning of the epidemic (e.g., Conway et al., 1989). One can only conclude that AIDS is more widespread than is being reported officially, even in the U.S. where the reporting network is relatively firmly in place.

10 The data reported by Judson (1989) that 10% to 20% of those who voluntarily seek antibody testing do not return to receive their results, that after a year only 64% of seropositive blood donors revealed their test results to their primary sexual partners, and that 55% to 60% of homosexual men in New York City are estimated to be already infected will coalesce to augment fear in most observers. There are many individuals who are unaware of their seropositivity and others who know but choose not to reveal it to those with whom they may have intimate contact. It is a crime in more than half the states in the United States to fail to inform a lover of one's seropositivity.

11 A second retrovirus capable of producing AIDS was detected in 1986 in West Africa, but it is not identifiable with the usual antibody laboratory tests now in use (Clavel et al., 1987). This discovery implies that previous work on potential vaccines and treatments for the original virus may not be applicable to AIDS cases stemming from the second HIV. Recent popular media reports describe a possible new fatal AIDS virus, undetectable by current HIV testing, may have emerged (Cowley, 1992). Identification of infected individuals and blood supplies is presently impossible.

12 The very visible case of the late Kimberly Bergalis, who contracted the virus from her dentist, Dr. John Acer, during a molar extraction in his Florida office in 1987 incites fear. Her infection was the first documented case of a patient acquiring HIV from a health professional during the course of routine care. At least four other patients of Dr. Acer's have also been infected. The exact mechanism of infection remains unclear, which, of course, only heightens the anxieties of the public. Their perception of infection risk in routine dental care is now unquestionably heightened.

13 Another widely reported case was that of 16-year-old Allison Gertz, who contracted the infection from a one-night sexual encounter with a man she had met at the popular club Studio 54 in New York City. Despite professionals' reassurances about the fragility of the virus and examples of partners of infected individuals who have not become infected after repeated unprotected intercourse, the Allison Gertz case convinced the general public that it is indeed possible to be infected in just one exposure to the virus.

14 The possibility of "revenge sex," known HIV-infected individuals deliberately attempting to infect as many unsuspecting partners as possible, strikes terror in everyone both on a personal basis and as an outrage to society. The case of the male homosexual "Patient O" was described by Shilts (1987), who documented the many infections transmitted by Gaetan Dugas. Shilts gave other examples of intentional infections, as did Krajick (1988), who provided a chilling account of an infected man who insisted on infecting his wife to keep other men away and to allow them to continue to "have sex forever and never use condoms" (p. 54).

The case of "C.J." in Dallas ultimately turned out to be a hoax, but until then C.J. was considered to be a "phone terrorist." A woman called disc jockey Willis Johnson at radio station KKDA and described her efforts to "murder" as many men as possible by seeking them out for sex. She claimed to have been infected by a man and now was attempting to kill as many men as possible via unprotected sexual relations. For months Dallas and surrounding communities were consumed by fear, and an episode of the Phil Donahue show was devoted to the case. A persuasive letter from C.J. describing her activities and motivation was published in *Ebony* magazine. Eventually the deception was discovered to be the combined efforts of two young women, but this case suggests that there may be other individuals who are indeed carrying out such pogroms.

15   Comments by Masters and Johnson in their most recent book, *Heterosexual Behavior in the Age of AIDS* (Masters, Johnson, & Kolodny, 1988), regarding the ease of being infected by casual contact have astounded the scientific community because of their likelihood of increasing the public's fears (Quinn, 1988).

16   Individuals who have engaged in past risky behaviors may dwell on those indiscretions, feel guilt, and ultimately become extremely phobic about possibly having been infected (Jager, 1988a). In a sense, their fear incubates over time.

17   Although it probably is no surprise to nonprofessionals, psychologists have recently shown that people do not always tell the truth when discussing their history with prospective sexual partners (Cochran, 1988). Deceptions occur with regard to numbers of previous partners, drug use history, antibody testing and its results, and experiences of bisexuality. The usefulness of the recommendation commonly offered by AIDS educators to quiz prospective lovers about their past is negated by the high likelihood that prospective lovers may be motivated to lie.

18   Fear of AIDS exists and persists in knowledgeable health professionals. Dr. Lorraine Day, a San Francisco surgeon, lectures to physicians on the risks of being infected by seropositive patients. Contrary to most experts, she believes the virus can become air borne during surgery and could be inhaled or transmitted even through contact with unbroken skin. Dr. Day has resigned from the San Francisco hospital where she treated many HIV-infected patients because of those perceived risks despite the present CDC Universal Guidelines for infection control (Clark, 1989).

Gerbert, Maguire, Badner, Altman, and Stone (1989) discussed why the fear of AIDS continues in health care workers given our current levels of knowledge. They suggested four major reasons: (a) The risk is indeed real. (b) Standard infection control procedures cannot eliminate the possibility of accidents. (c) There exist barriers to full and adequate communication between the scientific and administrative authorities and the practitioners. (d) Humans tend to distort cognitively the probabilities of risk in life-threatening situations by overweighing events with very low probability in their decision making. Gerbert et al. concluded that it is misleading to compare AIDS risks with those of hepatitis B because for the latter a vaccine is available, the mortality rate is lower, and there is no social stigma. They argued that "only proof that the risk is non-existent would eliminate health care professionals' perception of grave risk. This, of course, is not the case" (p. 44).

MANIFESTATIONS OF FRAIDS

Mainstream American society offers innumerable examples of the excessive fear of AIDS from its members. Discrimination against AIDS patients in housing; in employment; and socially from friends, neighbors, and family is a daily occurrence (Blendon & Donelan, 1988). Infected children are banned from schools and churches. A Florida family with three infected children was forced to leave their community because of the arson fire of their home. "Gay bashing" incidents are increasing (Exler, 1987; Herek & Berrill, 1990) and "sick" jokes about AIDS are frequently being shared among friends (Dundes, 1987). According to Dundes, AIDS jokes are popular because they involve two taboos (homosexuality and a deadly disease) and because the anxiety level among the general public about contracting the disease remains high.

In terms of clinical matters, the calls to AIDS information hotlines have increased dramatically (Salt et al., 1989). HIV antibody testing centers are being swamped with requests from individuals with low-risk life-styles (e.g., couples in long-term monogamous relationships and middle-age heterosexual women) and repeat clients who return for testing each week. One man arrived at a San Diego testing center with a bag over his head and insisted on remaining covered because of his suspicion that they had cameras everywhere to observe him.

D'Augelli (1989) assessed the fears of professional nursing personnel, which included not eating in a restaurant that had a waiter with AIDS (43%), not going to a dinner party where one of the guests had AIDS (54%), and believing that one could be infected by sharing meals or eating utensils (52%). Their "AIDS phobias" correlated significantly with homophobic attitudes.

Homophobia has been reported in physicians and nurses (Douglas, Kalman, & Kalman, 1985) and in heterosexual freshman university students (D'Augelli & Rose, 1990) and is obviously related to the unrealistic fear of AIDS. However, it should be clear that FRAIDS and homophobia are not a single attitude or factor. Bouton et al. (1987) found a correlation of only .55, accounting for about 30% of the variance, between scores on a fear of AIDS scale and a homophobia scale (the two scales had reliabilities of .80 and .89, respectively).

Professionals such as physicians, nurses, dentists, and their aides who may come into contact with the bodily fluids of possibly infected patients exhibit serious and strong fears of AIDS despite their technical knowledge and training in safety procedures (Fribourg, 1989; Wallack, 1989). CDC statistics as of March 31, 1991, indicate that reported cases of AIDS among health care workers have appeared most frequently among nurses (1,358), followed by health aides (1,101), technicians (941), physicians (703), therapists (319), dentists and hygienists (171), and surgeons (47). A "miscellaneous" category of health workers including social workers, administrators, and others contained an additional 1,680 cases (Kantrowitz et al., 1991). Gerbert et al. (1989) maintained that there is "no doubt that fear of AIDS among health care professionals is pervasive" (p. 42).

Among the consequences is the trend for medical staffs to move away from geographical areas with many AIDS cases (Cockcroft, 1989), to consider leaving the field of medical technology and regretting having chosen a profession that would involve handling HIV-positive samples (Gauch, Feeney, & Brown, 1990), to refuse to treat AIDS patients (Gerbert et al., 1989; Richardson, Lochner, McGuigan, & Levine, 1987), to choose a career specialty that will reduce their contacts with AIDS patients (Strunin, Culbert, & Crane, 1989), and to overestimate the personal risks in treating infected patients (D'Augelli, 1989; Strunin et al., 1989). The calls for and controversy about mandatory preoperative HIV antibody testing for all patients could be considered a manifestation of FRAIDS (Hagen, Meyer, & Paulker, 1988; Weiss & Thier, 1988).

The stigmatization of AIDS patients by physicians themselves (Kelly, St. Lawrence, Smith, Hood, & Cook, 1987a; Treiber, Shaw, & Malcolm, 1987) and by nurses (D'Augelli, 1989) is likely to be perpetuated for generations of health care providers to come because negative and judgmental attitudes have been detected in current medical students (Kelly, St. Lawrence, Smith, Hood, & Cook, 1987b) and nursing students (Kelly, St. Lawrence, Hood, Smith, & Cook, 1988). Imperato, Feldman, Nayeri, and DeHovitz (1988) found that medical students' misperceptions of the risks in various treatment procedures remained unchanged after the students received accurate information in a lecture. Scientific facts did not modify attitudes and fears.

Similar uninformed and negative attitudes have been found in mental health care providers by Knox, Dow, and Cotton (1989). They assessed mental health technicians/aides (54% of their sample), counselors (20%), nurses (15%), social workers (7%), and psychologists (4%), the majority of whom preferred not to care for AIDS patients and were excessively concerned about casual contacts.

The effects of professionals' FRAIDS include a lowering of the quality of care to their patients (Katz et al., 1987; Klonoff & Ewers, 1990), and negative personal consequences as well. Providers feel personally at risk for AIDS (Clever & Omenn, 1988; Cooke, 1988; Wallack, 1989) and report exceptional stress (Klonoff & Ewers, 1990; Link, Feingold, Charap, Freeman, & Shelov, 1988), high anxiety (Treiber et al., 1987), and nightmares (Cooke, 1988).

NEGATIVE CONSEQUENCES OF THE FEAR OF AIDS

The most obvious consequence of the fear of AIDS is the belief that one has AIDS when, in fact, it is not so. Many clinical reports are now available documenting factitious or pseudo-AIDS cases (e.g., Jacob et al., 1987, 1989; Mahorney & Cavenar, 1988; Miller et al., 1985; Miller et al., 1986; O'Brien & Hassanyeh, 1985; Rapaport & Braff, 1985; Windgassen & Soni, 1987). Such individuals are subjecting themselves to unnecessary psychiatric distress, such as overwhelming anxiety and hopeless depression, and chemical and psychological treatments. There have been suicides by men who erroneously thought they were infected. Bor and Miller (1989) noted that "worries about AIDS often conceal other problems" (p. 808), presumably relationship or intimacy issues. Salt et al. (1989) suggested that the concerns about AIDS allow some individuals to avoid obtaining professional help for sexual dysfunctions, such as premature ejaculation or impotence.

Insurance discrimination is a subtle but potent consequence of the AIDS crisis. Health and life insurance companies are denying and canceling coverage of AIDS patients or individuals who are deemed to be at high risk. Of course, this discrimination could be a function more of the fear of reduced profits than the fear of AIDS. Such discrimination of AIDS patients and their right to medical care has produced an unprecedented flood of litigation, according to a study conducted for the U.S. Public Health Service and released in January 1992. Professor Lawrence Gostin, the author of the report, pointed out, "There is still a basic fear, often an irrational fear, in society that is being litigated in the courts. The problem is many of the judges are reinforcing and perpetuating the stereotypes" (cited in Kong, 1992, p. A-1).

Changes in sexual activity in the dating world have occurred in *both* directions. One survey of 449 single persons between the ages of 18 and 34, conducted for Abbott Laboratories, found that because of FRAIDS, 28% of men and 46% of women were abstaining from sex with new partners (United Press International, 1987). At the opposite extreme is the heterosexual man quoted by Krajick (1988) who proclaimed, "If anything, I'm more desperate about getting laid. There's so much fear of AIDS around that in a few years, no one will want to have sex at all. I want to get it while I can" (p. 56). Thus, both celibacy and promiscuity are possible direct consequences of the fear of AIDS.

The *New York Times* News Service (1989) reported on the trend for women to hire private investigators who check the backgrounds of men they have met and begun to date. The Inter-Tect agency in Houston charges $500 for this service and will verify information within a week on financial and marital history. Of particular interest to the clients is whether a man may have had past gay relationships. Sociologist Bernard Beck of Northwestern University is quoted in this report as saying that "trust is viewed as a naive sentimentality" (p. A-2). Professional background investigations are supplementing what

Gerald Friedland of the Albert Einstein College of Medicine has called "ophthalmic virology" to determine a prospective sexual partner's HIV serostatus (Booth, 1988).

Other relationship disruptions that can result from FRAIDS might include a fear of commitment to a person whose past may not have been completely disclosed. Others in near panic have "dumped confessions" of past sexual or drug use indiscretions on unsuspecting spouses or lovers. In the absence of any indications that such individuals have indeed been exposed to the virus, such revelations may be counterproductive. Perhaps as a result of stereotypic sex role training, some women have reported that because of the threat of AIDS, they will not have sexual relations with men unless they are romantically "swept away" (Krajick, 1988). Obviously, that strategy can be a risky way to cope with the terror of possible infection from an unknown, untested partner.

Neraal (1988) listed four irrational types of reaction to the fear of HIV infection:

> (1) Denial of danger, contra-phobic behaviour patterns, in which risky sexual contacts are actively sought, to a strangely suicidal readiness to take risks, (2) Phobic fear of contamination with extreme avoidance behaviour, (3) Paranoid reactions with mounting delusional fears, the overcoming of which is attempted through draconian measures for control and restriction aimed at AIDS sufferers and the main risk groups, and (4) Hypochondriacal anxieties of being HIV infected, or having AIDS, in spite of repeated negative blood-test results. (pp. 107–108)

The fear of AIDS has given rise to a variety of suggestions for social restrictions for controlling the spread of AIDS. Hogan (1989) examined 12 possibilities: quarantine, the tattooing of infected persons, a computer data bank of all individuals' serostatus, prohibition of marriage between an infected person and a noninfected person, testing as a prerequisite for a marriage license, denial of employment, prohibition of parenthood, mandatory public education campaigns including provision of condoms, use of an AIDS card to document one's serostatus, motivational campaigns stressing the rewards of prevention and the horrors of acquiring AIDS, intensive educational programs, and no social restrictions (laissez faire). His 57 participants included young, working males; middle-aged married women; female college students; and young adult male homosexuals. Their recommendations of these possible social restrictions produced "a negatively accelerated growth function of increasing levels of threat" (p. 255). As the perceived threat to society increased, a greater amount of social restriction was necessary, participants believed. Ethical considerations did intervene as a constraint against the most imposing levels of restriction; however, it appears that these participants were willing to sacrifice a certain amount of social freedom for the larger benefit to society.

Franzini, Dexter, and Straits (1992) surveyed 429 university students about any social or sexual behavior changes they may have made in the previous 12 months in response to the "AIDS crisis." The five most frequently endorsed rational and appropriate changes were not having sex on the first date (48.2%), being more selective in choosing a sexual partner (45.5%), having condoms readily available (44.0%), knowing one's partner better (43.4%), and having fewer sex partners (43.4%). However, the authors considered some of the reported changes to be "irrational" because they were unrelated to any known modes of infection transmission. The five most commonly reported such changes were using paper toilet seat covers (34.7%), avoiding places where there are gay men (14.1%), avoiding social contacts with gay men (13.9%), not donating blood (12.8%), and avoiding using public toilets (12.6%). Of course, self-report surveys are always subject to distortion because of social desirability pressures, faulty memory, and response sets, and they do not tap the emotional reactions that accompany the behaviors in question.

TREATMENT SUGGESTIONS FOR THE YOUNG

Students' fears of AIDS and risk behaviors present a somewhat unique picture relative to health professionals and the general public. Because of AIDS education programs and the degree of accurate information available in the university setting, surveys are showing that students' knowledge about the facts of AIDS has steadily increased in recent years to a high level and that they have more and more positive attitudes toward safer sex behaviors (Fisher & Misovich, 1990). Nevertheless, because of their "illusion of invulnerability," they have actually *decreased* the safety of their own behaviors. In a cogent display of inconsistent logic, the students believe that their sexual partners are more and more at risk for AIDS, but they themselves are not.

Bruce and Bullins (1989) found that students' major sources of information about genital herpes were, in decreasing order, magazines, television, classes, newspapers, and friends (all greater than 50%). Only 18.3% reported doctors as an information source. The authors concluded that these sources "are not sufficient to dispel myths and misconceptions about the infection" (p. 267) of herpes. We might expect the same to be true with regard to obtaining information about AIDS.

Bruhn (1989) provided guidelines for counseling persons with the fear of AIDS and noted that fear will not in itself motivate all individuals to change their habits. Regarding treatment he recommended,

> It is necessary to understand the societal sources of the client's fear as well as the client's unique social and cultural milieus. Treatment and prevention goals need to be realistic and tied to current medical knowledge. The public must continually be reminded to seek facts from creditable sources. Unfortunately, fear is perpetuated by the media. (p. 455)

One way to implement the recommendations of Bruce and Bullins (1989) and Bruhn (1989) is to maximize the opportunity for counseling when young people see a physician. Hingson et al. (1990) found that 80% of the teenagers in their survey had seen a physician in the preceding year, but only 13% of those had discussed AIDS. Those teenagers who did discuss AIDS were more likely to have refused sex with someone because of FRAIDS, more likely to have used condoms if they did have sex, and more likely to ask partners to use condoms.

Standard methods of psychotherapy and behavior therapy can be applied in treating FRAIDS. For example, systematic desensitization would seem to be the treatment of choice for unwarranted excessive fears. Assertive role plays were successfully used by Franzini, Sideman, Dexter, and Elder (1990) to teach students to request personal history information about previous partners and to ask for safer sex behaviors, including condom use. (See Seeley, 1988, for some amusing but fear-reducing suggestions on the latter topic.)

Some more innovative techniques have been attempted and are worthy of further exploration. For example, Salt et al. (1989) introduced paradoxical interventions for this fear. Greenblat, Katz, Gagnon, and Shannon (1989) applied a series of interactive simulations (ENCOUNTERS) to teach communication skills and stress management in friends and families of seropositive individuals. Exposure to AIDS-related drama (Probart, 1989) and even rock music (Kotarba, Williams, & Johnson, 1991) has been tried as a vehicle for AIDS education and intervention. Fear reduction was not assessed directly in these studies, but it is a reasonable prediction that might be examined in future work.

Another suggestion for reaching teenagers has been offered by national newspaper columnist Susan White (1992). She suggested exploiting television to encourage changes in teenagers' risky behaviors. White explains that we should use the television "which has filled them with the wonders of sex to fill them with the fear of AIDS" (p. C-7).

However, Leventhal, Meyer, and Gutmann (1980), in discussing compliance with high-blood-pressure regimens, offered several reasons why fear arousal might be inappropriate in communications about risk. First, high-fear messages may not be more effective in producing behavior changes than low-fear messages. Second, high-fear messages are likely to promote anger or suspicion of manipulative motives. Third, a possible consequence is a fatalism in individuals who perceive themselves as helpless against the danger. Finally, there could be psychological denial of the danger (although this is not probable in AIDS risk communication). Because of these possible effects, high-fear messages are dysfunctional and not to be recommended.

Pierce and VanDeVeer (1988) implied that governments may initiate inappropriate programs in an effort to do something about the AIDS problem to assuage citizens' fears, even though the new policy actually has little potential to slow the epidemic. Fitzpatrick and Milligan (1987) also adopted a political stance, suggesting that the British government has been promoting a fear and safe sex campaign as just another way to repress homosexuals and that there is relatively little risk to heterosexuals. They concluded with the following politically conservative but socially unrealistic and unappealing recommendation: "Celibacy is the only lifestyle that can promise to deliver you from all fear of AIDS" (p. 38).

REFERENCES

Adame, D. D., Taylor-Nicholson, M. E., Wang, M., & Abbas, M. A. (1991). Southern college freshman students: A survey of knowledge, attitudes, and beliefs about AIDS. *Journal of Sex Education and Therapy, 17,* 196–206.

AIDS danger stalks millions worldwide. (1991, December 1). *The Desert Sun,* p. A-14.

Albrecht, G. L., Levy, J. A., Sugrue, N. M., Prohaska, T. R., & Ostrow, D. G. (1989). Who hasn't heard about AIDS? *AIDS Education and Prevention, 1,* 261–267.

Altamura, C. A., Mauri, M. L., Coppola, M. T., & Cazzullo, C. L. (1988). Delusional AIDS and depression. *British Journal of Psychiatry, 153,* 267–269.

Becker, M., & Joseph, J. (1988). AIDS and behavioral change to reduce risk: A review. *American Journal of Public Heath, 78,* 394–410.

Blendon, R. J., & Donelan, K. (1988). Discrimination against people with AIDS. *New England Journal of Medicine, 319,* 1022–1026.

Booth, W. (1988). Heterosexual AIDS: Setting the odds. *Science, 239,* 597.

Bor, R., & Miller, R. (1989). Psychotherapeutic interventions for patients with the delusion of having AIDS. *American Journal of Psychiatry, 146,* 808.

Bor, R., Perry, L., Jackson, J., & Miller, R. (1989). Strategies for counselling the "worried well" in relation to AIDS. *Journal of the Royal Society of Medicine, 82,* 218–220.

Bouton, R. A., Gallaher, P. E., Garlinghouse, P. A., Leal, T., Rosenstein, L. D., & Young, R. K. (1987). Scales for measuring fear of AIDS and homophobia. *Journal of Personality Assessment, 51,* 606–614.

Brandt, A. M. (1988). AIDS in historical perspective: Four lessons from the history of sexually transmitted diseases. *American Journal of Public Health, 78,* 367–371.

Bruce, K. E. M., & Bullins, C. G. (1989). Students' attitudes and knowledge about genital herpes. *Journal of Sex Education and Therapy, 15,* 257–270.

Bruhn, J. G. (1989). Counseling persons with a fear of AIDS. *Journal of Counseling and Development, 67,* 455–457.

Callero, P. L., Baker, D. V., Carpenter, J., & Magarigal, J. (1986). Fear of AIDS and its effects on the nation's blood supply. In D. A. Feldman and T. M. Johnson (Eds.), *The social dimensions of AIDS* (pp. 227–232). New York: Praeger.

Chodof, P. (1987). Fear of AIDS. *Psychiatry, 50,* 184.

Clark, C. (1989, October 4). Doctors get warning on AIDS risk. *San Diego Union,* pp. B-1–B-2.

Clark, C. (1991, November 4). New definition of who has AIDS could triple the official caseload in county. *San Diego Union,* p. B-3.

Clavel, F., Mansinho, K., Chamaret, S., Guetard, D., Favier, V., Nina, J., Santos-

Ferreira, M.-O., Champalimaud, J.-L., & Montagnier, L. (1987). Human immunodeficiency virus type 2 infection associated with AIDS in West Africa. *New
England Journal of Medicine, 316,* 1180–1185.

Clever, L. H., & Omenn, G. S. (1988). Hazards for health care workers. *Annual
Review of Public Health, 9,* 273–303.

Cochran, S. D. (1988, August). *Risky behavior and disclosure: Is it safe if you ask?*
Paper presented at the annual convention of the American Psychological Association, Atlanta, GA.

Cockcroft, A. (1989). AIDS/HIV counselling in occupational health. *AIDS Care, 1,* 97–
103.

Can you rely on condoms? (1989, March). *Consumer Reports,* pp. 135–141.

Conway, G. A., Colley-Neimeyer, B., Pursley, C., Cruz, C., Burt, S., Rion, P., &
Heath, C. W. (1989). Underreporting of AIDS cases in South Carolina, 1986 and
1987. *Journal of the American Medical Association, 262,* 2859–2863.

Cooke, M. (1988). Housestaff attitudes towards the acquired immunodeficiency syndrome. *AIDS and Public Policy, 3,* 59–60.

Cowley, G. (1992, July 27). Is a new AIDS virus emerging? *Newsweek,* p. 41.

D'Augelli, A. R. (1989). AIDS fears and homophobia among rural nursing personnel.
AIDS Education and Prevention, 1, 277–284.

D'Augelli, A. R., & Rose, M. L. (1990). Homophobia in a university community:
Attitudes and experiences of heterosexual freshmen. *Journal of College Student
Development, 31,* 484–491.

Douglas, C. J., Kalman, C. M., & Kalman, T. P. (1985). Homophobia among physicians and nurses: An empirical study. *Hospital and Community Psychiatry, 36,*
1309–1311.

Dundes, A. (1987). At ease, disease—AIDS jokes as sick humor. *American Behavioral
Scientist, 30,* 72–81.

Evans, G. A., & Gill, M. J. (1988). Factitious AIDS. *New England Journal of Medicine, 319,* 1605–1606.

Exler, A. (1987, April 2–15). Gay bashings grow. *The Edge,* p. 8.

Falkner von Sonnenburg, F. J., & Eichenlaub, D. (1988). AIDS—medical and epidemiological bases. In H. Jager (Ed.), *AIDS phobia* (pp. 13–33). Chichester, England:
Ellis Horwood Limited.

Fenton, T. W. (1987). AIDS-related psychiatric disorder. *British Journal of Psychiatry,
151,* 579–588.

Fisher, E. (1986). How to combat the AIDS—and FRAIDS—epidemics. *Michigan Medicine, 85,* 93–95.

Fisher, J. D., & Misovich, S. J. (1990). Evolution of college students' AIDS-related
behavioral responses, attitudes, knowledge, and fear. *AIDS Education and Prevention, 2,* 322–337.

Fitzpatrick, M., & Milligan, D. (1987). *The truth about the AIDS panic.* London:
Junius.

Franzini, L. R. (1987, July). AIDS fear spawns symptoms. *American Health, 6,* 12.

Franzini, L. R., Dexter, K. E., & Straits, K. (1992). *Social and sexual behavior
changes made as a result of the AIDS crisis.* Manuscript submitted for publication.

Franzini, L. R., Sideman, L. M., Dexter, K. E., & Elder, J. P. (1990). Promoting AIDS
risk reduction via behavioral training. *AIDS Education and Prevention, 2,* 313–321.

Fribourg, S. (1989). Health care professionals and fear of AIDS. *Journal of the American Medical Association, 262,* 2680.

Gauch, R. R., Feeney, K. B., & Brown, J. W. (1990). Fear of AIDS and attrition among medical technologists. *American Journal of Public Health, 80,* 1264–1265.

Gayle, H. D., Keeling, R. P., Garcia-Tunon, M., Kilbourne, B. W., Narkunas, J. P., Ingram, F. R., Rogers, M. F., & Curran, J. W. (1990). Prevalence of the human immunodeficiency virus among university students. *New England Journal of Medicine, 323,* 1538–1541.

Gerbert, B., Maguire, B., Badner, V., Altman, D., & Stone, G. (1988). Why fear persists: Health care professionals and AIDS. *Journal of the American Medical Association, 260,* 3481–3482, 3485.

Gerbert, B., Maguire, B., Badner, V., Altman, D., & Stone, G. (1989). Fear of AIDS: Issues for health professional education. *AIDS Education and Prevention, 1,* 39–52.

Goodman, E., & Cohall, A. T. (1989). Acquired immunodeficiency syndrome and adolescents: Knowledge, attitudes, beliefs, and behaviors in a New York City adolescent minority population. *Pediatrics, 84,* 36–42.

Greenblat, C. S., Katz, S., Gagnon, J. H., & Shannon, D. (1989). An innovative program of counseling family members and friends of seropositive haemophiliacs. *AIDS Care, 1,* 67–75.

Hagen, M. D., Meyer, K. S., & Paulker, S. G. (1988). Routine preoperative screening for HIV: Does the risk to the surgeon outweigh the risk to the patient? *Journal of the American Medical Association, 259,* 1357–1359.

Herek, G. M., & Berrill, K. T. (1990). Anti-gay violence and mental health. *Journal of Interpersonal Violence, 5,* 414–423.

Hingson, R., Strunin, L., & Berlin, B. (1990). Acquired immunodeficiency syndrome transmission: Changes in knowledge and behaviors among teenagers: Massachusetts statewide surveys, 1986 to 1988. *Pediatrics, 85,* 24–29.

Hogan, T. (1989). Psychophysical relation between perceived threat of AIDS and willingness to impose social restrictions. *Health Psychology, 8,* 255–266.

Holmes, K. K., Karon, J. M., & Kreiss, J. (1990). The increasing frequency of heterosexually acquired AIDS in the United States, 1983–88. *American Journal of Public Health, 80,* 858–862.

Imperato, P. J., Feldman, J. G., Nayeri, K., & DeHovitz, J. A. (1988). Medical students' attitudes towards caring for patients with AIDS in a high incidence area. *New York State Journal of Medicine, 88,* 223–227.

Jacob, K. S., John, J. K., Verghese, A., & John, T. J. (1987). AIDS-phobia. *British Journal of Psychiatry, 151,* 412–413.

Jacob, K. S., John, J. K., Verghese, A., & John, T. J. (1989). The fear of AIDS: Psychiatric symptom or syndrome? *AIDS Care, 1,* 35–38.

Jäger, H. (Ed.). (1988a). *AIDS phobia.* Chichester, England: Ellis Horwood Limited.

Jäger, H. (1988b). AIDS—psychosocial aspects. In H. Jager (Ed.), *AIDS phobia.* (pp. 35–46). Chichester, England: Ellis Horwood Limited.

Judson, F. N. (1989). What do we really know about AIDS Control? *American Journal of Public Health, 79,* 878–882.

Kamlana, S. H., & Gray, P. (1988). Fear of AIDS. *British Journal of Psychiatry, 153,* 129.

Kantrowitz, B., Springen, K., McCormick, J., Reiss, S., Hager, M., Denworth, L.,

Bingham, C., & Foote, D. (1991, July 1). Doctors and AIDS. *Newsweek,* pp. 48–52, 54, 56.

Katz, I., Hass, R. G., Parisi, N., Astone, J., & McEvaddy, D. (1987). Lay people's and health care personnel's perceptions of cancer, AIDS, cardiac, and diabetic patients. *Psychological Reports, 60,* 615–629.

Kegeles, S. M., Adler, N. E., & Irwin, C. E. (1988). Sexually active adolescents and condoms: Changes over one year in knowledge, attitudes and use. *American Journal of Public Health, 78,* 460–461.

Kelly, J. A., St. Lawrence, J., Hood, H. V., Smith, S., & Cook, D. J. (1988). Nurses' attitudes toward AIDS. *Journal of Continuing Education in Nursing, 19,* 78–83.

Kelly, J. A., St. Lawrence, J., Smith, S., Hood, H. V., & Cook, D. J. (1987a). Stigmatization of AIDS patients by physicians. *American Journal of Public Health, 77,* 789–791.

Kelly, J. A., St. Lawrence, J., Smith, S., Jr., Hood, H. V., & Cook, D. J. (1987b). Medical students' attitudes toward AIDS and homosexual patients. *Journal of Medical Education, 62,* 549–556.

Klonoff, E. A., & Ewers, D. (1990). Care of AIDS patients as a source of stress to nursing staff. *AIDS Education and Prevention, 2,* 338–348.

Knight-Ridder News Service. (1992, January 18). AIDS in U.S. spreading most rapidly among heterosexuals, agency says. *San Diego Union,* p. A-6.

Knox, M. D., Dow, M. G., & Cotton, D. A. (1989). Mental health care providers: The need for AIDS education. *AIDS Education and Prevention, 1,* 285–290.

Kong, D. (1992, January 19). AIDS virus produces "a flood of litigation." *San Diego Union,* pp. A-1, A-23.

Kotarba, J. A., Williams, M. L., & Johnson, J. (1991). Rock music as a medium for AIDS intervention. *AIDS Education and Prevention, 3,* 47–49.

Krajick, K. (1988, May). Private passions and public health. *Psychology Today, 22,* 50, 54, 56, 58.

Lamboi, S. E., & Sy, F. S. (1989). The impact of AIDS on state public health legislation in the United States: A critical review. *AIDS Education and Prevention 1,* 324–339.

Lawlor, B. A., & Stewart, J. T. (1987). AIDS delusions: A symptom of our times. *American Journal of Psychiatry, 144,* 1244.

Leventhal, H., Meyer, D., & Gutmann, M. (1980). The role of theory in the study of compliance to high blood pressure regimens. In R. B. Haynes, M. E. Mattson, & O. E. Tillmer (Eds.), *Patient compliance to prescribed antihypertensive medication regimes: A report to the National Heart, Lung, and Blood Institute.* Washington, DC: U.S. Department of Health and Human Services.

Link, R. N., Feingold, A. R., Charap, M. H., Freeman, K., & Shelov, S. P. (1988). Concerns of medical and pediatric house officers about acquiring AIDS from their patients. *American Journal of Public Health, 78,* 455–459.

Lipkin, B. (1988). Pseudo-AIDS, AIDS panic, or AIDS phobia. *British Journal of Psychiatry, 152,* 425.

Lippert, G. P. (1986). Excessive concern about AIDS in two bisexual men. *Canadian Journal of Psychiatry, 31,* 63–66.

Mahorney, S. L., & Cavenar, J. O. (1988). A new and timely delusion: The complaint of having AIDS. *American Journal of Psychiatry, 145,* 1130–1132.

Masters, W. H., Johnson, V. E., & Kolodny, R. C. (1988). *Crisis: Heterosexual behavior in the age of AIDS*. New York: Grove Press.

McDonald, J., & Wafer, K. (1989). Munchausen syndrome masquerading as AIDS-induced depression. *British Journal of Psychiatry, 154*, 420–421.

McKusick, L., Conant, M., & Coates, T. (1985). The AIDS epidemic: A model for developing intervention strategies for reducing high-risk behavior in gay men. *Sexually Transmitted Diseases, 12*, 229–233.

Miller, D., Green, J., Farmer, R., & Carroll, G. (1985). A "pseudo-AIDS" syndrome following from fear of AIDS. *British Journal of Psychiatry, 146*, 550–551.

Miller, F., Weiden, P., Sacks, M., & Wozniak, J. (1986). Two cases of factitious acquired immune deficiency syndrome. *American Journal of Psychiatry, 143*, 1483.

Muir, M. A. (1991). *The environmental contexts of AIDS*. New York: Praeger.

National Academy of Sciences. (1988). *Confronting AIDS: Update 1988*. Washington, DC: National Academy Press.

Negy, C., & Webber, A. W. (1991). Knowledge and fear of AIDS: A comparison study between White, Black, and Hispanic college students. *Journal of Sex Education and Therapy, 17*, 42–45.

Neraal, T. (1988). The irrational element in the fear of AIDS infection: Management of AIDS phobia in an 11-year-old boy. In H. Jager (Ed.), *AIDS phobia* (pp. 107–113). Chichester, England: Ellis Horwood Limited.

New York Times News Service. (1989, December 10). In high-risk age of AIDS, women snoop to conquer as caution replaces trust. *San Diego Union*, p. A-2.

O'Brien, G., & Hassanyeh, F. (1985). AIDS-panic: AIDS-induced psychogenic states. *British Journal of Psychiatry, 146*, 91.

O'Brien, L. S. (1987). Not a case of pseudo-AIDS. *British Journal of Psychiatry, 151*, 127.

Palca, J. (1991). The sobering geography of AIDS. *Science, 252*, 372–373.

Petit, C. (1988, June 15). 11-year incubation found for AIDS. *San Francisco Chronicle*, p. A-4.

Pierce, C., & VanDeVeer, D. (1988). *AIDS: Ethics and public policy*. Belmont, CA: Wadsworth.

Probart, C. K. (1989). A preliminary investigation using drama in community AIDS education. *AIDS Education and Prevention, 1*, 268–276.

Puckett, S. R., & Emery, A. R. (1989). *Managing AIDS in the workplace*. Reading, MA: Addison-Wesley.

Quinn, B. (1988). Fear, anger, and the hope of redemption in the age of AIDS. *New York State Journal of Medicine, 88*, 661–664.

Rapaport, M., & Braff, D. L. (1985). AIDS and homosexual panic. *American Journal of Psychiatry, 142*, 1516.

Riccio, M., & Thompson, C. (1987). Pseudo-AIDS, AIDS panic or AIDS phobia? *British Journal of Psychiatry, 151*, 863.

Richardson, J. L., Lochner, T., McGuigan, K., & Levine, A. M. (1987). Physician attitudes and experience regarding the care of patients with acquired immunodeficiency syndrome (AIDS) and related disorders (ARC). *Medical Care, 25*, 675–685.

Robinson, E. N., & Latham, R. H. (1987). A factitious case of acquired immodeficiency syndrome. *Sexually Transmitted Diseases, 14*, 54–57.

Salt, H., Miller, R., Perry, L., & Bor, R. (1989). Paradoxical interventions in counselling for people with an intractable AIDS-worry. *AIDS Care, 1*, 39–44.

Seeley, D. (1988, October). 10 ways to tell a man he has to wear a condom. *New Woman*, pp. 103–104.

Segal, M. (1988). Pseudo-AIDS, AIDS panic, or AIDS phobia. *British Journal of Psychiatry, 152,* 424–425.

Shilts, R. (1987). *And the band played on.* New York: St. Martin's Press.

Skurnick, J. H., Johnson, R. L., Quinones, M. A., Foster, J. D., & Louria, D. B. (1991). New Jersey high school students' knowledge, attitudes, and behavior regarding AIDS. *AIDS Education and Prevention, 3,* 21–30.

Stevenson, M. R., & Stevenson, D. M. (1990). Beliefs about AIDS among entering college students. *Journal of Sex Education and Therapy, 16,* 201–204.

Strunin, L., Culbert, A., & Crane, S. (1989). First year medical students' attitudes and knowledge about AIDS. *AIDS Care, 1,* 105–110.

Thomas, E. (1985, September 23). The new untouchables: Anxiety over AIDS is verging on hysteria in some parts of the country. *Time,* pp. 24–26.

Treiber, F., Shaw, D., & Malcolm, R. (1987). Acquired immune deficiency syndrome: Psychological impact on health personnel. *Journal of Nervous and Mental Disease, 175,* 496–499.

Tyson, E., & Fortenberry, J. D. (1987). Fraudulent AIDS: A variant of Munchausen's syndrome. *Journal of the American Medical Association, 258,* 1889–1890.

United Press International. (1987, July 16). Women more likely to abstain from sex because of AIDS fear. *San Diego Tribune,* p. A-16.

Vernon, A., Hoagland, M. H., & Perlman, E. J. (1987). AIDS wrongly diagnosed. *Journal of the American Medical Association, 258,* 2063–2064.

Walker, S. L. (1992, January 11). USAir class relaxes white knuckles. *San Diego Union,* pp. C1–2.

Wallack, J. J. (1989). AIDS anxiety among health care professionals. *Hospital and Community Psychiatry, 40,* 507–510.

Wein, B. (1987, June). Sex in the age of AIDS. *New Woman,* pp. 123–124, 126, 128, 130.

Weiss, R., & Thier, S. O. (1988). HIV testing is the answer—What's the question? *New England Journal of Medicine, 319,* 1010–1012.

White, S. (1992, January 4). TV has crucial role in war against AIDS. *San Diego Union,* p. C-7.

Windgassen, E., & Soni, S. D. (1987). AIDS panic. *British Journal of Psychiatry, 151,* 126–127.

Winslow, R., Rumbaut, R. G., & Hwang, J. (1989). AIDS, FRAIDS, and quarantine: Student responses to pro-quarantine initiatives in California. *Journal of Applied Social Psychology, 19,* 1453–1478.

Winslow, R., Rumbaut, R. G., & Hwang, J. (1990). AIDS-phobia and political reaction in California. *Archives of Sexual Behavior, 19,* 517–530.

Wu, A. W., Kennedy, C. J., & Paradise, M. (1988). Factitious false-positive test for HIV. *Journal of the American Medical Association, 259,* 1647.

Chapter Five

Responses from the Street: ACT UP and Community Organizing Against AIDS

Valeria Fabj
Matthew J. Sobnosky

On March 10, 1987, author and playwright Larry Kramer was invited to speak at the Gay and Lesbian Community Center in New York City because of his reputation as an outspoken critic of the government, the media, the medical establishment, and even the gay community for their response to the acquired immune deficiency syndrome (AIDS) epidemic. Kramer brought his characteristic stridency to his speech. He spoke about the type of care people with AIDS could expect to receive in the United States. Kramer had recently returned from Houston, Texas, where he had met with Dr. Peter Mansell, who ran the Institute for Immunological Disorders, a hospital especially for people with AIDS that has since closed. Kramer told his audience about some of the problems Mansell and others faced in trying to treat people with AIDS. According to Kramer, for example, Mansell had discovered that many complications associated with AIDS were better treated at significantly reduced cost at home. The only problem, according to Mansell, was that most insurance companies do not pay for home care and outpatient treatment. "The very insurance companies that are threatening to take away our insurance because we cost them too much won't pay for cheaper treatment," observed Kramer. "That doesn't make much sense, does it?" (Kramer, 1989, p. 130).

What made even less sense, said Kramer, was the Food and Drug Administration's (FDA's) policy on drugs used to treat AIDS. Kramer told the audience that several drugs for treating AIDS that had already passed early safety tests had proved promising in early trials. The FDA, however, was refusing to approve the drugs for testing on people with AIDS. "[Dr. Mansell] cannot get near the FDA," Kramer said. "He showed me the protocols that he submits, and he showed me how they're sent back—the FDA asking for one sentence rewritten, three words revised—nothing substantial—each change causing a delay of six to eight months" (Kramer, 1989, p. 130). Kramer included this characterization of the FDA from Ann Fettner of the *Village Voice*: "It is a bureaucratic mess, they aren't even computerized, things 'are likely to get stuck in the mailroom,' says Duke University economist Henry Graboswki—which means that much of our pharmaceutical talent diddles with refinements of approved drugs while many that are desperately needed are put on hold" (pp. 130–131). Kramer highlighted the tragic irony of the FDA's policies: "A new drug can easily take ten years to satisfy FDA approval" (pp. 130–131) He drove home the absurdity of the lengthy approval process by contrasting it with the urgency facing people with AIDS: "Ten years! Two-thirds of us could be dead in less than five years" (p. 131).

In his speech that evening, Kramer also accused gay organizations of failing to show leadership in the AIDS crisis. Gay organizations, he charged, were remaining silent or fragmented in response to FDA and government inaction. He attacked particularly the Gay Men's Health Crisis (GMHC), an AIDS advocacy group he helped to found. GMHC was, he said, "the only AIDS game in town in this country" (Kramer, 1989, p. 133). Despite its obvious opportunity for leadership, however, Kramer believed GMHC's response to the AIDS crisis to that point had been "tragically weak" (p. 134). Kramer contrasted the political ineptitude of GMHC with the effectiveness of other groups of advocates:

> This morning's front page of the *New York Times* has an article about two thousand Catholics marching through the halls of Albany today. On the front page of the *Times*. With their six bishops (including one whom we know to be gay). Two thousand Catholics and their bishops marching through the halls of government. That's advocacy! (p. 134)

Kramer asked his audience, "Why are we so invisible, constantly and forever! What does it take to get a few thousand people to stage a march!" (p. 135). Maybe, he reasoned, the time had come for more direct action. He asked the audience, "Do we want to start a new organization devoted solely to political action?" (p. 135). That question was answered with a clear yes when the AIDS Coalition to Unleash Power (ACT UP) was formed 2 days later. Kramer explained that his speech was followed by "much discussion" and "a decision to hold another meeting, two days later" (p. 137). About 300 people attended the meeting and established ACT UP (p. 137).

In the 5 years since it was founded, ACT UP has grown tremendously.[1] ACT UP/NY is still the largest ACT UP chapter in the United States, but there are now ACT UP chapters in most major American cities, in smaller cities and towns across the United States, as well as in Berlin, London, and Paris and other cities overseas. In some cities, such as San Francisco, existing AIDS advocacy organizations reformulated themselves as ACT UP. In others, as in New York, ACT UP represents a new group for AIDS advocacy. Most individual ACT UP chapters are loosely linked with other AIDS advocacy groups and each other through the nationwide AIDS Coalition to Network, Organize and Win (ACT NOW).

In this chapter, we examine the communication efforts of ACT UP in responding to the AIDS crisis. We first offer an overview of ACT UP's strategies for communicating with its various audiences. After a brief look at ACT UP's best known tactics, we focus on three areas that have received little attention in other examinations. The first area deals with ACT UP's communication about treatment and support for people with AIDS. The second area deals with ACT UP's efforts to promote safer sex and drug use to help stop the spread of AIDS. Finally, we consider ACT UP's recent efforts to embrace a broader agenda for social reform as the ultimate solution to the AIDS crisis.

OVERVIEW

ACT UP defines itself as "a diverse, nonpartisan group united in anger and committed to direct action to end the AIDS crisis" (ACT UP/NY Women and AIDS Book Group, 1990, p. 245). From its inception, ACT UP has attracted attention through its public demonstrations and the high level of visibility it maintains. One key element of that visibility is the group's logo, "Silence = Death," printed in white letters under a pink triangle.[2] The ubiquitous logo appears on posters, T-shirts, buttons, and stickers; as graffiti on sidewalks, walls, and bridges; and even as part of an art exhibit about AIDS at the New Museum of Contemporary Art in New York City.

[1]We realize that there is no central organization to ACT UP and that chapters exist independently of each other. Here, however, we use the acronym "ACT UP" to refer to both individual chapters and chapters collectively, as a matter of convenience. We hope that we do no violence to individual ACT UP chapters in the process.

[2]The "Silence = Death" logo did not originate with ACT UP, but had been developed several months before ACT UP was formed by a group of six gay men who, calling themselves the Silence = Death Project, produced posters with the logo for display throughout New York City. The members of the Silence = Death Project were present at the founding meeting of ACT UP and lent their design to ACT UP for signs at its second demonstration, held at New York City's main post office on April 15, 1987 (Crimp & Rolston, 1990).

In addition to the ubiquitousness of the "Silence = Death" logo, ACT UP chapters have maintained visibility through many high-profile demonstrations. ACT UP's first public demonstration took place on March 24, 1987, during the morning rush hour on Wall Street, and this set the tone for many ACT UP actions to come. The target for the demonstration was the FDA, because of its foot dragging on approving new drugs for treating people with AIDS. Demonstrators hanged in effigy FDA Commissioner Frank Young and passed out leaflets titled, "AIDS IS EVERYBODY'S BUSINESS," which detailed the group's complaints with the FDA's handling of the AIDS crisis. Demonstrators also tied up traffic for several hours. The demonstration, and the arrests that accompanied it, attracted the attention of the network newscasts. When Young promised to speed up the drug approval process 2 weeks later, CBS news anchor Dan Rather credited the ACT UP demonstration (Crimp & Rolston, 1990, pp. 28, 29).

Perhaps the most controversial actions taken by ACT UP occurred at its "Stop the Church" demonstration at St. Patrick's Cathedral in New York in December 1989. From its inception, ACT UP/NY had targeted Catholic Archbishop John Cardinal O'Connor for criticism. O'Connor, they argued, uses his authority to prevent education about safer sex generally, and condom distribution particularly, in Catholic schools, hospitals, shelters, and other charities in New York City. O'Connor's influence, however, extends beyond obedient Catholics, ACT UP argued. According to ACT UP,

> As soon as he came to New York, he formed a close alliance with his fellow reactionary, Mayor Koch, whose policies were consistently informed by the cardinal's "moral" positions. This means, for one thing, that in the public schools, where 85 percent of the students are people of color, AIDS education has been a just-say-no harangue—antigay, antisex, antilife. . . . (p. 131)

The impact of this position is clear: "Statistics show that the vast majority of students are sexually active and many use drugs. Preaching abstinence denies their reality and will ultimately deny many of them their lives" (Crimp & Rolston, 1990, p. 131).

In response to O'Connor's unwavering opposition to education about safer sex and condom distribution, ACT UP planned "Stop the Church," a demonstration to coincide with O'Connor's saying morning mass on Sunday, December 10, 1989. According to ACT UP, "Our demo scenario called for a legal picket around St. Patrick's, culminating in a mass 'die-in,' a tactic of playing dead in the streets often used by ACT UP to symbolize what the target was doing to us" (p. 136). In addition, "affinity groups" (small groups of ACT UP protesters who act independently) "secretly planned civil disobedience inside the cathedral while O'Connor said mass" (Crimp & Rolston, 1990, p. 136). The protests inside the cathedral drew most media attention during "Stop the

Church." Media coverage of the demonstration focused on activists inside the cathedral who staged a "die-in" in the aisles, shouted during the service and the sermon, chained themselves to the pews, and threw condoms. Reports noted that one protester discarded a consecrated host during communion (e.g., Magnuson). In all, 111 protesters were arrested during "Stop the Church" (Kistenburg, 1991, p. 14).

Closer analysis of "Stop the Church" provides important insight into the operation of ACT UP. First, discussion among ACT UP members, both before and after "Stop the Church," provides an example of how ACT UP functions. Actions are discussed and analyzed from a variety of points of view both before and after they are undertaken. ACT UP avoids traditional organization and often requires its membership to reach consensus on issues and actions, rather than putting issues to a vote.[3] This approach ensures that members take ownership over group actions and is attractive to some members. One lesbian activist, for example, explains that ACT UP's process of decision making and the commitment to action have kept her involved in a group about whose politics she is ambivalent. She explains,

> Everything was run democratically, and people go up and said what they thought. I could get up and say what I thought. They wanted to end the AIDS crisis, period, and if you had a good idea they would listen. No one spouted rhetoric; there was no party line. They had great ideas for actions without any pre-set idea of the right way to do things. They thought tabling was a new idea. (ACT UP/NY Women and AIDS Book Group, 1990, p. 235)

At the same time, other ACT UP members charge that decentralized decision making has paralyzed the group at times. In San Francisco, for example, when ACT UP split into two factions, some members cited paralysis brought on by the necessity of consensus as a reason. Hank Wilson, a San Francisco activist, is quoted in the *Advocate*, a national gay and lesbian news magazine, as saying, "I left because I want to get some stuff done. . . . I don't want to see the group paralyzed by process" (O'Loughlin, 1990, p. 48).

Clearly, such issues were sharpened in discussions of "Stop the Church." "It had been difficult to build consensus in ACT UP about 'Stop the Church,'" admit Crimp and Rolston (1990, p. 140), because members knew that the Church would not change its position and feared that media coverage of the action "would misrepresent the target of the demonstration as Catholics and Catholicism, rather than the church hierarchy's impact on all of us through the power illegally granted them by the state" (p. 140). Further evidence of some

---

[3]Different ACT UP chapters use different decision-making structures, Most, however, eschew traditional hierarchical approaches in favor of some type of consensus building (e.g., "AIDS and Politics: Transformation of Our Movement" in ACT UP/NY Women and AIDS Book Group, 1990; Nussbaum, 1991; Sullivan, 1990).

members' ambivalence about the action is also apparent in the way ACT UP members talk about "Stop the Church." Crimp and Rolston, for example, refer to planned actions by affinity groups inside the church as "secret," implying that these actions were undertaken separately from the planned demonstration outside the church.

Reaction among ACT UP members to the protest also yields insight into how ACT UP members define success and failure. Some ACT UP members expressed reservations about the success of the action. "I think we fucked up seriously," said one. "[T]here were 4500 people out there who didn't get their message across, and that is a problem" (Handelman, 1990, p. 116). Crimp and Rolston (1990) claimed that discussion afterward saw the event as a success, however, in that it demonstrated the lengths to which ACT UP is willing to go to "save lives" and represented an effective coalition "with other activist movements dedicated to the rights of health care and control over our own bodies" (p. 140), because the action had been planned with prochoice group Women's Health Action and Mobilization (WHAM!).

Furthermore, members viewed the publicity the event generated as positive, despite its negative tone. One demonstrator from inside the Church stated,

> I thought the 'Stop the Church' action was enormously successful . . . because what it did was get the issues into the public conversation, and that was our aim— not to change people's minds in the hierarchy of the church, not to make people think something in particular, but to start the conversation, to get these issues talked about. And that's what we did enormously successfully. (Kistenburg, 1991, pp. 20, 21)

Internal controversies are by no means limited to the action at "Stop the Church." Some argue, in fact, that ACT UP courts controversy and visibility, even when these do not contribute to the group's cause. One fan at a baseball game at Shea Stadium in New York, for example, called ACT UP's baseball-themed messages about AIDS and safe sex ("NO GLOVE, NO LOVE" and "AIDS IS NO BALL GAME") on banners "totally inappropriate" at an event like a baseball game (Salholz, 1988, p. 42). Even some gay activists go to great lengths to distance themselves from ACT UP's more extreme tactics. The *Advocate*, for example, reported that a Denver gay activist referred to protesters at an ACT UP demonstration as "a bunch of immature babies" after one protester had reportedly said of critics, "I hope their kids die" (Walter, 1990, p. 26).

Others, both within and outside of ACT UP, disagree with criticisms of the group's more extreme demonstrations. Kramer, for example, attributes much of the group's effectiveness as an advocate for change to the extreme tactics it uses. He puts it simply: "Surely ACT UP has taught everyone that you don't get anything by being nice, good little boys and girls. You do not get more with honey than with vinegar" (Kramer, 1989, p. 290). Activist Peter Staley (1991) is even more blunt: "The ability to hate us for what some regard as offensive tactics while ignoring the fact that we have improved, extended, and saved lives is shocking and despicable" (p. 98).

The most visible dimension of ACT UP is its commitment to public demonstrations to focus attention on government inaction to the AIDS crisis (e.g., Crimp & Rolston, 1990); on what ACT UP sees as price gouging by pharmaceutical companies who refuse to provide drugs to treat AIDS at affordable prices (e.g., Crimp & Rolston, 1990); on the medical establishment, which refuses to consider alternative treatments for AIDS and human immunodeficiency virus (HIV) infection (Lederer, 1990); or on the FDA, which refuses to speed up the drug approval process and insists on giving some people with AIDS placebos in order to provide control groups for experimental drugs (Nussbaum, 1991). Some ACT UP chapters have also boycotted Philip Morris and its subsidiary, Miller Beer, for the company's financial support of North Carolina Senator Jesse Helms, a strong opponent of much of ACT UP's agenda.

There is another dimension to ACT UP that is just as important as demonstrations to the organization's fight against AIDS. This dimension, which receives substantially less media attention than ACT UP's sensational demonstrations, focuses on the personal battle that everyone must fight to prevent the spread of AIDS. The real success of ACT UP, according to Kramer, is that "ACT UP has succeeded in forcing the system to finally let the people AIDS is happening to have a major voice in what is being done to us" (1989, p. 286). To ensure that this new voice is informed, ACT UP provides information to help people take control of their lives. ACT UP provides information about treatment and support, about safer sex and other behaviors to reduce the spread of AIDS, and about what we all need to do about AIDS.

TREATMENT AND SUPPORT

Historically, the first goal of ACT UP was to increase access to new drugs for people with AIDS. The group was formed as a reaction to the sluggish response of the medical establishment to the AIDS crisis. Activists recognize that people with AIDS cannot afford to wait for drugs to be approved by the FDA when their survival often depends on the availability of those drugs. Although ACT UP stages demonstrations against the establishment, it also works on the personal level in helping HIV-positive people and people with AIDS regain control over their lives. To do so, the group offers information about support groups, information about new and experimental drugs, as well as medical advice and suggestions for how to talk to doctors about AIDS.

ACT UP argues that "health care delivery is stratified (rich to poor), fragmented (lacking in an overall plan), and specialized (different doctors for different body parts) rather than centering on the individual as a whole person" (ACT

UP/NY Women and AIDS Book Group, 1990, p. 69). As a result, doctors are often misinformed about AIDS (especially in the case of women patients) and about how to best treat illnesses related to AIDS. One of the recommendations that ACT UP/NY's Women and AIDS groups makes, for example, is for "respect on the part of clinicians for the patient's participation in her own health care and willingness to provide care regardless of which therapies a patient chooses or refuses, including alternative therapies such as acupuncture, macrobiotics, or herbal remedies" (ACT UP/NY Women and AIDS Book Group, 1990, p. 70).

Such an approach requires information about various treatments and therapies. One of the most important sources for information about AIDS is ACT UP's Treatment + Data Committee. Kramer (1989) claims that "ACT UP's Treatment + Data Committee has learned more than most scientists and doctors" (p. 286) about AIDS and how to treat it. ACT UP believes that the best way for HIV-positive people and people with AIDS to regain control over their lives is to inform themselves about HIV, AIDS, and the variety of available treatments. Armed with information, people can then make knowledgeable decisions regarding their medical treatment, even when those decisions challenge the authority and expertise of physicians.

ACT UP's message to people to take control of their own lives often takes the form of direct attacks on the medical community, especially doctors. A videotape titled "Doctors, Liars, and Women" produced by women in ACT UP suggests that we cannot blindly accept information about AIDS just because it comes from a doctor. The videotape was made in response to an article that had appeared in *Cosmopolitan* in which the risk to women of contracting AIDS through "normal" heterosexual intercourse was minimized. In the videotape, women from ACT UP confront the doctor who wrote the article. ACT UP describes it this way: "We show a group of women from ACT UP's Women's Caucus confronting Dr. Gould [the author of the *Cosmopolitan* article] with the information that the 'evidence' in his article was not only out of date, but also inaccurate. By challenging his authority with our knowledge, we make it clear that we are the experts" (ACT UP/NY Women and AIDS Book Group, 1990, p. 216).

SAFER SEX AND DRUG USE

The second thrust of ACT UP's outreach is also related to helping people to take control of their own lives but in this case takes the form of efforts to reduce the transmission of AIDS through unsafe sex and the sharing of dirty needles.

Safer Sex

The issue of safer sex is addressed both in large demonstrations and in information provided to communities and to individuals. ACT UP stresses that safer sex needs to be practiced by all men and women: gay, lesbian, bisexual, and heterosexual. No one is exempt from the threat of AIDS and no one is safe unless he or she practices sex responsibly. Thus, ACT UP rejects the designation of high- and low-risk groups and argues instead that *behaviors* are high or low risk. ACT UP argues, "It's not who you are that puts you at risk, it's what you do" (ACT UP/NY Women and AIDS Book Group, 1990, p. 114). Consequently, ACT UP provides the community with clear messages about how to make "what you do" safer. What distinguishes the information ACT UP provides from most other information about safer sex is (a) the explicit language ACT UP uses to describe sexual acts and (b) ACT UP's commitment to communicate its message in any way possible.

Perhaps ACT UP's best known demonstration focusing on safer sex occurred at Shea Stadium on "Women's Day," May 4, 1988, when ACT UP decided to target men and to make them feel responsible for practicing safer sex (a responsibility usually placed on women in heterosexual relationships). ACT UP members bought 400 tickets to the game, which allowed them to flash their messages on the electronic billboard (Kistenburg, 1991, p. 11); they also held banners with explicit messages and distributed a flier entitled "AIDS IS NO BALL GAME." The flier used the language of the game:

SINGLE Only **one** woman has been included in government-sponsored tests for new drugs for AIDS.
DOUBLE Women diagnosed with AIDS die **twice** as fast as men.
TRIPLE The number of women with AIDS has **tripled** as a result of sexual contact with men in New York City since the 1984 World Series.
THE
GRAND Most men **still** don't wear condoms.
SLAM

The entire demonstration was summarized in their slogans: "NO GLOVE NO LOVE" and "DON'T BALK AT SAFER SEX." Another poster, a graphic depiction of an erect penis accompanied by the slogan "MEN, USE CONDOMS OR BEAT IT" was developed for AIDS and Women Day, but was not used at demonstration sites "for obvious reasons." The slogan, however, has appeared at other ACT UP demonstrations and on stickers and T-shirts (Crimp & Rolston, 1990, pp. 63–65).

In his analysis of ACT UP, Gamson (1989) explains that the choice to demonstrate in a forum such as a baseball stadium is deliberate and strategic. First, events such as baseball games represent traditional American values and are therefore considered "safe" from AIDS, which "only attacks others." These settings allow ACT UP members to seize control "of symbols that traditionally exclude gay people or render them invisible, and take them over, endowing them with messages about AIDS" (Gamson, p. 362). Appropriation of a symbol like baseball allows activists to redefine AIDS. Gamson explains,

"They reclaim them . . . and make them mean differently. In so doing, they attempt to expose the system of domination from which they reclaim meanings and implicate the entire system in the spread of AIDS" (p. 362). Thus, ACT UP is able to coopt existing symbols like a baseball game to force people to face the existence of AIDS and the fact that AIDS is an issue that concerns them personally.

Clearly, there is a measure of shock value in ACT UP's messages and in the places in which they are delivered, but ACT UP argues that sometimes shock is important and necessary to force people to confront issues they find unpleasant or frightening. More important, however, we need to realize that ACT UP members do not see shock as an end in itself, but only as a means to get their message across. The demonstrators at Shea Stadium, for example, minimized the shock of their messages somewhat by couching them in the language of baseball. Typically, there is a clear connection between the target of ACT UP demonstrations and their messages. Demonstrations on Wall Street borrowed from the language of business and finance. Similarly, attacks on New York City Mayor Edward Koch borrowed Koch's famous slogan, "How'm I doin'?" (Crimp & Rolston, 1990). In all these instances, activists communicated shocking statistics and slogans in a clear and sometimes even grimly humorous way. If people are shocked, it is because the facts and statistics are shocking. Media coverage of ACT UP frequently misses this point. ACT UP uses theatrics and shocking messages because they work.

The explicit messages used in the demonstration at Shea Stadium are representative of the messages ACT UP uses in its community outreach through fliers, literature, and group presentations. Here, the main purpose of the explicit language is to be as clear as possible and to reach as many people as possible. Since many HIV-positive people and people with AIDS live on the margins of American society and lack access to educational and medical resources, they do not always understand technical terms used in medical discussions of risk behaviors. Thus, ACT UP materials use language from the streets, words that are graphic rather then euphemistic and that frequently offend middle-class sensibilities.

An example of such language can be found in Cynthia Chris's graphic explanation of safer sex for women in

> Safe sex can include penetration of a woman's vagina (cunt, pussy) or anus (asshole) by her partner's fingers or penis (cock, dick) or by a dildo. She may enjoy oral sex: 'going down' on one's partner may consist of mouth to vulva contact (cunnilingus, eating pussy), mouth to penis contact (fellatio, giving head) or mouth to anus contact (annilingus, rimming). . . . All of these activities can be performed safely, so that blood, semen, and vaginal fluids do not enter your or your partner's bloodstream through the mouth, vagina, anus, cuts or other openings in the skin. (ACT UP/NY Women and AIDS Book Group, 1990, p. 20)

The article also explains how to perform many sexual acts safely, how to use a condom, and how to use a dental dam (complete with explanation of what a dental dam is and how one can be made). Clearly, members of ACT UP are more concerned with describing behaviors in accurate, understandable terms than with observing conventions for public discussions about sex.

Not only is the language used accessible to people, but the information is distributed so as to reach as many people as possible. Because conventional public safety announcements are made through television, on billboards, and in pamphlets distributed at schools and health care centers, they are not generally explicit. Furthermore, they are not always useful to the people who might need them most: people who do not read or do not understand English (especially the technical terms for sexual organs and practices) and people who do not have access to health care. ACT UP tries to solve this problem by going into communities to organize talks about AIDS, distribute pamphlets, or simply talk to people in the streets about AIDS.

Frequently, these outreach efforts take unusual forms. Yannick Durand, who works with the Brooklyn AIDS Task Force (BATF), describes how her group reaches out to people in the Haitian community:

> It just doesn't work to bring Haitians, or for that matter most non-middle-class people, together just to talk about AIDS. At BATF, we have a lot of activity groups. For women there might be groups for sewing, knitting, or skill building. For teenagers, we have pizza parties, drawing groups, and so on. AIDS information is conveyed, but it's not the main focus. People love our activities groups who would never go on an AIDS program, but they end up very well informed about AIDS. (ACT UP/NY Women and AIDS Book Group, 1990, p. 89)

This approach to community outreach reflects a different understanding of ACT UP's commitment to "any means necessary" in the fight against AIDS. Most people, including health care workers, see little connection between women's social circles or teen pizza parties and AIDS prevention. Members of ACT UP, however, see reaching people with messages about safer behaviors as a key element in the fight against AIDS and are willing to try alternative routes to reach people with their messages.

The basic message ACT UP provides on the issue of safer sex is that people need to take control of their lives. This message empowers people, giving them practical advice and solutions to problems they face, rather than talking down to them, preaching to them, or imposing foreign value systems on them to change their sexual behavior. Cynthia Chris describes safer sex as follows:

> Safer sex is a way of taking control of, and taking responsibility for, one's sexual behavior. It allows us to protect ourselves and our partners against the transmission

of HIV. . . . Safer-sex practices recognize that sex is not only intercourse between a woman's vagina and a man's penis. Sex can involve any part of the body. It may be heterosexual, gay, or lesbian and it may take place in monogamous relationships or among a number of partners. (ACT UP/NY Women and AIDS Book Group, 1990, p. 19)

A similar message is echoed in the words of Monica Pearl:

> The only way we are going to get through the AIDS crisis is by taking care of ourselves and each other. This means not only educating ourselves but agitating for information and consideration. Organize teach-ins around the issues of safer sex; don't let anyone tell you to stop being sexual or to have sex that isn't safe . . . have sex—and do it safely. (ACT UP/NY Women and AIDS Book Group, 1990, p. 190)

ACT UP believes that everybody is entitled to information about safer sex, including minors. Unfortunately, activists argue, we often deny teens the information they need about sex in a misguided attempt to protect them from unpleasant information or because of a mistaken belief that talking about sex will lead automatically to promiscuity. The irony of this practice is not lost on activist Rachel Lurie:

> On the verge of adulthood, teenagers are not allowed information that will shape the types of adults they could become. Instead adult society restricts the information given to teens and then punishes them for making the wrong choices, never thinking that the answer is to give teenagers more information in the first place. Nowhere is this contradiction more evident than in the area of teenage sexuality. (ACT UP/NY Women and AIDS Book Group, 1990, p. 135)

At any time, such a position is shortsighted. In the age of AIDS, it is potentially deadly. To rectify this lack of information, ACT UP members distributed safe sex literature, condoms, and dental dams outside of New York high schools. Often, these actions drew attention as a protest against the New York Board of Education for not providing explicit information about safe sex to the students. The most important feature of the action, however, was to provide public school students with the information they need (Crimp & Rolston, 1990).

Safer Drug Use

ACT UP's commitment to help people take control of their own lives also extends to actions toward intravenous drug users. AIDS is spreading rapidly among intravenous drug users, who frequently share needles. Not surprisingly, ACT UP is very involved in trying to stop the spread of the disease among these individuals. Therefore, to its call for safer sex ACT UP adds a call for intravenous drug users to use clean needles. This effort takes two directions. First,

ACT UP teaches intravenous drug users how to clean dirty needles and provides them with necessary materials, such as bleach.

Second, and more important, ACT UP tries to provide intravenous drug users with clean needles through needle exchange programs. ACT UP members realize that the best way to help intravenous drug users avoid AIDS and other health risks is through drug treatment, including counseling and recovery programs. ACT UP recognizes, however, that current demand for such programs outstrips supply by a wide margin. In general, argues one activist, "There are so few drug treatment slots that those who want to quit drugs are often on waiting lists for months before they can begin treatment" (ACT UP/NY Women and AIDS Book Group, 1990, p. 126). Until enough money is allocated by the government (federal, state, and local) for wider access to drug treatment programs, ACT UP sees no alternative route to stop AIDS except providing clean needles and information about how HIV is spread to intravenous drug users. Because needle exchange programs are still illegal in many areas, participants in needle exchange programs may face legal action, including arrest and prosecution.

Even where needle exchange is legal, it is controversial because many believe that it encourages drug use. ACT UP counters this charge with two arguments. First, needle exchange programs require that intravenous drug users exchange a dirty needle for every clean needle they receive. Therefore, the number of needles available to intravenous drug users remains constant. Second, in the words of activist Yolanda Serrano, "It is not the needle that gets people to use drugs; it's the high" (ACT UP/NY Women and AIDS Book Group, 1990, p. 126). According to ACT UP, the reality we must face is that most intravenous drug users will continue using drugs regardless of whether they have clean needles. In the face of death, the threat of social disapprobation or even of arrest and prosecution is not sufficient to deter action. San Francisco activist Patricia Case explains her involvement in a street-based needle exchange project there: "I started doing this so that I could sleep at night 20 years from now" (ACT UP/NY Women and AIDS Book Group, 1990, p. 127). Case, who had a job giving HIV antibody tests, explains that she "couldn't give out one more positive test result without starting to give out needles" (ACT UP/NY Women and AIDS Book Group, 1990, p. 127). Obviously, ACT UP will not solve the drug problem that faces America by providing clean needles for intravenous drug users. It can, however, enable intravenous drug users to take control of one aspect of their lives, thereby playing a small part in preventing the spread of HIV through the intravenous use of drugs.

THE BROADER AGENDA

Clearly, a common thread links ACT UP's commitment to providing people with information on AIDS treatment and support, safer sex, and intravenous drug use. That thread—the desire to help people take control of their lives—has a third strand as well. ACT UP also calls for all of us to take responsibility for the AIDS crisis and to realize that AIDS is not only (or even primarily) a medical problem, but also an economic and a social problem. At the heart of ACT UP's message is that many of the AIDS deaths thus far have been needless. We have all sat by quietly while more than 100,000 Americans have died from complications related to AIDS and millions more have been infected with HIV. To counter this complacency, ACT UP struggles to bring the issue of AIDS into the lives of every American, pointing out that no one is safe and that AIDS is everybody's problem. At the same time, ACT UP also tries to raise the general awareness that AIDS is growing most rapidly among minorities and women and that the lack of resources allocated to the research and prevention of AIDS as well as to treatment for people with AIDS points to sexist and racist tendencies in American society.

One way ACT UP tries to show that AIDS is everybody's problem is by "invading" places that are considered "safe," places that people usually do not associate with AIDS. This technique was used in their demonstration at Shea Stadium, in their "Stop the Church" demonstration at St. Patrick's Cathedral in New York, in their disruption of Judge David Souter's confirmation hearings (O'Neil, 1990), and in their interruption of the evening news programs at CBS and PBS to protest the Persian Gulf war by yelling "Fight AIDS not Arabs!" (Bull, 1991). It is also used (although on a smaller scale) when San Francisco activists place "Touched by a Person with AIDS" stickers in places like phone booths (Gamson, 1989), when New York activists paint graffiti such as the "Silence = Death" logo on sidewalks, or when Boston activists place stickers announcing "The AIDS Crisis Is Not Over" all around the city. All these actions have a strong shock value, but the shock is not limited to the words they use—rather it is the shock of seeing what is considered "safe" contaminated by AIDS and the realization that "safe" does not exist anymore.

The demarcation of AIDS as an economic and social problem underscored by racist and sexist tendencies forces ACT UP to address concerns that go beyond the fight against AIDS. Although this is perhaps the most ambitious of ACT UP's causes, it is also the most difficult to tackle and has created conflict in the group. In fact, there are people in ACT UP who believe that the group should focus solely on AIDS treatment and prevention and not on broader social issues that might water down the group's effectiveness.

This difference in approach emerges from a discrepancy that exists between ACT UP's definition of itself and the reality of ACT UP's membership and program. Despite its claims about diversity, for example, members of ACT UP are mostly White, male, gay, and middle class (see, e.g., "Reproductive Rights and AIDS: The Connections" and "AIDS and Politics: Transformation of Our Movement" in ACT UP/NY Women and AIDS Book Group, 1990). Women in the AIDS activist movement charge that "the white, gay, AIDS

activist movement [including ACT UP] initially embraced a single issue strat-
egy (getting new drugs into bodies) and didn't consider the needs of women,
intravenous drug users . . . and children" (ACTUP/NY Women and AIDS
Book Group, 1990, p. 202). Over the 5 years of its existence, however, ACT
UP has diversified its membership. According to ACT UP/NY, "Lesbian, bisexual, and straight women, and women and gay men of color joined the gay
AIDS activist movement to get our concerns on the agenda" (ACT UP/NY
Women and AIDS Book Group, 1990, p. 202). As a result, ACT UP now
comes closer to its announced goal of diversity in its membership.

ACT UP's increasing diversity is related to a change in the group's focus.
ACT UP's original goal was simple: freeing up the process by which new AIDS
treatments were made available to people with AIDS. Thus, early demonstrations were directed at the FDA and drug manufacturers, who controlled the
process of drug approval. Currently, however, ACT UP is broadening the focus
of its efforts to address issues that on the surface seem only tangentially related
to AIDS activism. Some in ACT UP view this move as highly positive and a
natural result of the rapid spread of AIDS among groups of people who have
been marginalized in contemporary America, especially women and people of
color. Such a move begins to address issues that are at the heart of the AIDS
crisis—sexism and heterosexism, which discourage education about safer sex
and condom use; racism, which limits access to health care among people of
color; and class oppression, which ensures that pharmaceutical manufacturers
and government laboratories continue to pursue profits, permitting high prices
for AIDS treatment. Until these issues are addressed, argue activists, no solution to the AIDS crisis will be found (see, e.g., "How Do Women Live?" in
ACT UP/NY Women and AIDS Book Group, 1990).

Other activists, most notably long-time ACT UP leader Peter Staley, see a
threat in ACT UP's move to embrace a broader reform agenda. Staley sees a
sharp contrast between early ACT UP members, most of whom either were
HIV positive or had lost someone to AIDS, and newcomers, many of whom
have a history of activism and commitment to a broader social agenda. According to Staley (1991),

> A rift has occurred between those of us who joined as a matter of survival and those
> who joined seeking a power base from which their social activism could be ad-
> vanced. The common denominator that was missing was the crisis mentality—the
> view that time was our ultimate enemy. Defeating racism, sexism, and homophobia
> will take decades at best and become a never-ending fight at worst. Successfully
> countering the antiabortionists or America's imperialist tendencies will take more
> time than people with AIDS have. (p. 90; see also Wachter, 1992)

Despite differences of opinion about tactics, however, members of ACT
UP still agree that almost any action (short of violence) aimed at ending the

AIDS crisis is justified. Staley (1991) sums up the group's commitment this way:

> If saving lives meant going to jail, we'd do it. If it meant sitting down to a candle-light dinner with Tony Fauci [of the National Institute of Allergies and Infectious Diseases, often an ACT UP target] through four bottles of wine and a quiet debate, we'd do it. If it meant kissing ass or kicking ass, we'd do it. (p. 98)

Staley's willingness to take almost any action is echoed by Crimp and Rolston (1990), who say that "there aren't any barriers we won't cross—with the exception of our pledge to nonviolence—in order to help save lives" (p. 140). Still, overall, ACT UP does call for greater social awareness while fighting the prevalent belief that people with AIDS somehow deserve to have AIDS because they are gay, intravenous drug users, or prostitutes.

ACT UP fights the classification of children, hemophiliac individuals, and even heterosexual persons as innocent victims but all other people with AIDS as "guilty" and affirms the innocence of all people with AIDS. Thus, ACT UP takes it upon itself to speak for those who cannot speak, whose words are insignificant in today's society because they are people of color, intravenous drug users, prostitutes, or prisoners. The group fights to inform people of color of the dangers of AIDS; to provide clean needles for intravenous drug users; to encourage prostitutes to practice safer sex and to change the depiction of prostitutes as "'pools of contagion,' 'reservoirs of infection,' and 'vectors of transmission' who are 'selling death' to the supposedly pure, innocent heterosexuals" (ACT UP/NY Women and AIDS Book Group, 1990, p. 179), and provide education about safer sex, clean needles, condoms, and dental dams to people in prisons. ACT UP fights to make people aware that AIDS is spreading rapidly in all these communities and that people of color, intravenous drug users, prostitutes, and prisoners who have AIDS die much faster than other people with AIDS.

This call for greater awareness is united with a call for action, for people to get involved in fighting AIDS, sexism, racism, and discrimination, although not necessarily through acts of civil disobedience. Rachel Lurie explains that "activism and direct action can take many forms. Writing a letter to the editor, leafletting at a shopping mall, setting up an information table outside a high school, coming out at work or to a family member are all forms of direct action that create change" (ACT UP/NY Women and AIDS Book Group, 1990, p. 212). Certainly this form of activism is very different from the kind of theatrical demonstrations organized by ACT UP and covered by the media, and it is certainly less confrontational and less focused than many of the activities for which the group is known. Whether this form of activism is effective is more difficult to measure, but few people within the movement object to it as long as it does not interfere with what they see as the more direct ways of fighting AIDS.

A final assessment of ACT UP as an agent of social change is difficult. Certainly, the group has met with both successes and failures in its actions. Dr. Robert M. Wachter (1992) suggests that "the pressures brought to bear by AIDS activists on researchers, health officials, and pharmaceutical industry have led to important changes in the course of the epidemic" (p. 129). These changes include increased access for people with AIDS to drugs that have not been fully approved by the FDA; a lower price for zidovudine (AZT), the antiviral drug approved for use against AIDS; and increased funding from the federal government for research on HIV and AIDS. In addition, ACT UP empowers its members, especially those with AIDS. Kramer (1989) explains, "ACT UP gives me my greatest energy, and my greatest commitment to staying alive. Each week I go to meetings, tired at the end of a long day, and emerge euphoric. I now know more than ever the empowerment that comes from activism" (p. 290). Kramer's feeling of empowerment is shared by others, for whom ACT UP is an alternative to passive acceptance of the disease.

ACT UP has also met with some success in its efforts at promoting safer sex and intravenous drug use. At the very least, ACT UP demonstrations and actions have called the public's attention to the need for vigorous action to prevent the spread of AIDS, especially among groups who have been excluded from AIDS education efforts, such as people of color, women, sexually active teens, prisoners, prostitutes, and other marginalized groups. When ACT UP members distribute condoms to teens at schools, they give some students the opportunity to exercise control over their sexual behaviors and reduce the spread of AIDS. When an ACT UP chapter sets up a needle exchange, they ensure that at least some intravenous drug users can help prevent the spread of AIDS. Of course, it is impossible to determine exactly how many people are served by these programs; however, it is undeniable that ACT UP is having an impact on these communities.

At the same time that ACT UP has enjoyed a great deal of success, its actions have generated a great deal of criticism, both within and outside the group. Staley (1991) accuses the group of "arrogance" and an unwillingness to listen to constructive criticism of its actions:

> In today's ACT UP, the prevailing view is that we can do no wrong. The perpetrators of an action simply present their glorious feat to wild applause from our members. Any constructive criticism is frequently countered by personal attacks. Criticism, constructive or not, is simply dismissed with the adage, 'Everybody's always hated us, so we can't let that stop us now.' (p. 98)

ACT UP has always walked a fine line with its tactics. On one hand, the visibility of demonstrations has contributed greatly to the group's success. On the other hand, ACT UP runs a very real risk of alienating those people whose support is necessary if the group is to function effectively.

It should not be surprising to find that the basic problem facing ACT UP is focus. As this chapter illustrates, the group is struggling to find a direction and to focus on either helping people with AIDS and stopping the spread of the disease or trying to reform society by attacking what they see as the root of the problem regarding AIDS: social inequality. Are these two goals necessarily contradictory? Is the group trying to do too much by embracing the second and too little by limiting itself to the first? We do not have answers to these questions except to note that social movements often struggle with issues such as these and the path they choose to take often determines whether they are successful.

Regardless of the ultimate success or failure of ACT UP and the AIDS activism movement, many agree that it has changed forever the way medicine is done in America. No longer is medical research solely the province of the giant research institutes, big pharmaceutical manufacturers, the government, and major teaching and research hospitals. This, perhaps, will be ACT UP's most lasting legacy—that people who suffer from disease demand a voice in the way they are treated. Martin Delaney, executive director of Project Inform, a gay community foundation that provides AIDS treatment information to people with AIDS, offered this advice at the beginning of 1992:

> The hard truth is that the conservatism of the medical establishment aims to keep people wedded to treatment as we knew it in 1987. The best-informed [people with AIDS] are living longer, working longer, and living a better quality of life. But you won't learn how from newspapers, medical journals, TV, or sometimes even your own doctor. If you wait for the formal endorsement of the medical journals and societies before taking action, you will always be about two years behind the state of the art. Resolve in 1992 to get yourself informed and take charge of your own health. It's the only way. (p. 29)

As people who are affected by cancer, Alzheimer's disease, and other diseases follow the path of AIDS activists and ACT UP, they will continue to change the nature of medical care in the United States in profound ways.

REFERENCES

ACT UP/NY Women and AIDS Book Group. (1990). *Women, AIDS and activism.* Boston: South End Press.

Bull, C. (1991, February 26). Media watchers say day of desperation caught nation's eye. *Advocate,* pp. 14–15.

Crimp, D., & Rolston, A. (1990). *AIDS demo graphics.* Seattle, WA: Bay Press.

Delaney, M. (1992, February 11). AIDS front. *Advocate,* p. 29.

Gamson, J. (1989). Silence, death, and the invisible enemy: AIDS activism and social movement 'newness.' *Social Problems, 36,* 351–367.

Handelman, D. (1990, March 8). ACT UP in anger. *Rolling Stone,* p. 80.

Kistenburg, C. J. (1991, November). *ACTing UP: AIDS activism as performance.* Paper presented to the annual convention of the Speech Communication Association, Atlanta, GA.

Kramer, L. (1989). *Reports from the holocaust: The making of an AIDS activist.* New York: St. Martin's Press.

Lederer, B. (1990, October 24). A powerful blow for freedom of treatment choice. *Outweek,* p. 36.

Magnuson, E. (1989, December 25). In a rage over AIDS: A militant group targets the Catholic Church. *Time,* p. 33.

Nussbaum, B. (1991). *Good intentions: How big business and the medical establishment are corrupting the fight against AIDS, Alzheimer's, cancer, and more.* New York: Penguin.

O'Loughlin, R. (1990, November 6). San Francisco ACT UP splits into two chapters. *Advocate,* p. 48.

O'Neill, C. (1990, October 3). Gay women's groups pile on court nominee. *Outweek,* p. 18.

Salholz, E. (1988, June 6). Acting up to fight AIDS: A group's angry tactics. *Newsweek,* p. 42.

Staley, P. (1991, July 30). Has the direct action group ACT UP gone astray? *Advocate,* p. 98.

Sullivan, A. (1990, December 17). Gay life, gay death. *New Republic,* pp. 19–25.

Wachter, R. M. (1992). AIDS, activism, and the politics of health. *New England Journal of Medicine, 326,* 128–133.

Walter, D. (1990, June 5). Immature babies. *Advocate,* p. 26.

Part Two

AIDS: Communication, Education, and the Media

Chapter Six

Perceived Control in the Age of AIDS: A Review of Prevention Information in Academic, Popular, and Medical Accounts

David A. Brenders
Lisaanne Garrett

The scope and relentlessness of the acquired immune deficiency syndrome (AIDS) crisis have presented severe social, medical, psychological, and personal challenges to our society. The past decade has revealed that living in the age of AIDS is not merely a matter of public health. The greatest challenge of the AIDS era may be maintaining a sense of personal control of one's involvement in some of life's most meaningful experiences, namely love, sexuality, and the nurturing of committed interpersonal relationships. The personal challenge of AIDS is not only to avoid disease, but to remain healthy while not allowing the spectre of human immunodeficiency virus (HIV) infection to compromise one's sense of mastery of important life goals (Harowski, 1987).

Unfortunately, for many people, especially the young, the threat of AIDS can be seen as further curtailment of an ever limited domain of personal control. In an age when political cynicism, economic stagnation, and diminished prospects for the future seem foremost in the minds of many, AIDS poses an additional demoralizing threat to the person's final sphere of personal control, his or her ability to form and enjoy intimate relationships. In such an environment, the challenge posed by AIDS may seem overwhelming and foster a state of learned helplessness (Beck & Lund, 1981; Harowski, 1987; Seligman, 1990).[1]

Surveys report that young persons get most of their AIDS-relevant information from the mass media (television, newspapers, magazines, and radio) (Abraham, Sheeran, Abrams, Spears, & Marks, 1991; Edgar, Freimuth, & Hammond, 1988; Freimuth, Edgar, & Hammond, 1987). The work of Levine (1977, 1986) suggests that the mode of presentation employed by one segment of the mass media (television news) may actually encourage helplessness. Levine suggests that television news tends to demand that a story possess "action and drama" to provoke "an emotional response" from viewers (1986, p. 12). The "meta-message" embedded in this information is that

> Members of the general public are most often presented as helpless. . . . A dominant and repeated theme in local television news is that there is considerable unpredictability, chaos, and uncontrollability . . . and the general public cannot be expected to exert meaningful control. (1986, p. 18)

The meta-message of helplessness pervaded 71% of the national news broadcasts and 71.4% of the local news broadcasts Levine surveyed. She speculated on the implications of this finding:

> Might exposure to newscasts which dramatize the plight of crisis victims cultivate in viewers the sense that the environment is beyond human control? . . . If television news emphasizes crisis and catastrophe, the very situations in which individuals are rendered most helpless, might exposure to such depictions create an illusion that social change is impossible? (1986, p. 12)

With regard to AIDS, the consequences of helplessness are certainly as dire. Consider, for example, the description offered by Rigby, Brown, and Anagnostou (1989) of the Australian "Grim Reaper" AIDS campaign:

> The video showed a series of death-life figures ("Grim Reapers" with skeletal faces, each carrying scythes) wreaking destruction at bowling alleys with bowls aimed with deadly intent at the "pins" in the form of men, women, and children *unable to avoid the relentless onslaught.* (p. 146, emphasis ours)

Such information about AIDS may have unforeseen negative consequences (see also Edgar et al., 1988).

In this chapter, we explore one connection between AIDS prevention information and perceived control. Specifically, we examine the control-relevant

---

[1]Seligman (1990) argued that three factors exacerbate helplessness, namely, our ideas about the permanence, pervasiveness, and personalization of the causes to which we attribute helplessness. Thus, a disease that seems to be spreading through the population, admits to no cure, and is often blamed on "immoral" sexual practices seems to be a prescription for extreme helplessness.

implications of AIDS prevention information available in three literatures: the academic literature of social science, popular magazines, and selected medical journals.[2] The academic accounts of perceived control are applied to an analysis of the control-relevant implications of AIDS discussions in the popular literature. The medical literature is reviewed as a check on the veracity of popular accounts.

We begin by reviewing the literature of perceived control and helplessness as it relates to an individual's reaction to health threat. Next, information regarding young adults' knowledge of AIDS and attitudes toward prevention of AIDS are examined. These discussions form a basis for assessing the control-relevant impact of the attempts made by popular magazines to provide AIDS prevention education. Implications for health communication are then discussed.

PERCEIVED CONTROL AND HEALTH THREAT

The relationship between perceived control and reactions to challenging life events has been heavily investigated (Lefcourt, 1981, 1982, 1983, 1984). Numerous studies support the proposition that the belief that important life outcomes are attainable through personal effort yields perceptions and behaviors that are fundamentally at odds with those arising from a fatalistic orientation.

Learned Helplessness

The most general approach to the role of perceived control in adverse situations can be found in the concept of learned helplessness (Garber & Seligman, 1980; Seligman, 1975, 1990). In the paradigmatic case of learned helplessness, an organism learns that outcomes important to it are uncontrollable by the self. According to Seligman (1990), "Helplessness is that state of affairs in which nothing you choose to do affects what happens to you" (p. 5). As an ongoing condition, learned helplessness produces chronic motivational, cognitive, and affective deficits:

> Laboratory evidence suggests that when an organism has experienced trauma it cannot control, its motivation to respond in the face of later trauma wanes. Moreover, even if it does respond, and the response succeeds in producing relief, it has trouble learning, perceiving, and believing that the response worked. Finally, its

---

[2]The medical journals surveyed were the ones listed in *Magazines for Libraries* (Katz & Sternberg-Katz, 1989) as being of general medical interest. The popular magazines were gathered through a search of the *Reader's Guide to Popular Literature* from 1987 through 1991 using "AIDS (disease)" as the only limiting descriptor. We realize that the *Reader's Guide* does not adequately access some important periodicals, such as *Cosmopolitan*. Whenever possible, important articles (e.g., ones that sparked controversy) from such sources were accessed separately.

emotional balance is disturbed: depression and anxiety, measured in various ways, predominate. (Seligman, 1975, pp. 22–23)

Recent formulations of learned helplessness suggest that the presence and persistence of helplessness depend on the permanence, pervasiveness, and personalization of the explanation of uncontrollability (Seligman, 1990). Studies suggest that the helplessness-causing events need not be experienced firsthand, but may be acquired by vicarious experience or modeling (Breen, Vulcano, & Dyck, 1979; Brown & Inouye, 1978; DeVellis, DeVellis, & McCauley, 1978).

Cognitive Style and Coping with Threat

Lazarus and his associates (Coyne & Lazarus, 1980; Lazarus & Launier, 1978; see Silver & Wortman, 1980, for a review) described the transactional dynamics of coping in the face of threat. According to this approach, a person more or less continuously evaluates "judgments about demands and constraints in ongoing transactions with the environment on his or her resources and options for managing them" (Coyne & Lazarus, 1980, p. 150). This ongoing cognitive process is responsible for the person's experience of stress, the person's emotional state, and how the person responds to the situation.

This cognitive dynamic includes two components that Coyne and Lazarus (1980) termed primary and secondary appraisal. "Primary appraisal refers to the cognitive process of evaluating the significance of an encounter for one's well-being, answering the question 'Am I OK or in trouble?'" (Coyne & Lazarus, p. 151). As a result, the person may conclude that the circumstances are irrelevant, benign/positive, or stressful. Stressful evaluations come in three forms: (a) the person concludes that the harm/loss has already occurred, (b) the person concludes that a threat to future loss or harm exists, or (c) the person interprets the situation as a challenge rather than a threat to his or her future well-being. For Coyne and Lazarus, the difference between a threat and a challenge is an important one and involves "whether the person focuses on the potential for mastery and gain or the potential for harm" (p. 151).

Secondary appraisal concerns what the person feels that he or she can do about the stressful situation. In Coyne and Lazarus's (1980) words,

> Secondary appraisal refers to the person's ongoing judgments concerning coping resources, options, and constraints. . . . Essentially, secondary appraisal involves the evaluation of coping strategies with respect to their cost and probability of success. (p. 153)

Coping strategies include information seeking, inhibition of action, as well as intrapsychic calming (denial or thinking calming thoughts; Lazarus & Launier, 1978; Silver & Wortman, 1980).

The primary and secondary appraisal processes determine which of these coping strategies is finally used. For example,

> a high degree of uncertainty or ambiguity about a given outcome may result in decreased use of direct action and increased use of information seeking. If information is not available, the individual may resort to intrapsychic modes of coping [i.e., denial and emotional calming strategies]. Intrapsychic modes may also be used if direct action has been unsuccessful and/or if harm has already occurred or is judged as inevitable. (Silver & Wortman, 1980, p. 288)

Denial is not necessarily seen as a dysfunctional strategy, because persons who deny threats that they do not control may fare better than those who cannot. Optimal coping involves a flexibility or coping options tailored to the situation. As Coyne and Lazarus (1980) suggested, "the denial processes that allow a victim of myocardial infarction to cope with the coronary care unit can also have disastrous consequences if they delay or prevent the seeking of indicated treatment" (p. 152).

The work of Lazarus and his associates parallels that of other researchers in the area of health threat communication. Leventhal (in Beck & Frankel, 1981) also distinguished between coping with the emotional reactions to stress and the cognitive process involved with appraising and controlling danger. Beck and Frankel (1981) wrote,

> Leventhal (1971) stresses the necessity of convincing people that they are susceptible to the health threat and that it is potentially serious, yet he warns that "we risk arousing various forms of resistance to influence if we present communications that combine vivid information on a threat with clear information on one's vulnerability to it. This combination appears to stimulate loss of hope and feelings of resignation and inability to cope with danger" (1971; 1220). (p. 209)

When persons are faced with a health threat, the perception that they can do something about the threat is all important in guiding their actions. If they perceive themselves to be helpless, coping moves from instrumental action to withdrawal and calming strategies.

Protection Motivation Theory

The protection motivation theory (PMT) of Rogers (1975) includes most of the logic above (distinguishing between threat appraisal and coping appraisal) and specifies the dynamics of threat communications. These dynamics include (a) the severity of the threat, (b) the probability that the threat will occur if the person does not take corrective action, and (c) the efficacy of strategies available to meet the threat (Beck & Frankel, 1981). The concept of efficacy includes both *response efficacy* (will the response succeed in reducing the threat?)

and *self-efficacy* (can the person successfully implement the strategy?) (Prentice-Dunn & Rogers, 1986). Beck and Frankel (1981) described PMT as follows:

> Protection motivation theory predicts that people will be most likely to accept advice on how to protect themselves from a health threat when they can be convinced of the threat's seriousness and their susceptibility to it, and also persuaded that by following the recommended actions they will be able to control or avoid the health threat. (p. 210)

PMT also distinguishes between conditions that lead to a maladaptive response and those that lead to an adaptive response. That is, PMT assumes that maladaptive behavior also has rewards, while adaptive behavior is not without costs. Therefore,

> PMT assumes that protection motivation is maximized when (i) the threat to health is severe; (ii) the individual feels vulnerable; (iii) the adaptive response is believed to be an effective means for averting the threat; (iv) the person is confident in his or her abilities to complete successfully the adaptive response; (v) the rewards associated with maladaptive behavior are small; and (vi) the costs associated with adaptive responses are small. (Prentice-Dunn & Rogers, 1986, p. 156)

PMT predicts that if response efficacy or self-efficacy is low, threat communications may actually impede compliance with the appropriate recommendations. As Prentice-Dunn and Rogers (1986) suggested,

> It is assumed that if response efficacy and/or self-efficacy are high, then increases in severity and/or vulnerability will produce a positive main effect on intentions; on the other hand, if response efficacy and/or self-efficacy are low, increases in severity or vulnerability will either have no effect or a boomerang effect, actually reducing intentions to comply with the health recommendation. (p. 156)

Beck and Frankel (1981) summarized research on the protection motivation approach as suggesting that "the important factor in mediating the effects of health threat communications is not fear but the degree to which the communication depicts a real, but controllable threat" (p. 211). If threats are depicted as severe but coping responses are pictured as relatively ineffective,

> strong health threat communications may cause a helplessness reaction in certain individuals by emphasizing the danger and failing to emphasize clear ways in which to control the danger, thereby creating the expectation that the threat is beyond personal control. (Beck & Frankel, 1981, p. 211)

For example, Rippetoe and Rogers (1987) found that although high-vulnerability messages roused persons to actions, exposure to low-response-efficacy messages resulted in maladaptive coping modes such as helplessness, fatalistic acceptance, and reliance on religious faith. Exposure to low-self-efficacy messages also produced helplessness, Prentice-Dunn and Rogers (1986) found, but without the stoic acceptance conferred by a fatalistic orientation. Instead, persons in this condition "personalized or internalized blame for the danger" (Prentice-Dunn & Rogers, p. 159). Conversely, these researchers found that high-response efficacy and self-efficacy resulted in proactive avoidance of danger even when the risk of danger was perceived as small. Persons in this situation "adopted a precautionary strategy, thinking 'Why take the chance?'" (Prentice-Dunn & Rogers, p. 158).

Health Belief and Morin Models

Beck and Frankel (1981) and Prentice-Dunn and Rogers (1986) drew a parallel between PMT and the widely cited Health Belief model (HBM) (see Rosenstock, 1974). For example, the HBM components of perceived susceptibility and perceived severity were likened to PMT's severity and vulnerability dimensions. The HBM component of perceived benefits was likened to PMT's response efficacy, while HBM's perceived barriers to action was said to roughly parallel PMT's personal efficacy and reward–cost components (Prentice-Dunn & Rogers, 1986). However, Prentice-Dunn and Rogers (1986) pointed out that, "While the HBM was originated to predict health behavior, PMT was developed to explain the effects of fear-arousing communications on attitude change" (p. 157). Montgomery et al. (1989) found components of HBM, such as susceptibility, of little use in predicting health prevention in gay men, but did find self-efficacy to be valuable.

Similarities also exist between the PMT and HBM models and the Morin model (Miller, Booraem, Flowers, & Iversen, 1990). The components of the Morin model include

(a) the belief that AIDS is a personal threat, (b) a belief in prevention, (c) a belief in personal efficacy, (d) a belief in the possibility of satisfaction, and (e) a belief in the existence of peer support. (Miller et al., p. 14)

The PMT, HBM, and Morin formulations all stress the notion that knowledge of one's vulnerability is not a sufficient cue to action. Information that suggests high vulnerability to illness coupled with uncertain chances for avoiding the danger risks promoting dysfunctional coping strategies. As Beck and Frankel (1981) suggested, "Acceptance or rejection of health recommendations may not be so much a matter of being convinced of the seriousness of the threat, but of one's control over it" (p. 215).

PERCEIVED AIDS RISK AMONG ADOLESCENTS
AND COLLEGE STUDENTS

The notion that knowledge of AIDS does not necessarily promote changes in sexual behavior is becoming well documented (Abraham et al., 1991; Baldwin & Baldwin, 1988; Bowie & Ford, 1989; Brown & Fritz, 1988; Edgar et al., 1988; Flora & Thoresen, 1988; Freimuth et al., 1987; Kegeles, Adler, & Irwin, 1988; Miller et al., 1990; Roscoe & Kruger, 1990; Shayne & Kaplan, 1988; Wober, 1988). Many of these researchers used the HBM and/or the notion of self-efficacy (another way of conceptualizing perceived control) as a guide in parsing out various dimensions of AIDS-related attitudes.

In a survey of college students at the University of Maryland, Freimuth et al. (1987) found that although the students sampled were very knowledgeable about AIDS, and that many grossly overestimated the probability of acquiring HIV from a single unprotected sexual encounter, the majority of these students did not perceive a personal risk of acquiring the infection, and few reported any intention of being tested for HIV.

In a study of 7th- through 11th-grade students, Petosa and Wessinger (1990) used the HBM to study knowledge, attitudes, and behavioral intentions. Although AIDS knowledge was found to be fairly good (93% knew that women can infect men, and an average of 74% of the students realized that one can get the disease from an asymptomatic carrier) and knowledge of AIDS prevention strategies was also good (more than 90% knew about condom use and refraining from needle sharing), "one third of this sample did not intend to use condoms or avoid having sex with several people," and only 27% intended to abstain from sex (Petosa & Wessinger, p. 134). Susceptibility to AIDS was reported to be very high, but it is impossible to separate the risk of causal contacts from the risks of sexual contact in this study. Although an average of 43% of this sample reported that they "would be fearful of getting AIDS if someone in my classes had AIDS" (Petosa & Wessinger, p. 132), it may be erroneous to assume that this fear of the disease generalized to a risk of HIV from *their* sexual partner.

In a survey of Scottish teenagers and university students, Abraham et al. (1991) used the HBM to assess AIDS knowledge and attitudes toward the severity of AIDS and their vulnerability to it. The majority of respondents indicated that the consequences of AIDS would be very severe, but 85% did not feel personally vulnerable. Only 2% of this sample believed it was likely that they would be infected in the next 5 years.

Kegeles et al. (1988) found that although sexually active adolescents visiting a San Francisco health clinic saw the value of condom use, only 8% used condoms during every sexual encounter. Like many other researchers, Kegeles et al. concluded that adolescents do not "feel personally vulnerable to contracting diseases from their sex partners" (p. 461; see also Bowie & Ford, 1989).

The surveys cited above all attest to the fact that although adolescents and college students are well versed in the facts of AIDS and consider it to be a severe disease, the majority of them do not feel personally vulnerable to the disease. In addition, they are not adopting safe sex practices.

In the next section, attention is turned to a significant part of the information environment available for individuals' use in sexual decision making. This environment has implications for perceived control, as is established later.

HELPLESSNESS AND POPULAR ACCOUNTS ABOUT AIDS

In this section a selection of popular articles, culled from those available for access through the *Reader's Guide to Periodical Literature,*[3] is examined in terms of the perceived vulnerability, response efficacy, self-efficacy, and rewards and costs factors discussed in the previous sections. It is assumed that:

1 Without a sense of perceived vulnerability, health protection will not be perceived to be warranted.

2 High-vulnerability messages coupled with low-response efficacy and/or low self-efficacy are likely to produce high initial fear followed by helplessness and/or denial of risk.

3 As the costs of health protection are magnified, health prevention motivations are undermined.

4 High-response-efficacy and high-self-efficacy messages may be conducive to proactive behavior change even when vulnerability is perceived to be low.

The articles are examined in roughly chronological order to take into account trends in reporting and the introduction of new information.

1987: Fear and Loathing

The year 1987 saw a wide divergence in the reporting of heterosexual vulnerability to HIV/AIDS. Early benchmarks were three dramatic articles, two in *Time* ("The Big Chill: Fear of AIDS," Smilgis, 1987; "You Haven't Heard Anything Yet," Wallis, 1987) and one in the *Atlantic Monthly* ("Heterosexuals and AIDS," Leishman, 1987).

The *Time* article "The Big Chill: Fear of AIDS" used a combination of quotations and testimonials combined with moralistic quotations to dramatize the heterosexual threat of AIDS. Rather than merely suggesting that one's sex-

---

[3]We accessed every article available under the descriptor "AIDS (disease)" through the *Reader's Guide* for 1987 through 1991. From this list, a more select group of articles was chosen on the basis of their relevance to AIDS prevention. The resultant survey is admittedly impressionistic.

ual habits contribute to one's risk, the article blamed promiscuity as the *cause* of AIDS. Loss of previous sexual freedoms was emphasized. For example, Otis Bowen's comment "I can't emphasize too strongly the necessity of changing life-styles" (p. 50) was followed by the assertion that "To America in the 80's, that means rescinding the sexual revolution of the past quarter century" (p. 50). An Atlanta executive was quoted as saying, "We are paying for our sins of the 60's, when one-night stands and sex without commitment used to be chic" (p. 50). Erica Jong, a person presumably liberal on the subject of sexuality, was quoted as saying that "giving up sex altogether or joining a religious order" (p. 50) is easier than what it takes to negotiate safe sex. All heterosexual activity (including oral sex) without a barrier was described as "high risk."

These observations were followed by descriptions of heterosexuals who contracted AIDS after relatively few sexual encounters. The use of condoms was discussed, but the potential unreliability of condoms was highlighted. A discussion of condom advertising was followed by the lament, "What does all this leave to the imagination?" The article noted that most young Americans do not feel at risk. The article concluded that unless there is an increase in monogamy, abstinence, and acceptance of "tough new rules of the game" (p. 53) the casualties of AIDS will mount.

The *Atlantic Monthly* article, "Heterosexuals and AIDS" (Leishman, 1987), although more measured, also stressed vulnerability without stressing a recourse. The author suggested that a pool of HIV-positive persons one step removed from the primary risk groups is now forming. Therefore,

> Even if heterosexually transmitted cases continue to be a secondary feature of the epidemic in the United States, the crucial questions that men and women outside of monogamous relationship—and many people in them—must ask themselves are, Am I at any risk of exposure to the virus? and, more frightening, since ten years can pass before someone exhibits any visible sign of infection, Have I ever been exposed? (Leishman, p. 40)

Although much of the *Atlantic Monthly* article was taken up with explaining the facts of AIDS as then known and the psychology of denial, a major theme of the article concerned fearful testimonials of sexually active heterosexuals who were afraid they may have encountered an infected partner somewhere in their past. This was followed by the stories of former Lotharios who were fearful of both harboring the disease and of being tested.

As the preceding analysis suggests, such accounts depict high vulnerability, high uncertainty, and little in the way of response efficacy or personal efficacy. The *Time* article "The Big Chill: Fear of AIDS" seemed to suggest that the only answer to the AIDS threat is renouncing sex, or at least nonmonogamous sex (for those who consider sex to be a fundamental part of their life, this is tantamount to helplessness). The *Atlantic Monthly* article suggested that even this tactic cannot dispel the fear that it is already too late (this suggests total helplessness).

In the remaining articles that had a prevention focus, the news was pessimistic, but a variable amount of control was stressed. *Mademoiselle* discussed the possibilities of one's partner being a secret bisexual ("Is There a Man in Your Man's Life," Heller, 1987). *People* devoted an entire issue to a photo essay on people with AIDS, ominously titled, "Diary of a Plague in America" (Friedman & Van Biema, 1987). An essay in *Life*, "The Paranoia of a Modern Plague" (Wainwright, 1987), catalogued AIDS fears without offering any optimism. Amidst stories of female AIDS sufferers, an article in *Ladies Home Journal* (Salvatore, 1987) quoted Dr. Matilda Krim as saying, "We had a chance to contain the virus and we missed it. . . . Now the virus is out and will spread to the general population" (p. 186). Krim anticipated that by 1991, "ten to twenty million people will become infected" (p. 186). No mention was made as to whether these were national or international figures. A *Vogue* article (Orth, 1987) quoted Krim as asserting that "Across the U.S. one man in thirty is infected. . . . One never knows with any man" (p. 246). *Essence* (Edwards, 1987) offered that AIDS "strikes from the depths of something primal, something evil" (p. 77).

Not to be outdone in gloomy prognosticating, *The Futurist* (Cornish, 1987) speculated that in the near future, "Kissing, hugging, even handshaking may become less casual;" bowing will replace shaking hands as the preferred greeting; persons will avoid toilets and crowded restaurants; mothers will not let their children play outside for fear of their being exposed to contaminated materials; and that clothing styles will become more modest as persons "downplay sexuality"[4] (p. 2).

Other articles were more moderate in their approach. *McCalls* ("AIDS: What we know now," Zimmerman & Goldstein, 1987) reassured its readers that, "for the vast majority of women, the risk of becoming infected with the AIDS virus is now extremely small" (p. 145); articles in *McCleans* ("Confrontation and Concern About AIDS," Barber, 1987) and *Vogue* ("Playing it Safe," Asnes & Giese, 1987) echoed this belief. *U.S. News and World Report* (McAuliffe, 1987) reported that heterosexual AIDS is not exploding, but spreading. *Science News* (Edwards, 1987) found the facts of heterosexual AIDS "both hopeful and horrific."

Prevention information ran the gamut of response efficacy and self-efficacy as well. A *Vogue* article entitled "On the Difficulty of Asking a Man to Wear a

---

[4]Although we should breathe a sigh of relief that these possible futures have not come to pass, one is tempted to recall the observations of Bertrand Russell (Gardner, 1957) on the issue of the predictive power of the Great Pyramid: "It is a singular fact that the Great Pyramid always predicts the history of the world accurately up to the date of publication of the book in question, but after that date it becomes less reliable. Generally the author expects, very soon, wars in Egypt, followed by Armageddon and the coming of the Antichrist, but by this time so many people have been recognized as Antichrist that the reader is reluctantly driven to skepticism" (p. 181).

Condom" (Giese, 1987) catalogued how difficult it is to use a condom and to ask a man to use one. Although the author stressed the importance of safe sex, she apparently also believed that it is especially difficult and distasteful. Condoms were described as "a squeaky, rubbery, socklike contraption" (p. 273). A companion article, "The Offer You Can't Refuse," asserted that "now we have to prepare for romance as if for a surgical procedure" (p. 273). The article also recommended blowing up the condom before use to check for leaks, although the author conceded that "this will not always lend a festive air to foreplay."

However, an article in *Cosmopolitan* entitled "What Every Woman Must Know About Condoms" (Brenton, 1987) took a completely different tone. The article was subtitled "How to Buy Them, Get Your Man to Use—and Even Enjoy Them." The article contained positive and frank advice for negotiating condom use in a positive spirit, outlined very specific suggestions for condom use, and highlighted techniques for eroticizing condom use. As such, the article conveyed a completely different message about response and self-efficacy. It did not report that condoms sometimes leak, but rather elaborated the skills necessary to keep them from leaking; it did not report that men will resist wearing a condom, but rather highlighted ways of preventing or overcoming resistance. Rather than reporting that condoms kill romance, it elaborated ways that women may eroticize condom use.

Other articles chronicled changes in dating and courtship. *Jet* ("AIDS Fear Leads Many Singles to Marry," 1987) reported that fear of AIDS was encouraging singles to marry and changing the ways stars made love on television ("AIDS Scare Changes Way Stars Make Love," 1987). Other articles noted how AIDS was making persons more cautious about sex or leading to the avoidance of sex altogether (Edwards, 1987; Gillies, 1987; Paranoia of a Modern Plague, Wainright, 1987; "The New Sexual Morality," 1987).

By the end of 1987, information regarding heterosexuals' vulnerability to AIDS would be further confused. Six months after C. Evert Koop warned a U.S. House of Representatives committee that it was a matter of time before we learned whether or not a "heterosexual explosion" of AIDS would devastate the country, *Commentary* published an article by Fumento (1987) entitled "AIDS: Are Heterosexuals at Risk?" Fumento argued that because it is blood borne, AIDS "is a disease that is extraordinarily difficult to transmit or contract, even by the standards of other sexually transmitted diseases" (p. 22) and that "the media and other responsible authorities" like the Surgeon General and the Centers for Disease Control gravely understate the contribution of receptive anal sex in the spread of AIDS.

Fumento (1987) then reviewed the research of Dr. Nancy Padian, which suggested that one's chances of contracting AIDS from a single sexual contact with an infected partner are one in a thousand. Her study also suggested that female to male transmission is much more difficult than male to female. Fumento concluded,

In fact, the risk to the male, or penetrating, partner of acquiring AIDS in vaginal intercourse is so small that this alone could be enough to prevent any substantial heterosexual spread of the disease. Women, in other words, act as a "firebreak" against the spread of the virus. (p. 24)

Fumento also challenged the notion that the heterosexual spread of AIDS in Africa previsions its eventual heterosexual spread in the United States. He argued that factors such as the inadequate screening of blood; unsterilized needles; the scarification of men and declitorization of women; and the widespread, if taboo, practice of bisexuality make the African situation much different from the one in the United States.

Fumento (1987) also claimed that available evidence argues against the spread of AIDS outside high-risk groups (intravenous drug users, bisexuals, etc.) and the partners of individuals in such groups. Spread of the disease between heterosexuals not connected with high-risk activities is called "tertiary transmission." Fumento stated that such transmission "simply is not happening" (p. 25).

Fumento's (1987) conclusion was that various constituencies—gay rights groups, medical researchers, and groups promoting certain moral agendas (such as Christian fundamentalists)—have distorted the facts of heterosexual AIDS in the interest of "democratizing the disease." Fumento warns,

Every dollar spent, every commercial made, every health warning released, that does not specify promiscuous anal intercourse and needle-sharing as the overwhelming risk factors in the transmission of AIDS is a lie, a waste of funds and energy, and a cruel diversion. (p. 27)

Fumento would not be alone in positing a media overreaction to the heterosexual threat of AIDS.

1988: Is Heterosexual AIDS a Myth?

In 1988 an article in *Cosmopolitan* entitled "Reassuring News About AIDS: A Doctor Tells Why *You* May Not Be At Risk" by Dr. Robert Gould (1988) echoed some of Fumento's (1987) claims (the difficulty of heterosexual AIDS transmission; the noncomparability of the African experience; the hidden agenda of researchers, gay groups, and puritan moralists to create an unfounded heterosexual panic) but adds the extraordinary claim that "there is almost no danger of contracting AIDS through *ordinary* sexual intercourse" (p. 146).

In "Has the Threat Been Exaggerated?" (1988), *U.S. News and World Report*, while not quite as optimistic as Gould, quoted Gould's (1988) conclusion and went on to cite that the average person's chances of getting AIDS are one in a million:

Jeffrey Harris of the Massachusetts Institute of Technology has calculated that the chance of becoming infected in a single, random heterosexual encounter with a person who is neither gay nor uses i. v. drugs is about 1 in a million—a 1-in-1,000 chance of meeting someone who is infected multiplied by a 1-in-1,000 chance the virus will be transmitted in any single encounter between an infected person and a noninfected one.

The article pointed out that Black and Hispanic youths in the inner city are at much greater risk than the average population and that intravenous drug use alone cannot explain the situation.

The *New Republic* ("AIDS Now," 1988) suggested that a breakout of AIDS into the general population was probably unlikely, but it would "be hard to do less than the Reagan administration is doing [about AIDS prevention]" (p. 7). In "Experts Debate the Threat to Heterosexuals," (1988), *People* cited conflicting opinions on heterosexual AIDS. The article quoted Randy Shilts as follows: "This is never going to be a middle-class disease. . . . The whole media engaged in shameless hype about heterosexual AIDS. Now that it is not happening, no one will believe that there is a threat" (p. 108). According to Shilts, "AIDS is going to become a disease of the underclass" (p. 108).

This optimistic attitude toward the public's vulnerability to heterosexual HIV infection was soon shaken by dramatic news from the nation's best known sex researchers. On March 14th, *Newsweek* published an excerpt from Masters and Johnson's *Crisis: Heterosexual Behavior in the Age of AIDS* ("Sex in the Age of AIDS," 1988). Masters and Johnson also believed that the health establishment was engaged in a conspiracy of disinformation. However, these authors thought that the AIDS risk to heterosexuals was "deliberately presented in the most optimistic light when even a healthy degree of scientific skepticism would have produced a more realistic response" (p. 45). Masters and Johnson asserted that the general public's worst fears about AIDS may be coming true:

> the epidemic has clearly broken out into the broader population and is continuing, even now, to make its silent inroads of infection while many maintain an attitude of complacency, not realizing that they too are at risk. (p. 45)

Possibly more alarming than the hypothesized heterosexual spread of the virus was their conclusion that persons are at risk from nonsexual contact. Their prevention advice was also severe and included an enforced six-month abstinence from sex between an initial HIV test and follow-up confirmatory test. In addition, "to rely on condoms for truly safe sex—or even a reasonable approximation—is to blatantly disregard the facts" (p. 49). Realizing that the 6-month period of abstinence might be too great a temptation for some, they offer the "slightly less reliable plan" of following an initial negative antibody test with a strict regimen of condom use until the follow-up test proves negative.

However, these conclusions were soon challenged. The March 21st issue of *Newsweek* contained an article ("Storm Over Masters and Johnson," Seligman, 1988) quoting AIDS experts who declared that these researchers had done a "disservice" to the cause of HIV prevention by inspiring "confusion and hysteria." *U.S. News and World Report* ran a longer piece ("What the Press Release Left Out," Findlay & Silberner, 1988) that criticized the methodology of the studies Masters and Johnson used to support their claims, accusing their approach to be "slick marketing" but bad science. A companion piece ("Why Do We Fall for It?" Findlay & Silberner, 1988) accused both the Masters and Johnson (1988) work and the Gould (1988) *Cosmopolitan* article of being "extreme views not supported by the overwhelming weight of evidence" (p. 60). *Time* ran an article ("Just How Does AIDS Spread?", Grady, 1988) voicing some of the same criticisms. Nonetheless, the May issue of *Good Housekeeping* ran its own excerpt from *Crisis* ("AIDS: Worse Than We Think?", 1988), with a somewhat critical companion piece.

Outside these extremes, the prevention message that emerged in the popular media (aside from condom use) seemed to center on avoiding sex with someone who might be at high risk. In a February 22 article by Erika Goode entitled "I Love You, but Can I Ask You a Question" (1988), *U.S. News and World Report* declared the risk to heterosexuals to be small, but sufficient to put an end to one-night stands and encourage a "return of lingering courtship." The article quoted a series of experts on strategies to get to know one's partner's sexual history.

The strategy of lingering courtship and more discriminating partner selection received support from an influential article in the *Journal of the American Medical Association* by Dr. Norman Hearst and Dr. Stephen Hulley (1988), entitled "Preventing the Heterosexual Spread of AIDS: Are We Giving Our Patients the Best Advice?" Their conclusions made the front page of the April 22 edition of the *New York Times* and was incorporated in many popular articles on AIDS prevention.

Hearst and Hulley (1988) stressed the importance of knowing one's partner. They contended that available sources of AIDS prevention information

> do not make explicit the strategy that should be the foremost goal for most people. . . . The single most important recommendation to give our patients is this: avoid choosing a sexual partner who may be at high risk of carrying HIV. (p. 2428)

The reason for this conclusion was that available data suggested that one was at much greater risk of AIDS while having protected sex with a member of a high-risk group than while having unprotected sex with someone not in a risk group. Hearst and Hulley cited statistics that suggested that the chances of acquiring HIV in one unprotected sexual encounter with a person not in a high-risk group is 1 in 50 million. Over a period of 500 encounters (an average of 4 1/2 years of sex), the risk is 1 in 110,000. In contrast, the risk of HIV infection from one unprotected encounter with someone in a risk group is between 1 in 10,000 to 1 in 1,000. Using condoms reduces this risk to between 1 in 100,000 and 1 in 10,000. Over 500 encounters, however, the probability of HIV infection from protected sex with someone in a risk group becomes 1 in 210 to 1 in 21. Four and a half years of unprotected sex with a member of a risk group yields a probability of infection of 1 in 32 to 1 in 3. (Hearst and Hulley calculated the probability of HIV infection from one unprotected encounter with someone *known* to be HIV positive to be 1 in 500.) This analysis suggested that much of the current wisdom regarding HIV prevention was not warranted by the data. The best advice for HIV prevention, according to these authors, is to engage in a prolonged courtship:

> This means not only asking potential partners about their present and past behavior but also getting to know the person and his or her friends and family well enough to know whether to believe the answers. (p. 2430)

Hearst and Hulley (1988) also suggested that the usual advice such as monogamy and use of condoms may yield a false sense of security. According to their data, monogamous sex with someone at risk for HIV is much riskier than casual sex with persons outside of risk groups. As an example, they cited the plight of many prostitutes, who are at greater risk of HIV from their regular partner (who may be an intravenous drug user) than from their customers who are not in any risk group. The chances of acquiring HIV from an infected partner over a period of 500 encounters is calculated at 1 in 11 even with the use of condoms. Therefore promoting condom use in such circumstances is bad advice; such couples "should stop having vaginal intercourse" (p. 2431). Similarly, Hearst and Hulley did not believe that condom use is indicated for those outside risk groups. The preceding estimates and advice were based on data that suggested a low level of HIV infection in the heterosexual population. Hearst and Hulley conceded that "if circumstances change, then our advice may also need to change" (p. 2432).

Although their article was provocative and widely cited in the popular press, Hearst and Hulley (1988) did not reflect the views of all AIDS researchers. Replies to Hearst and Hulley's piece in the *Journal of the American Medical Association* focused on the difficulty of acquiring an accurate sexual history, especially as HIV "spreads beyond initially identified risk groups," wrote Padian and Francis (1988, p. 1879). These authors stated, "Individuals have more direct control over choosing whether to have sex and whether to wear (or have their partner wear) a condom than they do over obtaining a reliable sexual history" (p. 1879). Another letter pointed out that "in socioeconomically disadvantaged areas of New York, high-risk partners are virtually indistinguishable from low-risk partners" (Schulman, 1988, p. 1879). These themes would be taken up in popular articles as well.

Popular prevention articles began tentatively including Hearst and Hulley's (1988) advice. *Science* (Booth, 1988) summarized Hearst and Hulley's risk calculations but included a number of criticisms of the "know your partner" advice. *Essence* (Whigham, 1988) quoted Dr. Mathilde Krim as follows:

> If your partner is not infected then there is no risk. This is why when you look for a new boyfriend, you should look for a partner in life. If you choose one and stick to him, you'll lessen your chance of getting AIDS.

However, the same article stated that the rate of infection among "young sexually active people" is 1 in 250 and asserted that in inner cities the rate is 1 in 50.

The April issue of *Cosmopolitan* (Gardner, 1988) described every prevention strategy including greater selectivity, abstinence, condoms, dental dams, and mutual masturbation. A July *Cosmopolitan* survey ("Cosmo's Private Sex Survey," 1988) reported, "More women had only one sex partner with each passing year" from 1985 through 1987, and the percentage of women who didn't sleep with anyone that year rose from 6 to 9 percent" (p. 140). A July article in *Glamour* (Ellis, 1988) cited the Hearst and Hulley (1988) statistics and the need to select low-risk partners but also suggested condom use. A companion article ("And How Do Men Feel Now About Monogamy?", Mehlman, 1988) discussed the compensations of monogamy. *Psychology Today* (Roberts, 1988) reported a study that suggests that "dishonesty [including dishonesty about one's sexual history] is alarmingly frequent among both men and women" (p. 60). (This study was also reported in the June 1989 issue of *Mademoiselle,* Sanders, 1989.) The best way to overcome potential dishonesty was reported to be "waiting to have sex." Paul Eckman was quoted as saying that because intimate relations are hard for liars to maintain, "Sooner or later they're found out" (p. 216).

Ladies Home Journal ("Women & Sex: 1988," 1988) took a skeptical look at how much safe sex is actually practiced. "AIDS had generated an extraordinary amount of fear. But the actual use of safety measures—condoms and spermicides—is sporadic at best and absent in most cases" (p. 106).

The September issue of the *Utne Reader* explored various AIDS issues, including discussion of the unproductive moralistic bias in much AIDS information (Hooper, 1988), a call for prosex messages in the media and the elimination of the message that abstinence is the only solution (Levine, 1988), and discussion of the need for more mature attitudes toward sexuality (Elshtain, 1988).

1989–1991: AIDS Is a Disease
of the Disenfranchised

In June of 1988, *People* ran a story on a promiscuous HIV-positive man accused of knowingly spreading the disease (Tamarkin, 1988). However, by 1989 the low risk of HIV infection for heterosexuals outside risk groups had become a standard theme in AIDS prevention articles. On January 30th, *Time* ("How to block a killer's path," Langone, 1989) commented, "While the virus can sometimes be transmitted in heterosexual intercourse, the evidence does not indicate that AIDS is about to break out in a big way into the mainstream population" (p. 60). The article repeated the conclusion that AIDS is a disease of poverty. "It is conceivable that AIDS will fan out from the ghettos into the general population, but not likely. If the spread occurs, it will be slow" (p. 61). The best advice, according to *Time*, is condom use coupled with more discriminating partner selection:

> Heterosexuals can have a "very low risk of contracting AIDS" if they use condoms and take the time to learn enough about their sexual partners to avoid drug abusers or the promiscuous. (p. 62)

Ms. (Halpern, 1989) answered the question by repeating the current wisdom that AIDS "is becoming a poor person's disease" (p. 80) and the chance that the reader herself is infected is "not very great" (p. 84).

The lack of heterosexual fear of AIDS was highlighted in a May article in *Ms.* (Rafferty, 1989). The author was clearly uneasy about how the "lingering courtship" strategy of AIDS prevention was being implemented by the singles she surveyed. Declaring that, "The one night stand is down, but not out" (p. 51), the author suggested that, "The three-dates-before-sex rule has become all of five dates. We're still sleeping with people we haven't met yet" (p. 51). Most of the singles the author surveyed believed that dating only those in a comfortable socioeconomic class will protect them from AIDS. However, the author declared, "Sleeping only with those who fit a nonrisk profile is putting our health in the hands of strangers" (p. 55).

An Emerging Focus on Teenage Sexuality The focus of prevention advice centered increasingly on teenagers. *Seventeen* (Kolata, 1990) highlighted the case of Alison Gertz, a heterosexual teen who claims to have contracted AIDS from one sexual experience. The article cited teen sex as an emerging AIDS threat:

> Because of the way the AIDS virus is spreading in teenagers—and especially in teenage girls—Dr. Hein says that people who predict AIDS will remain mostly a problem for gay men and drug users who share needles are wrong. (p. 149)

The unstated implication of this assertion was that AIDS will spread through the teenage population through tertiary transmission. The article asserted that although abstinence is best, using a condom every time one has sex is "a matter of life and death."

Many articles stressed the need to talk to teens about sex and AIDS.[5] One of the reasons cited for parental communication was the inadequacy of other forms of sex education. The *Seventeen* article quoted a spokesperson for the Center for Population Options as saying, "People are arguing about sex education in some high schools where a kid has an 85 percent chance of being sexually active" (p. 150). One author in *Time* depicted the current approach as "just say no (or die)" ("Better Safe Than Sorry," Tift, 1991). An article in *Mother Jones* (Talbot, 1990) decried the federal government's campaign to "sell the nation's youth on the joys of sexual abstinence" (p. 42) through the "Sex Respect" high school campaign as "breathtakingly stupid." The author stated:

> The conservative morality campaigns of the 1980's have had virtually no impact on the nation's high rates of adolescent sexual activity. But these chastity crusaders have succeeded in limiting teenagers' access to contraceptives and information. As a result, the United States has by far the highest teenage pregnancy rate in the Western world. (p. 42)

Even *Christianity Today* (Neff, 1989) told parents that given that "Just under half of all youths who attend conservative churches have had sexual intercourse by the time they are 18" (p. 15), even sending their children to a Christian college is no guarantee against sexual experimentation. Therefore, the article urged parents to talk to their teens about sex.

Thus all of the above articles conceded that there is an adolescent "information gap" resulting from inadequate sex education in school and urged parents to discuss AIDS with children and adolescents.

1991: Reassurance, but Still No Consensus

Popular magazines in 1991 featured a number of AIDS-relevant issues, such as testing ("Should You Get an AIDS Test," Cimons, 1991, in *Essence*; "Facing the Test," Fraser, 1991, in *Vogue*) and how AIDS affects women ("HIV: The Global Crisis," Gillespie, 1991, in *Ms.*). The received wisdom on heterosexual AIDS risk was optimistic, but this optimism was not unanimous.

The April 1st issue of *Newsweek* ran an opinion piece by Robert Noble, an

---

[5]See "Time to Talk" (Ullman, 1989), "How the World is Selling Safe Sex: The Condom Conundrum" (Talbot, 1990), "Talking About AIDS" (Comer, 1991), and "Better Safe Than Sorry" (1991).

infectious disease physician, entitled, "There Is No Safe Sex" (Noble, 1991). Dr. Noble declared,

> Passing out condoms to teenagers is like issuing them squirt guns for a four alarm blaze. Condoms just don't hack it. We should stop kidding ourselves. . . . What am I going to tell my daughters? I'm going to tell them that condoms give a false sense of security and that sex is dangerous. (p. 8)

An article by Elmer-Dewitt in the November 25th issue of *Time* entitled, "How Safe Is Sex?" (1991), gave a much different picture. The article stated, "The risk to most American heterosexuals is still small, but it is real and growing" (p. 72). However, it also described the heterosexual risk of infection as so unlikely as to provoke skepticism regarding Magic Johnson's claim that he acquired the disease heterosexually. "'When a guy says he got it from a woman, we just nod,' says a nurse. 'It's probably not true, but that's the way most of them want to handle it. And that's fine'" (p. 73).

PERCEIVED CONTROL AND AIDS: HOW WELL DO POPULAR ACCOUNTS ACTIVATE HEALTH PROTECTION MOTIVATION?

The foregoing summary provides a picture of a significant portion of the information environment available to young heterosexuals during the period covered by the surveys of sexual attitudes and intentions discussed earlier in this chapter. In this section, the components of the protection motivation/helplessness model are applied to this impressionistic data.

In terms of perceived threat or vulnerability to illness, the information available in popular sources may not have provided a clear picture. Although popular articles often provided the best information available at the time of publication, the summary shows evidence for heterosexual confusion about AIDS. High-fear accounts in *Time* ("The Big Chill," 1987) and the *Atlantic Monthly* ("Heterosexuals and AIDS," Leishman, 1987) did not differentiate between the risk of acquiring the disease heterosexually and the risk of having already acquired the disease (which, according to Hearst and Hulley's [1988] figures, was very, very low at this time). In such cases, high fear may have actually blocked the motivation for testing and subsequent safe sex given the perceived futility of such measures. The testimonials of heterosexuals themselves in the *Atlantic Monthly* piece convey this impression, because many of them expressed both anxious vigilance with regard to new and possibly reassuring information about the disease and a resistance to knowing their own HIV status.

Early reports such as the one in *Time* ("The Big Chill," 1987) also employed moralistic language that may have encouraged resistance. Appeals to chastity, which ignore the fact that to many persons sexual abstinence may be seen as an extreme or unacceptable cost of prevention, encourage resistance or denial as the preferred coping option (Gochros, 1988). Those with extremist views of the threat to heterosexuals often cited this as part of their rationale. For example, in the controversial *Cosmopolitan* piece, Dr. Gould (1988) expressed his motivations for questioning the threat of AIDS to heterosexuals as follows:

> Some health officials have told me that although they cannot prove transmission of the virus does occur in heterosexual intercourse, they cannot rule out the possibility "and so let's be overly cautious—it can't hurt." But it can. The hurt exists in the continually mounting fear and false alarm that may make it difficult for any of us to enjoy sex. . . . We are once again being persuaded that sex is wrong, dirty, bad for us, even deadly. (p. 204)

Some prevention messages sounded as if sex, rather than HIV infection, were the underlying evil. Such an approach ("Renouncing the sexual revolution of the 60's", see Smilgis, 1987) only makes sense if one assumes that there is something essentially wrong with sexuality outside marriage, regardless of one's risk of sexually transmitted diseases. This strategy may be especially problematic when addressing teenage sexuality.

Moralistic exaggerations of the heterosexual AIDS risk not only obscure important facts in the attempt to fit the statements about the disease to the tenets of the moral code (see Hearst & Hulley, 1988, with regard to AIDS and monogamy vs. promiscuity), but also may trigger reactions that disqualify messages related to vulnerability. Much of the force of Fumento's (1987) argument of the myth of a heterosexual AIDS epidemic comes from the notion that it is in the interests of certain groups to propagate the myth. Just as in the case of the "reefer madness" exaggerations of the effects of marijuana a generation earlier, exaggerated claims of risk may taint any later claims with the suspicion that they are similarly exaggerated, as Shilts observed.

More recent information on the heterosexual risk of HIV infection is less dire but possibly more ambiguous. The low probability of infection may suggest that protective measures adopted in the present will be effective, but the characterization of heterosexual AIDS as a poor person's disease may suggest that such measures are unnecessary. Choosing one's partner more carefully may be more palatable for many than using condoms (Hearst & Hulley, 1988; Remafedi, 1988). However, discriminating partner choice is depicted as being fraught with difficulty by many reports and may be ineffective if tertiary transmission becomes common.

Some ambiguities regarding risk assessment may be abetted by the way popular magazines use vivid stories of those afflicted. Nisbett and Ross (1980) have shown that persons overestimate the weight of information if it is provided in terms of vivid, concrete information rather than as a pallid set of abstractions. This circumstance may make the facts of the stories appear more representative than they are.

For example, Fineberg (1988) noted that persons are required to weave their way through risk information that is sometimes daunting and ambivalent:

> The feeling conveyed to the public from responsible officials about AIDS in fact is ambivalent, both reassuring and alarming. . . . To the physician or epidemiologist schooled in the transmission of viral disease, the dual message is eminently sensible. The layperson runs an understandable risk of confusion. (p. 594)

Given the predilection of the popular media for vivid and emotional storytelling, the public may have a similar problem determining that the case of Kimberly Bergalis, a woman infected by her dentist, is a tragic fluke, whereas the case of Alison Gertz, a young woman who apparently became infected by one encounter with her only sexual partner, is evidence of personal risk.

Perhaps the greatest ambiguity regarding the response and self-efficacy of protective measures involves the available popular information regarding condom use. Although the early *Cosmopolitan* piece ("What Every Woman Must Know About Condoms," Brenton, 1987) highlighted both response and self-efficacy, most articles reinforced the difficulty of negotiation regarding condom use, the male's ability to use the condom correctly, and/or the reliability of the condom in preventing infection if it were to be used. Although some popular reports have suggested that condom sales are up substantially ("Membrane of the Year," Berkman, 1988, in *Discover*), the surveys summarized earlier suggest that many heterosexuals do not use them.

However, normalizing as well as sensualizing condom use may be of great benefit. As the discussion above suggests, persons may be willing to employ health protection measures in the face of low probability of illness if response efficacy and self-efficacy are high (the why-take-the-chance phenomenon described earlier). Therefore, decreasing people's perceptions that condom use will be difficult and ineffective may encourage condom use even in the face of ambiguous information about AIDS risk. Because many authors agree that the spread of heterosexual AIDS will be slow, dramatic changes in the perceived risk for heterosexuals are unlikely. Under such circumstances, lowering the perceived costs of condom use may have a greater effect than highlighting the danger of unprotected sex. Sensualizing condom use may do much to promote use in such situations.

The current situation with regard to AIDS and the heterosexual mainstream population can be compared to the economic phenomenon called the "tragedy of the commons" (Cross & Guyer, 1980). If the goal of AIDS prevention information is a change of behavior before a high rate of infected persons in the heterosexual community requires it, AIDS educators are going to have to contend with a situation wherein preventive measures perceived to be high in cost (abstinence, limiting partners, and consistent condom use) are coupled with the perception of little immediate gain for the person.

Psychologists Cross and Guyer (1980) described a similar phenomenon they called an "externality trap." For example, the personal costs associated with hanging on to an item of litter until the person finds a trash receptacle may be perceived as greater than the damage done to the area by throwing the item on the ground. This is especially the case when the area is already littered with many items. Thus, each person, in pursuing his or her individual self-interest, creates a collective problem. As Cross and Guyer summarized it, "The neighborhood is in a trap, not because any one individual is acting against the public interest, but because the public, as a collectivity, is acting against the public interest" (p. 30).

The answer to such situations is to (a) lower the personal cost of the prosocial behavior, (b) increase the rewards of the prosocial behavior, or (c) add to the costs to the antisocial behavior. In the case of safe sex, sensualizing condom use would reduce its perceived cost. Because "impression management" is also a potent motivator for most people, making safe sex consistent with group norms would be a way of rewarding it or adding to the costs of pursuing unsafe sex (Fisher, 1988). However, it is not clear from the academic literature how this goal might be speedily accomplished without invoking the *deus ex machina* of the magic of "Madison Avenue" (Fisher, 1988). Nonetheless, every popular article featuring condoms incrementally adds to the normative acceptance of safe sex.

Overall, popular articles on AIDS prevention began with a high level of helplessness that decreased as more reliable information became available. However, conflicting accounts of personal risk, the mixing of homilies with facts, and the reluctance of providing preventative strategies in a way that affirms sexuality are still barriers to personal control in the age of AIDS. Although recent accounts have been more temperate, there is still enough doubt and confusion to incite the fears of the worried well as well as encourage the complacency of those wishing to depersonalize their risk.

The depersonalization of AIDS for the majority of heterosexuals may have unfortunate consequences for the community as well. Depicting AIDS as afflicting mainly the poor and disenfranchised may blunt the compassion of the majority of the real suffering of people at risk.

Psychologist Martin Seligman, originator of the theory of learned helplessness, has a prescription that applies to the worried well. In a recent work, *Learned Optimism*, Seligman (1990) declared that "Young people today are ten times likelier to suffer severe depression than their grandparents were, and depression takes a particularly heavy toll among women and among young men" (p. 282). This epidemic of depression, caused by increased feelings of helplessness, has arisen commensurate with the rise of the notion that the self is the center of all things. Asserts Seligman, "The epidemic of depression stems from the much-noted rise in individualism and the decline in the committment to the common good" (p. 286). Therefore, devoting our collective energies to help those afflicted by AIDS may not only benefit those at risk, but also provide what is missing for many of the worried well. This may be the best prevention strategy of all.

REFERENCES

Abraham, C., Sheeran, P., Abrams, D., Spears, R., & Marks, D. (1991). Young people learning about AIDS: A study of beliefs and information sources. *Health Education Research, 16,* 19–29.

AIDS fear leads many singles to marry. (1987, February 23). *Jet,* p. 31.

AIDS now. (1988, February 29). *The New Republic,* p. 7.

AIDS scare changes way stars make love on TV. (1987, September 28). *Jet,* pp. 58–59.

Asnes, M., & Giese, J. (1987, June). Playing it safe: The new sexual landscape. *Vogue,* pp. 226–227, 272–274.

Baldwin, J. D., & Baldwin, J. I. (1988). Factors affecting AIDS-related sexual risk-taking behavior among college students. *Journal of Sex Research, 25,* 181–196.

Barber, J. (1987, June 15). Confrontation and concern about AIDS. *McClean's,* pp. 40–41.

Barry, L. (1990, July/August). Of jungle juice and getting loose: The timeless ritual of teenage sex. *Utne Reader,* pp. 90–97.

Beck, K. H., & Frankel, A. (1981). A conceptualization of threat communications and protective health behavior. *Social Psychology Quarterly, 44,* 204–217.

Beck, K. H., & Lund, A. K. (1981). The effects of health threat seriousness and personal efficacy upon intentions and behavior. *Journal of Applied Social Psychology, 11,* 401–415.

Berkman, S. (1988, January). Membrane of the year. *Discover,* pp. 78–79.

Booth, W. (1988). Heterosexual AIDS: Setting the odds. *Science, 239,* 579.

Bowie, C., & Ford, N. (1989). Sexual behavior of young people and the risk of HIV infection. *Journal of Epidemiology and Community Health, 43,* 61–65.

Breen, L. J., Vulcano, B., & Dyck, D. G. (1979). Observational learning and sex roles in learned helplessness. *Psychological Reports, 44,* 135–144.

Brenton, M. (1987, May). What every woman must know about condoms. *Cosmopolitan,* pp. 108, 112, 118.

Brown, I., & Inouye, D. K. (1978). Learned helplessness through modeling: The role of perceived similarity in competence. *Journal of Personality and Social Psychology, 36,* 900–908.

Brown, L. K., & Fritz, G. K. (1988). AIDS education in the schools: A literature review as a guide for curricular planning. *Clinical Pediatrics, 27,* 311–316.

Cimons, M. (1991, May). Should you get an AIDS test? *Essence,* pp. 24, 29, 129.

Comer, J. P. (1991, February). Talking about AIDS. *Parents Magazine,* p. 186.

Cornish, E. (1987 November/December). AIDS and the year 2000. *The Futurist,* pp. 2, 46.

Cosmo's private sex survey. (1988, July). *Cosmopolitan,* pp. 140–143.

Coyne, J. C., & Lazarus, R. S. (1980). Cognitive style, stress perception, and coping. In I. L. Kutash & L. B. Schlesinger (Eds.), *Handbook on stress and anxiety* (pp. 144–158). San Francisco: Jossey-Bass.

Cross, J. G., & Guyer, M. J. (1980). *Social traps.* Ann Arbor: University of Michigan Press.

DeVellis, R. F., DeVellis, B. M., & McCauley, C. (1978). Vicarious acquisition of learned helplessness. *Journal of Personality and Social Psychology, 36,* 894–899.

Edgar, T., Freimuth, V. S., & Hammond, S. L. (1988). Communicating the AIDS risk to college students: The problem of motivating change. *Health Education Research, 3,* 59–65.

Edwards, A. (1987, September). Don't get around much anymore. *Essence,* pp. 77, 131, 133–134.

Edwards, D. (1987, July 25). Heterosexuals and AIDS: Mixed messages. *Science News,* pp. 60–61.

Ellis, R. (1988, July). The fears and facts of sex now. *Glamour,* pp. 154–156.

Elmer-Dewitt, P. (1991, November 25). How safe is sex? *Time,* pp. 72–74.

Elshtain, J. (1988, September/October). Why we need limits. *Utne Reader,* pp. 52–55.

Experts debate the threat to heterosexuals. (1988, March 14). *People,* pp. 107–108.

Findlay, S. (1988, February 29). Has the threat been exaggerated? *U.S. News and World Report,* pp. 58–59.

Findlay, S., & Silberner, J. (1988, March 21). What the press release left out. *U.S. News and World Report,* pp. 59–60.

Fineberg, H. V. (1988). Education to prevent AIDS: Prospects and obstacles. *Science, 239,* 592–596.

Fisher, J. D. (1988). Possible effects of reference group-based social influence on AIDS-risk behavior and AIDS prevention. *American Psychologist, 43,* 914–920.

Flora, J. A., & Thoresen, C. E. (1988). Reducing the risk of AIDS in adolescents. *American Psychologist, 43,* 965–970.

Fraser, L. (1991, June). Facing the test. *Vogue,* pp. 96–102.

Freimuth, V. S., Edgar, T., & Hammond, S. L. (1987). College students' awareness and interpretation of the AIDS risk. *Science, Technology and Human Values, 12,* 37–40.

Friedman, J., & Van Biema, D. (1987, August 31). AIDS: A diary of the plague in America. *People,* pp. 61–64, 67–70, 73–79.

Fumento, M. (1987, November). AIDS: Are heterosexuals at risk? *Commentary,* pp. 21–27.

Garber, J., & Seligman, M. E. P. (Eds.). (1980). *Human helplessness: Theory and applications.* New York: Academic Press.

Gardner, B. (1988, April). Would you believe heavy petting, masturbation, vibrators, *hot* music, and other passionate play toys—all pinch hitting for bedding new partners in the age of AIDS! *Cosmopolitan,* pp. 235–237.

Gardner, M. (1957). *Fads and fallacies in the name of science.* New York: Dover.

Giese, J. (1987, June). On the difficulty of asking a man to wear a condom. *Vogue,* pp. 226–227.

Gillespie, M. A. (1991, January/February). HIV: The global crisis. *Ms.,* pp. 16–22.

Gillies, B. (1987, September). How has AIDS changed your sex life. *Cosmopolitan,* pp. 140, 144.

Gochros, H. L. (1988). Risks of abstinence: Sexual decision making in the AIDS era. *Social Work, 33,* 254–256.

Goode, E. E. (1988, February). I love you, but can I ask you a question? *U.S. News and World Report,* p. 85.

Gorman, C. (1988, March 21). Outbreak of sensationalism. *Time,* pp. 58–59.

Gould, R. (1988, January). AIDS: A doctor tells why you may not be at risk. *Cosmopolitan,* pp. 146–147, 204.

Grady, D. (1988, March 21). Just how does AIDS spread. *Time,* pp. 60–61.

Halpern, S. (1989, May). AIDS: Rethinking the risk. *Ms.,* pp. 80–87.

Harowski, K. J. (1987). The worried well: Maximizing coping in the face of AIDS. *Journal of Homosexuality, 14,* 299–306.

Hearst, N., & Hulley, S. B. (1988). Preventing the heterosexual spread of AIDS: Are we giving our patients the best advice? *Journal of the American Medical Association, 259,* 2428–2432.

Heller, A. (1987, July). Is there a man in your man's life? *Mademoiselle,* pp. 134–135.

Hooper, J. (1988, September/October). Sex and circulation: Why media hypes hetero risk. *Utne Reader,* pp. 69–70.

Katz, B., & Sternberg-Katz, L. (1989). *Magazines for libraries* (6th ed.). New York: Bowker.

Kegeles, S. M., Adler, N. E., & Irwin, C. E. (1988). Sexually active adolescents and condom use: Changes over one year in knowledge, attitudes and use. *American Journal of Public Health, 78,* 460–461.

Kolata, G. (1990, May). Teenagers and AIDS. *Seventeen,* pp. 148–151.

Langone, J. (1989, January 30). How to block a killer's path. *Time,* pp. 60–62.

Lauerson, N. (1987, November). Safe sex: A doctor answers your questions. *Cosmopolitan,* pp. 284–287.

Lazarus, R. S., & Launier, R. (1978). Stress related transactions between person and environment. In L. A. Pervin & M. Lewis (Eds.), *Perspectives in interactional psychology* (pp. 287–327). New York: Plenum Press.

Lefcourt, H. M. (Ed.). (1981). *Research with the locus of control construct: Vol. 1. Assessment methods.* New York: Academic Press.

Lefcourt, H. M. (1982). *Locus of control: Current trends in theory and research* (2nd ed.). Hillsdale, NJ: Erlbaum.

Lefcourt, H. M. (1983). *Research with the locus of control construct: Vol. 2. Developments and social problems.* New York: Academic Press.

Lefcourt, H. M. (1984). *Research with the locus of control construct: Vol. 3. Extensions and limitations.* New York: Academic Press.

Leishman, K. (1987, February). Heterosexuals and AIDS. *Atlantic Monthly,* pp. 39–49, 52–58.

Leventhal, H. (1971). Fear appeals and persuasion: The differentiation of a motivational construct. *American Journal of Public Health, 61,* 208–224.

Levine, G. F. (1977). Learned helplessness and the evening news. *Journal of Communication, 27,* 100–105.

Levine, G. F. (1986). Learned helplessness in local TV news. *Journalism Quarterly, 63,* 12–23.

Levine, J. (1988, September/October). Beware of setting limits. *Utne Reader,* pp. 56–60, 62–63.

Masters, W. H., Johnson, V. E., & Kolodny, R. C. (1988, March 14). Sex in the age of AIDS. *Newsweek,* pp. 45–46, 47–50, 52.

Masters, W. H., Johnson, V. E., & Kolodny, R. C. (1988, May). AIDS: Worse than we think? *Good Housekeeping,* pp. 164–165, 266–271.

McAuliffe, K. (1987, August 17). AIDS and 'straights': Unsettling questions. *U.S. News and World Report,* p. 34.

Mehlman, P. (1988, July). And how do men feel now about monogamy? *Glamour,* pp. 157–158.

Miller, T. E., Booraem, C., Flowers, J. V., & Iversen, A. E. (1990). Changes in knowledge, attitudes, and behavior as a result of a community-based AIDS prevention program. *AIDS Education and Prevention, 2,* 12–23.

Montgomery, S. B., Joseph, J. G., Becker, M. H., Ostrow, D. G., Kessler, R. C., & Kirscht, J. P. (1989). The health belief model in understanding compliance with preventive recommendations for AIDS: How useful? *AIDS Education and Prevention, 1,* 303–323.

Neff, D. (1989, September 22). Will your child get AIDS? *Christianity Today,* p. 15.

Nisbett, R., & Ross, L. (1980). *Human inference: Strategies and shortcomings of social judgment.* Englewood Cliffs, NJ: Prentice-Hall.

Noble, R. (1991, April 1). There is no safe sex. *Newsweek,* p. 8.

Orth, M. (1987, October). Across the U.S., one man in thirty is infected. Vogue, pp. 246, 248.

Padian, N. S., & Francis, D. P. (1988). Preventing the heterosexual spread of AIDS [letter to the editor]. *Journal of the American Medical Association, 260,* 1879.

Petosa, R., & Wessinger, J. (1990). The AIDS education needs of adolescents: A theory-based approach. *AIDS Education and Prevention, 2,* 127–136.

Prentice-Dunn, S., & Rogers, R. W. (1986). Protections motivation theory and preventive health: Beyond the health belief model. *Health Education Research, 1,* 153–161.

Rafferty, M. (1989, May). Fearless flying: Singles on the prowl. *Ms.,* pp. 51, 54–55.

Remafedi, G. J. (1988). Preventing the sexual transmission of AIDS during adolescence. *Journal of Adolescent Health Care, 9*(2), 139–143.

Rigby, K., Brown, M., & Anagnostou, P. (1989). Shock tactics to counter AIDS: The Australian experience. *Psychology and Health, 3,* 145–159.

Rippetoe, P. A., & Rogers, R. W. (1987). Effects of components of protection motivation theory on adaptive and maladaptive coping with a health threat. *Journal of Personality and Social Psychology, 52,* 596–604.

Roberts, M. (1988, December). Dating, dishonesty, and AIDS. *Psychology Today,* p. 60.

Rogers, R. W. (1975). A protection motivation theory of fear appeals and attitude change. *Journal of Psychology, 91,* 93–114.

Roscoe, B., & Kruger, T. L. (1990). AIDS: Late adolescents' knowledge and its influence on sexual behavior. *Adolescence, 25*(97), pp. 39–48.

Rosenstock, I. M. (1974). The health belief model and preventive health behavior. *Health Education Monographs, 2,* 354–386.

Salvatore, D. (1987, October). How AIDS affects us all. *Ladies Home Journal,* pp. 119–121, 183–192.

Sanders, L. (1989, June). The worst lie of all: What they'll say for sex. *Mademoiselle,* pp. 216.

Schulman, K. (1988). Preventing the heterosexual spread of AIDS [letter to the editor]. *Journal of the American Medical Association, 260,* 1879.

Seligman, J. (1988, March 21). Storm over Masters and Johnson. *Newsweek,* pp. 78–79.

Seligman, M. E. P. (1975). *Helplessness: On depression, development, and death.* San Francisco: Freeman.

Seligman, M. E. P. (1990). *Learned optimism.* New York: Knopf.

Shayne, V. T., & Kaplan, B. J. (1988). AIDS education for adolescents. *Youth and Society, 20,* 180–208.

Silver, R. L., & Wortman, C. B. (1980). Coping with undesirable life events. In J. Garber & M. E. P. Seligman (Eds.), *Human helplessness: Theory and applications* (pp. 279–340). New York: Academic Press.

Smilgis, M. (1987, Feb. 16). Big chill: fear of AIDS. *Time,* pp. 50–56.

Talbot, D. (1990, January). How the world is selling safe sex: The condom conundrum. *Mother Jones,* pp. 38–44, 46–47.

Tamarkin, C. (1988, June 27). Love and death in Key West. *People,* pp. 38–40, 43.

The new sexual morality. (1987, November). *Ebony,* pp. 52, 54, 56.

Tift, S. E. (1991, January 21). Better safe than sorry. *Time,* pp. 66–67.

Ullman, L. (1989, September). Time to talk. *Seventeen,* pp. 112–113.

Wainwright, L. (1987, August). The paranoia of a modern plague. *Life,* p. 11.

Wallis, C. (1987, February 16). You haven't heard anything yet. *Time,* pp. 54–56.

Whigham, M. (1988, April). AIDS: What's your risk. *Essence,* pp. 20, 112–113.

Wober, J. M. (1988). Informing the British public about AIDS. *Health Education Research, 3,* 19–24.

Women and sex: 1988. (1988, August). *Ladies Home Journal,* pp. 105–110.

Zimmerman, D. R., & Goldstein, K. (1987, April). AIDS: What we know now. *McCalls,* pp. 143–147.

Chapter Seven

AIDS in the Media: Entertainment or Infotainment

Nina Biddle
Lisa Conte
Edwin Diamond

On November 14, 1991, when the cohosts of "NFL This Weekend," a nightly sports news show on Cable channel ESPN, expressed their reactions to basketball star Earvin (Magic) Johnson's earlier announcement that he has the human immunodeficiency virus (HIV), no one really expected any new light to be shed on the topic of acquired immune deficiency syndrome (AIDS). But neither were they prepared for the depth of the misunderstanding conveyed. The cohosts were discussing the coming weekend's professional football schedule:

"Many 'open wounds' are incurred by players during a football game," Blue Blazer No. 1 began. "Perhaps the National Football League should require mandatory testing for the AIDS virus."

Blue Blazer No. 2 concurred: "If a player tests positive, maybe it would be a good thing to remove him from the team and get him out of the league." Pause. Break for commercial.

So much for the nation's education on how AIDS is spread. The cohosts failed to mention that, in fact, viruses live in moist, interior places and exposure to air, light, cold, or heat kills them instantly, making the passage of a virus between open wounds virtually impossible. Unfortunately, for the past 10 years, this type of misinformation has been all too common in the media.

For the past 8 years, our News Study Group at New York University has been examining the way mainstream television, newspapers, and magazines have covered the AIDS epidemic. We have found that although major constituencies—the federal government, local officials, gay activists, and medical authorities—contributed to some of the misunderstanding and confusion, journalism has also added its own share of contradictory practices and ambivalent attitudes. For the first half of the AIDS Decade (1981–1991), journalists spoke too often in euphemisms and evasions; by being squeamish about their coverage in the initial stages of the epidemic, journalists added another layer of confusion to an already complex medical narrative (Diamond, 1991).

In more recent years, AIDS coverage has improved in some ways and faltered in others. The media euphemisms are gone—the mainstream press speaks of "anal intercourse" now, not "intimate contact"; the words "semen" and "vaginal discharge" are used in place of "body fluids." Despite these needed reforms, unsafe journalistic practices continue. We have found that AIDS and its victims are disproportionately presented in the mainstream media through biographical details, in the entertaining-while-informing style of *People* magazine and all its imitators in print and on television. As projected *People*-style, the face of AIDS is usually middle- or upper-class, White, famous or soon to be a "celebrity," and implicitly heterosexual or "innocent." Such a portrait, of course, is at odds with the statistics of the AIDS epidemic, which show that HIV-positive men and women are, in the main, homosexuals and drug-abusers. As of March 1, 1992, the statistics of the Centers for Disease Control on people with AIDS were as follows: 56% are homosexual and bisexual men; 19% are male and female intravenous drug users; 6% are heterosexual; 2% are blood transfusion recipients; and 1% are hemophiliacs. The remainder are combinations of the above, with a predominance of homosexuals who are intravenous drug users.

Any number of examples can be cited to illustrate the phenomenon we term medical infotainment—the media's tendency to overcover celebrity AIDS cases while often skimping on coverage of the more prevalent ones. In this chapter, we examine three of the most widely reported cases to date: movie actor Rock Hudson; Kimberly Bergalis, a young woman in Florida who was raised to celebrity status through the coverage she received; and super athlete Magic Johnson. They are examples of how AIDS victims and HIV carriers are disproportionately represented by the media, how misinformation about the AIDS epidemic has spread and continues to spread through both error and omission, and how the media still shies away from frank discussion of topics that may be distasteful to a mainstream public.

ROCK HUDSON: STAR TREATMENT

Rock Hudson had long embodied the masculine, handsome, clean-cut, all-American screen star who played opposite Elizabeth Taylor and Doris Day in his films. On July 25, 1985, however, he became known, literally overnight, for something else: Hudson was the first celebrity to publicly announce he had AIDS.

That summer, Hudson's publicists initially said he was being treated for inoperable liver cancer at the American Hospital in Paris. Two days later they acknowledged that he was dying of AIDS and that he had been diagnosed a year earlier. Hudson died October 2, 1985. By the summer of 1985, nearly 6,000 people had already died of AIDS nationwide and close to 12,000 had been diagnosed with the HIV virus. Despite these figures, press coverage of AIDS had been minimal until Hudson made his announcement.

The media's reaction to the news that July conformed to an already established pattern. As the journalist James Kinsella (1989) explained in his book *Covering the Plague—AIDS and the American Media,* AIDS coverage rises and falls on the wave of media and audience identification with the victim. Each peak comes about as a result of news that seems to make AIDS a threat for either the media's major audience or for journalists themselves (Kinsella, p. 4). Kinsella called this the "personal threat rule." Thus, during the early years of the epidemic, AIDS disappeared and reappeared in the news depending on whether the disease seemed to be approaching the heterosexual community.

When Rock Hudson's diagnosis of AIDS became known, ABC News gave Hudson and AIDS-related stores 7 min and 20 s, an unprecedented amount of time in the history of the epidemic (Kinsella, 1989). Within days, media coverage of AIDS tripled nationwide, and small-town publications covered AIDS for the first time. Yet there was relatively little information about the basics of AIDS: how it is acquired, how it is transmitted, how much of its stigma is related to mainstream attitudes about homosexuals. Most of the coverage was personal information about the celebrity: Rock Hudson was the focus, not AIDS. Stories were by turns conservative, tentative, caring, and admiring: "Rock Hudson Being Treated for AIDS" (Hall & Rovner, 1985), "A Star Gets AIDS" (Cohen, 1985), "Facing Reality with Rock Hudson" (Johnson, 1985), "AIDS Strikes a Star" (Gelman & Reese, 1985), and "Rock Hudson AIDS Case Sends a Message" ("Rock Hudson AIDS Case," 1985). The press was clearly concerned about Hudson in a way it hadn't been about any other AIDS case.

In the manner of celebrity articles, the focus more often than not was on Hudson's achievements and glamour image: "Hudson rose to sophisticated leading-man status in the '50s and '60s, starring in dozens of films," (Hall, 1985a, Section B, p. 1) for example. More substantive issues, such as his double life, were not explored. Hudson's declining physical appearance was described for extra effect: "The 6 foot 4 actor looked almost unrecognizably hollow cheeked and emaciated" (Gelman & Reese, 1985, p. 65). A presumably eager public was told how friends and colleagues were reacting: Doris Day was praying, Linda Evans had no comment, Susan St. James would take no phone calls, Carol Burnett was inaccessible, and the cast of "Dynasty" was stunned (Hall & Rovner, 1985).

Although the coverage of Hudson's case offered little in terms of medical information or education, it spurred other AIDS-related stories using Hudson as their lead or news peg. Hudson's visit to Paris for treatment with the experimental drug HPA-23 produced articles in major dailies and magazines on drug treatments abroad and Food and Drug Administration regulations: "Search for an AIDS Drug Is Case History in Frustration" (Altman, 1985), "AIDS Program in Paris Gives Hope to Americans" (Prial, 1985), "AIDS Exiles in Paris" (Clark & Coleman, 1985), and "Ill Treatment" ("Ill Treatment," 1985). These resulting articles were more informational, but they still refrained from specifically addressing the modes of transmission of AIDS.

In fact, almost the same identical cursory "AIDS paragraph" would appear in article after article about Hudson or AIDS, as in this example from the *Washington Post*: "AIDS, a usually fatal illness that destroys the body's natural immune system, has most often struck homosexuals, abusers of injectable drugs, and, to a lesser degree, recipients of blood and blood products" (Hall & Rovner, 1985, Section A, p. 1). These perfunctory descriptions did not mention sexual transmission, let alone what specific activities allowed the virus to be spread.

Granted, the media were coving a film star and not a medical convention. There were additional reasons, however, for the press's reticence in exploring these issues. First, the media had received limited information about AIDS from the scientific and medical communities. Second, their position also reflected the federal government's attitude toward AIDS. Ronald Reagan had never mentioned AIDS in public until Hudson was diagnosed. Third, television news in particular did not want to offend the dinner-time American public with terms like "anal sex" and "oral sex."

But Hudson's news lifted the lid on other AIDS news. Coverage of Ryan White, the young hemophiliac in Indiana who contracted the HIV virus from tainted blood, increased dramatically once Hudson's story broke. White first appeared on national television on July 30, 5 days after the first news stories about Hudson (Kinsella, 1989, p. 187).

Mainstream news outlets, such as the *Washington Post,* also started writing about how the new interest in AIDS was affecting homosexuals: "Sympathy in the Gay Community: Hudson Illness Expected To Put Spotlight on AIDS" (Hall, 1985b). Articles were empathetic toward homosexuals: "Gays yesterday also said they had grown weary of bearing most of the burden of fundraising on the disease, and bearing most of the abuse that the public aims at them" (Hall, 1985b, Section G, p. 1). Columnist Richard Cohen described indirectly the media's AIDS problems: "The Hudson story reflects the country's confusion about homosexuality. We're not sure whether we're dealing with a scandal or tragedy" (1985, Section A, p. 23). Cohen also wrote about the "familiar and reassuring face that Hudson put on homosexuality" (Section A, p. 23).

The well-publicized story of Rock Hudson may have helped bring awareness that AIDS was more prevalent than previously thought. But it was probably a horror-movie type of awareness: scary at the time, and soon forgotten. AIDS, too, receded from the mainstream media for a while.

KIMBERLY BERGALIS: FEATURE FODDER

Kimberly Bergalis was neither a film star nor a celebrity. She was cast into the public eye because she was young, White, heterosexual, and a virgin—and she had acquired AIDS. Bergalis was the embodiment of one of the mainstream public's worst fears.

Bergalis ignited a national debate over AIDS testing when she became the first known case of a patient contracting the HIV virus from a health care worker. She was diagnosed with the disease in December 1989. As the story was reported, she contracted the virus from her dentist, Dr. David Acer, during a tooth extraction. Acer was bisexual; he died in September 1990. When hundreds of his patients were later tested, four more discovered they were infected with the same strain of HIV. These were patients who, like Bergalis, reportedly had no other AIDS risk factors in their lives (Lambert, 1991).

Bergalis quickly became a familiar face through which the widest public could identify with AIDS. She was the girl next door who shocked the reticent public into—as the media now told it—realizing that anyone could get AIDS. Both Bergalis and her family made a point of testifying to her virginity. Along with this shock of recognition came its companion, hysteria, fueled largely by the type of coverage the Bergalis case received.

Cast variously in the press as both AIDS "hero" and AIDS "martyr," Bergalis became feature fodder for the media. In October 1990, *People* magazine ran a cover story on Bergalis. The article inside began: "The weather in Fort Pierce, on Florida's east coast, was sunny and unseasonably warm on a recent September afternoon. But inside her parent's three-bedroom house, 22-year-old Kimberly Bergalis lay shivering on the family room sofa, worn out from a trip to the beach just a block away" (Johnson & Grant, 1990, p. 72). The reader was taken into her house and, with a mix of literary license and flair, under her skin.

Nine months later, in July 1991, *Newsweek* ran *its* cover story: "Doctors With AIDS." The story began, "It is 80 degrees in the Florida dusk, but Kimberly Bergalis huddles under a quilt on the couch in her family's living room" (Kantrowitz, 1991, p. 49). A photograph of Bergalis accompanied the story. The caption lifted a line from the close of her letter to Florida health officials: "I'm dying guys. Goodbye" (Kantrowitz, p. 48).

The story line was set: the innocent victim, the uncaring medical establishment, the evil dentist. The human-interest narrative had taken root early and continued to grow.

Headlines picked up Bergalis's personal plight: "A Life Stolen Early"

(Johnson & Grant, 1990), "Kim's Brave Journey" (Johnson & Grant, 1991), "AIDS Heroes and Villains" (Ehrenfeld, 1991), and "The Accuser" (Weisberg, 1991). The tone and dramatic content of the "Kim coverage" often overshadowed any primary AIDS information in the stories. Like Hudson, Bergalis could have been a vehicle for the press to convey scientific information, but, for the most part, it again appeared to be a missed opportunity.

In the October 1990 *People* article (Johnson & Grant, 1990), the young woman's father, George Bergalis, was quoted as saying, "Her sickness would have been easier to accept if she'd been a slut or a drug user. But she had everything right" (Johnson & Grant, p. 77). According to George Bergalis, there were innocent and guilty AIDS victims. His statements, and the others like it that followed, to some degree became a media subplot further detracting from the calm dissemination of information.

The Bergalises alliance with the conservative Congressman William Dannemeyer (R., California) also drew much media attention. Dannemeyer, who announced his candidacy for the U.S. Senate in 1992, sponsored a bill named after Bergalis. (As Jacob Weisberg [1991] wrote in *The New Republic*, the Republicans "finally found an AIDS patient they could embrace" [p. 14].) The Kimberly Bergalis Patient and Health Provider Protection Act of 1991 would require the testing of doctors and dentists for HIV and hepatitis B. Those infected would not be allowed to perform invasive surgical procedures without informing their patients and receiving written consent (Weisberg, 1991).

Backers of the legislation brought Bergalis to Washington in September 1991, hoping that a direct appeal from the now famous "victim" of AIDS would bolster chances of eventual passage. Bergalis, frail in both voice and physical appearance, evoked sympathy from the press. Several accounts personalized the drama of the event. *Time* magazine, for example, called her 15-second message "shattering" and ran a photograph of her with the caption "Innocent victim: Bergalis appeals to Congress" ("Anguished Testimony," 1991, p. 27). The *New York Times* coverage was full of sympathy: "Kimberly Bergalis, wearing pale flowers in the strands of short, sandy-colored hair she has remaining after her treatment for AIDS, was wheeled to the witness table in Congress today to utter 15 seconds of testimony" (Hilts, 1991, p. A8). A large photograph of Bergalis accompanied the story. Jeffrey Levi, policy director of the AIDS Action Council, told the *New York Times*, "Her case is being used by some of the right-wing forces to rekindle some of the fear that has always been lurking under the surface about AIDS" (Hilts, p. A8).

The dramatic coverage further evolved as Bergalis and her family added their own fuel to the press's fire. In the April 1991 letter to Florida health officials, which her family released to news organizations 2 months later, Bergalis described the physical symptoms she endured and the emotional pain she and her family experienced and again professed her "innocence." "Do I blame myself? I sure don't. I never used IV drugs, never slept with anyone and never had a blood transfusion. I blame Dr. Acer and every single one of you bastards" ("I Blame," 1991, p. 52). The story gained new life in the press. Bergalis was a reminder to the public that "anyone" can be at risk, an exaggerated conclusion for the press and the general public to have reached.

Some journalists stood apart from the hype. "How many health care workers in the United States are thought to have transmitted the AIDS virus to patients?" asked a *New York Newsday* editorial ("Editorial," 1991). "Exactly one—ever." Almost 34,000 Americans had been diagnosed with AIDS so far that year. In the words of former Surgeon General C. Everett Koop, the risk of contracting AIDS from a health care worker is practically nonexistent: "so remote that it may never be measured" (Hilts, 1991, p. A8). Media accounts also noted that dozens of medical groups, led by the American Medical Association, refused to comply with the Centers for Disease Control's request to draw up lists of procedures that pose a threat to patients because, the medical groups maintained, no measurable threat existed.

However, these statements usually came in the form of rebuttals to discussions of possible restrictions on medical professionals and assertions that patients were at risk. On September 25, 1991, ABC News combined its coverage of a National Commission on AIDS report with the story of Bergalis's arrival in Washington, treating both sources as equally authoritative.

The Bergalis case raised some important questions concerning the public's education on AIDS. Unfortunately, hysteria seemed to have prevailed over what limited education had taken place up to that point.

MAGIC JOHNSON: "AMERICA FINDS A HERO"

Just before Bergalis's death in December 1991, the media found another celebrity AIDS case—Magic Johnson.[1] In the space of 20 days in late 1991, the coverage of the Magic Johnson HIV story went through at least three phases, by now each one maddeningly predictable.

The first stage was surprise: America, including the media, in shock. Television offered repeated tape replays of the news conference called by the Los Angeles Lakers basketball team and the National Basketball Association at which Johnson announced his retirement as well as his determination to be a spokesperson and role model in the fight against AIDS. Then, Johnson, poised and smiling, appeared on his friend Arsenio Hall's late-night talk show, to receive a standing ovation. There were the headlines with the expected word plays: "Tragic Magic" in *New York Newsday*; "Magic's Message" in *Newsweek*; and in *Sports Illustrated*, just the single word "Magic" on the

---

[1]Edwin Diamond has files and a set of videocassettes on the Magic Johnson AIDS story that he will share with anyone who wishes to write him at New York University—News Study Group, 10 Washington Place, New York, NY 10003.

cover. Inside *Sports Illustrated* was a 28-page package of articles and photographs, including a contribution from Johnson himself, written with the help of a *Sports Illustrated* editor ("I'm still the same happy-go-lucky guy I've always been," Johnson said.

Then came Stage 2: "America Finds a Hero," as *People* put it (November 25, 1991). Johnson was instantly accorded superhero status for coming forward to acknowledge the new fact of his medical life. "His Huge Heart Will Lead Fight," the headline over a sports column promised in the *New York Daily News*. Everyone quickly climbed aboard the Magic tour without knowing exactly where it was going; this included George Bush, who asked Johnson to serve on the President's National Advisory Commission on AIDS.

In a matter of days, hope and hype gave way to second, third, and fourth thoughts. The subject shifted from saint Magic to sinner Johnson. In the attempt to strike the right "reflective" note, some misleading information was passed on from press to public. The medical writer B. D. Colen in *Newsday*, for example, wrote that the "tragedy of Magic Johnson serves to demonstrate, in a way never before demonstrated, that anyone can get AIDS. Neither sexual orientation, physical fitness, social class nor fame can provide protection from this viral infection." Narrowly presented, this lesson in internal medicine was correct. The trouble was, Magic Johnson wasn't "anyone." He was a man of 32 with a specific sexual history. Although he didn't boast of 20,000 1-hr stands, as fellow NBA athlete Wilt Chamberlain did, "Everyman" Johnson did say that when he "traveled around the NBA cities, I was never at a loss for female companionship."

Furthermore, the Lakers, the league, and Johnson's agent all tried to ensure that no one thought Johnson was homosexual, bisexual, or an intravenous drug user. As Dr. Arthur W. Caplan, a bioethicist at the University of Minnesota rather dryly told the *Boston Globe*, Johnson's "attractiveness as a spokesman will evaporate instantaneously" if it turned out that he had acquired the HIV virus by some other route than heterosexual intercourse (Palmer, 1991, p. 1).

These hard-eyed efforts at media spin control eventually backfired, as they usually do. When Johnson declared in *Sports Illustrated*, "I did my best to accommodate as many women as I could" from the time he put on a Lakers uniform in 1979, the press pack had something new to pursue. Columnists began to ask about all the women, in Los Angeles and in the other cities on the NBA circuit, with whom Johnson had—in his words—"unprotected sex." Did they test positive for HIV? And who infected them with the virus? (Transmission from men to women is more typical than from women to men.)

Thus the third stage of the trajectory of the Johnson HIV news. The story moved out from a magic circle of friends and business associates. The good notices turned sour and mean spirited. Sports columnist David Anderson (1991) wrote in the *New York Times* that Johnson has been "hailed as hero, when hedonist might be a better word." Anderson suggested that it was "hardly courageous" for Johnson to go public because "he had no choice. He knew he couldn't possibly cover up a sudden retirement." The next day, also in the sports pages of the *Times*, columnist Robert Lipsyte (1991) wondered whether Johnson wasn't "exactly the worst kind of role model for young men." He had dropped out of college, had fathered a child out of wedlock (Johnson has a young son living with the boy's mother in Michigan), and had "been sexually promiscuous without protection."

After shock, hero hype, and second thoughts, the media's final act was equally predictable. The supermarket papers produced the inevitable women who claimed to be among Johnson's sexual partners. Many members of the public had little difficulty dismissing the tabloid stories on the grounds that someone can be found to say anything when paid enough money; sometimes, simply having their picture in the paper is sufficient. Should protracted lawsuits alleging disease or death arise, however, the mainstream press and the Johnson fans will have a harder and harder time standing firm. How he fares in the public eye over time will depend on which Johnson the public sees, the saint or the sinner.

SUMMING UP: AIDS NEWS AND "PEOPLE" NEWS

The AIDS story line has moved erratically, as we have seen, with elements of information and entertainment intermixed. At times the level of excitement in some of the coverage has made it hard to determine where medical urgency ends and the media's own commercial considerations begin. Media coverage of AIDS has significantly increased during the last 10 years. Both the national media and the smaller news outlets cover the subject now; the AIDS narrative is no longer confined to alternative newspapers and publications intended for a homosexual audience, as it was in the early 1980s.

And yet, considering the tragedy of AIDS, coverage is still disappointing. By March 1, 1992, about 135,000 Americans had died from AIDS—a figure based only on cases reported to the Centers for Disease Control—and more than 1,000,000 had been infected with the HIV virus. But much of the media continues to focus disproportionately on the dramatic, resulting in infotainment sometimes and uninformed hysteria other times. This is due partly to the media's need to find new sensations rather than offer more of the same. Sadly, the fact that many mainstream readers and viewers have an appetite for such material makes it easier for much of the media to avoid learning the lessons they might have learned after 10 years of the AIDS experience.

REFERENCES

Altman, L. K. (1985, July 30). Search for AIDS drug is case history in frustration. *New York Times,* p. C1.

Anguished testimony. (1991, October 7). *Time,* p. 27.

Clark, M., with Coleman, F. (1985, August 5). AIDS exiles in Paris. *Newsweek,* p. 68.

Cohen, R. (1985, July 27). A star gets AIDS. *Washington Post,* Section A, p. 23.

Diamond, E. (1991). *The media show: The changing face of the news, 1985–1990.* Cambridge, MA: MIT Press.

Editorial. (1991, October 8). *New York Newsday.*

Ehrenfeld, T. (1991, October 14). AIDS heroes and villains. *Newsweek,* p. 10.

Gelman, D., & Reese, M. (1985, August 5). AIDS strikes a star. *Newsweek,* p. 65.

Hall, C. (1985a, July 24). Hudson gravely ill. *Washington Post,* Section B, p. 1.

Hall, C. (1985b, July 27). Sympathy in the gay community: Hudson illness expected to put spotlight on AIDS. *Washington Post,* Section G, p. 1.

Hall, C., & Rovner, S. (1985, July 26). Rock Hudson being treated for AIDS. *Washington Post,* Section A, p. 1.

Hilts, P. J. (1991, September 27). AIDS victim urges Congress to enact testing bill. *New York Times,* p. A8.

I blame every one of you bastards. (1991, July 1). *Newsweek,* p. 52.

Ill treatment. (1985, August 7). *Wall Street Journal,* p. 16.

Johnson, H. (1985, July 28). Facing reality with Rock Hudson. *Washington Post,* Section A, p. 3.

Johnson, B., & Grant, M., with Sider, D. (1990, October 22). A life stolen early. *People,* pp. 72–78.

Johnson, B., & Grant, M. (1991, October 14). Kim's brave journey. *People,* pp. 44–45.

Kantrowitz, B. (1991, July 1). Doctors and AIDS: Should patients and doctors have the right to know each other's HIV status? *Newsweek,* p. 49.

Kinsella, J. (1989). *Covering the plague—AIDS and the American media.* New Brunswick, NJ: Rutgers University Press.

Lambert, B. (1991, December 9). Kimberly Bergalis is dead at 23; symbol of debate over AIDS tests. *New York Times,* p. D9.

Palmer, T. (1991, November 13). Magic's impact tied to infection source. *Boston Globe,* p. 1.

Prial, F. J. (1985, July 31). AIDS program gives hope to Americans. *New York Times,* p. A10.

Rock Hudson AIDS case sends a message. (1985, August 5). *U.S. News and World Report,* p. 12.

Weisberg, J. (1991, October 21). The accuser: Kimberly Bergalis, AIDS martyr. *The New Republic,* p. 12.

Chapter Eight

Crisis in Communication: Coverage of Magic Johnson's AIDS Disclosure

J. Gregory Payne
Kevin A. Mercuri

Our idea was to have Magic answer questions from kids about his health, his future and his fears, and tell them what he thought was important to know. We felt we could inform kids—and help them to feel better about what had happened to Magic Johnson. This part was important. He was their hero. He could show them how a hero behaves. He could show us all. ("Magic, TV and Kids," 1992, p. 8).

Four months after the shocking November 7th, 1991, announcement by Earvin "Magic" Johnson that he was infected with the human immunodeficiency virus (HIV), *TV Guide* heralded "A Conversation with Magic" (1992), a special featuring the "basketball superstar . . . and a dozen kids in a frank discussion about AIDS" (p. 8).

Since his announcement, Johnson's condition has been a focal point of in-depth stories in newspapers, magazines, and special programs on television throughout the world. And while millions previously had acknowledged the disease's deadly verdict with the deaths of Rock Hudson, Halston, Ryan White, and others, the news that Magic Johnson was HIV positive spawned open dis-

We extend our appreciation to the Division of Communication Studies at Emerson College and the Political News Study Group for assisting in the preparation of this chapter. Specifically, our thanks to Jeremy Milner for his work as a primary research associate. In addition, Aktina I. Daigle was invaluable in the final preparation of the manuscript, as was Christopher Mann. Jane Borrowman provided her expertise in preparing the graphs on newspaper coverage. And to the admirals of the ship of state, our special thanks to Diego Salazar and Karen Asaro for their loyalty and support.

cussion among people of all ages on the dangers of acquired immune deficiency syndrome (AIDS).

Dialogue on transmission of and protection against the virus widened to include groups previously prone to believe the disease would never strike them or strike down superstar athletes like Magic Johnson. The day after his announcement, Johnson began what has characterized his actions since the November announcement: a proactive campaign against the spread of AIDS. In a highly emotional moment, Johnson appealed to young people to practice safe sex in a special appearance on November 8, 1991 on the late-night talk show of his friend Arsenio Hall.

Even though the initial coverage of the announcement reflected shock, sympathy, and compassion for Johnson's condition, subsequent stories in both the print and electronic media took on a less sympathetic tone. Johnson's hero status was called into question. National coverage included details of Johnson's fast-paced life-style, outlining in vivid detail wild parties and numerous group sexual encounters with the NBA superstar. There also was speculation and innuendo in news reports that perhaps Johnson had not contracted the virus through sexual encounters involving women. According to such speculation, the NBA superstar was bisexual and had contracted the AIDS virus through homosexual contact, a charge that Johnson repeatedly has denied in various articles and interviews.

Johnson's character and his superstar status have withstood such attacks in the mediated reality presented to millions. Last winter he not only participated in the NBA All-Star game, he won the coveted Most Valuable Player Award, once again dazzling his fans. Furthermore, his Nickelodeon cable television special that aired nationally in March 1992 received positive reviews, and there are plans for the show to be rerun and available on cassette for classroom use throughout the country. Since November 1991, Johnson has traveled throughout the country speaking to young people on the perils of AIDS. His appearance on the 1992 Olympic Dream Team in Barcelona further emphasized his optimistic outlook toward his AIDS condition.

The developments of the Johnson AIDS story in the mediated reality presented to the public provoke several intriguing questions: Were there notable differences in print coverage of the story during the initial weeks following the announcement, the intense period of impression formation for the public? Intrinsically, did such coverage reflect a particular tone or bias? What effect, if any, did the HIV-positive revelation have on Johnson's ethos or image as presented in such coverage? Were there notable turning points in the evolution of the story that helped shape the public's opinion of Johnson?

PURPOSE

In an effort to shed light on these and other queries, we conducted an analysis of the coverage of the Johnson AIDS revelation adopting a method similar to that previously used to examine questions regarding the press coverage of Jesse Jackson in the 1984 presidential campaign (Payne, Ratzan, & Baukus, 1989). Given our interest in noting any regional differences in print coverage, we examined selected print media during the first month after Johnson's disclosure. The *New York Times,* the *Boston Globe,* the *San Francisco Examiner,* the *Denver Post,* and *USA Today* were chosen because of their regional as well as editorial value.

Content analyses were performed in the following areas

1 The *number of column inches* generated on the Johnson story over the first month.

2 *Topics* of stories on Johnson.

3 The *tone* of coverage and the degree of bias toward or against Johnson.

4 The *mediated image,* formed by defining characteristics and descriptive references found in the coverage (i.e., Johnson referred to as a "superstar," "hero," and "AIDS advocate"). Such a mediated image ultimately can shape the story's impact, including, for example, evaluative titles or connotations (positive or negative) by the writer or publication that seek to instill a certain image or tone. Such coverage often reflects an opinion or bias through the use of value-laden words, or represents a reporter's penchant to offer an "enlightened opinion," rather than just presenting the facts.

Following a discussion of the results of the analysis, we will apply such fact-rich material to a paradigm in an effort to reveal possible phases of press coverage during the first month after Johnson made his announcement.

METHOD

We examined each of the aforementioned newspapers' daily editions from November 8th (the day after Johnson's announcement) through December 8th. During this initial month, the press coverage centered on Johnson's actual announcement, as well as development and enrichment of the important mediated reality context from which to further view, understand, and render judgments concerning this dramatic event.

In a pilot study, independently coded and cross-examined results of the stories were tabulated by a trained coding team to ensure consistency in categorization. Coders consisted of senior and graduate communication students with training in research methods and familiarity with the process and techniques of content analysis. All coders attended multiple training sessions to guarantee familiarity with the operational definitions of the categorical variables and the rules of classification used in the study. Sample stories were coded and discussed to ensure the reliability of coding procedures.

RESULTS

The total column inches of stories generated are shown in Figures 1 and 2. After brief discussion of the overall coverage of the Johnson HIV story, the topics, tone, and mediated image found in the coverage are summarized for November 8th, 9th, 10th, and the weeks thereafter.

Total Coverage of the Johnson Story

Of the newspapers analyzed in this study, the *Boston Globe* provided the most coverage of Johnson's condition during the month after his announcement. In contrast, the *Denver Post* provided its readers with the least coverage on Johnson's HIV status. It should be pointed out that the majority of the *Globe's* coverage occurred in the first few days of the story's evolution and was placed predominantly in the sports section, reflecting Johnson's leadership of the Boston Celtics' arch-rival basketball team, the Los Angeles Lakers.

The *San Francisco Examiner*, on the other hand, featured more front-page coverage than any other paper. In contrast to the *Globe*, the focus of *Examiner* stories was on the AIDS issue rather than Johnson's NBA career. The *Examiner's* coverage also tended to be more feature oriented rather than short wire-service copy, which characterized other newspapers' approach to the Johnson story. The paper with the most diverse AIDS-related coverage was *USA Today*, which varied its reporting to include Johnson's announcement as well as the impact on condom sales, and other areas of society affected by the AIDS epidemic.

November 8 Daily Editions

Topic All the newspapers we examined conveyed the "American hero" theme in the first day of coverage of Johnson's HIV-positive status. Front-page features included the following headlines: "The NBA's Goodwill Ambassador" (*Globe*), "A Hero Exits With a Smile" (*Examiner*), "His Was the Name of the Game" (*USA Today*).

In contrast to the pessimism that typically permeates AIDS coverage, Johnson's announcement was cast in an optimistic context regarding his future. The *Denver Post,* in reporting on basketball teammate James Worthy's reading a letter from Johnson to Lakers fans at a crowded Forum in Los Angeles, wrote, "The message was pure Magic, straight from the heart and filled with remarkable good humor and positive outlook that have marked his amazing acceptance of cruel truth" ("The gift of Magic remains with us," p. 10).

Also evident in the first day's coverage was speculation that the end of Johnson's stellar basketball career, brought on by the HIV disclosure, would indeed translate into a beginning of another superstar effort: Johnson emerging as a major spokesperson for AIDS awareness. The *Globe* reported Johnson

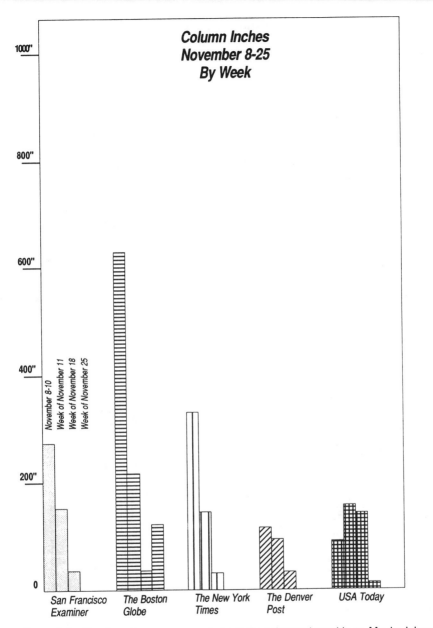

Figure 8-1 Number of newspaper column inches devoted weekly to Magic Johnson's disclosure that he is HIV positive in the month following the disclosure.

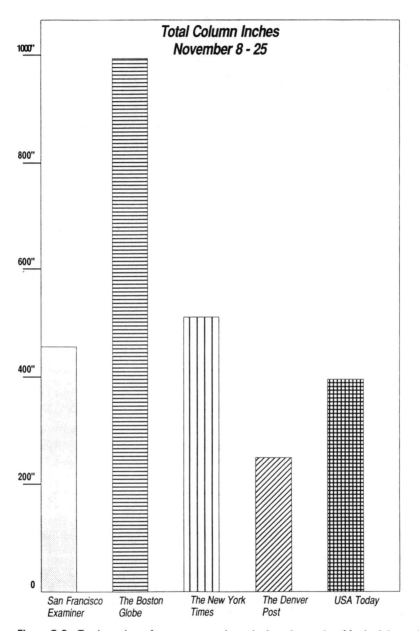

Figure 8-2 Total number of newspaper column inches devoted to Magic Johnson's disclosure that he is HIV positive in the month following the disclosure.

would be the "NBA's goodwill ambassador" ("Star, 'Healthy Now,' to Speak Out About Illness to Youth," p. 1), thereby furthering understanding of the AIDS crisis among people of all ages.

Tone   In contrast to the positive tone that characterized coverage in each of the other papers, the *Denver Post* introduced doubt and concern about Johnson's revelation and wondered about its potential effect on his ethos. On the same day in which the *Globe* predicted an immediate transformation from superstar to superspokesperson, the *Post* suggested that the ultimate judgment was still out as to Johnson's future status within the public. A *Post* article by Mark Kiszia entitled, "Will Illness Smear His Reputation?" posed the following question to Denver readers:

> And now he is HIV positive, a dangerous affliction many people still regard as punishment for sins of sex or drugs. After the initial shock subsides, will sports fans offer Johnson sympathy or disdain? (p. 1D)

In contrast, the *Examiner's* coverage left no doubt about Johnson's ethos or his future. From this day forward his would be characterized by a "New Life," with new potential and new energy joining AIDS activists and thousands of the *Examiner's* readership—San Franciscans infected with the HIV virus. Clearly evident in the *Examiner's* coverage was the theme that Johnson's HIV status would have a positive component: "The word is now out. AIDS is not just a disease involving homosexuals, bisexuals, and intravenous drug users. It is a disease that affects us all, even NBA superstars." Evident throughout the *Examiner's* coverage was the implicit theme that Johnson's HIV status further supports the claim that government and society must do more to combat the AIDS menace.

Mediated Image   The most common descriptive reference, or mediated image, of Johnson on the initial day of coverage echoed that found in the *New York Times's* description of Johnson as "a courageous man," a "hero," and an "idol." Such terms dramatically contrast the "victim" image that typically characterize AIDS-related stories on less famous individuals.

November 9 Daily Editions

Topic   Second-day coverage of Johnson's HIV status focused on the positive ramifications of such an announcement. Stories echoed the theme that Johnson was the ideal rhetorical icon, communicating the AIDS message to various audiences.

All the newspapers we examined featured stories on Johnson's appearance on the Arsenio Hall show the evening after his press conference. The primary topic of articles examined was Johnson's rhetorical promise: His safe sex message, writers concluded, could translate into millions of lives—especially those of young people—being saved from AIDS.

The most fervent voice of this particular theme, as one might expect given its large gay community, was the *San Francisco Examiner*. In an article entitled "A Message That Works Its Own Kind of Magic" (p. 1), numerous people on the street praised Johnson for his decision to be an advocate for AIDS prevention. One reader even cited a divine impetus for the entire incident: "I am sorry about Magic, but I guess it is true, God always sends a messenger. He will be able to do things that no one else can do" (p. D3). In addition, Joan Ryan, columnist for the *Examiner*, credited Johnson for "stripping the disease of its shame" (p. D3).

In seeking to assess the shock and sadness brought on by Johnson's announcement, the *Los Angeles Times* ("Carrying the Suffering in His Strong Arms," p. 1) included a quote from Major Tom Bradley, who compared Johnson's revelation to the shooting of President Kennedy in terms of its impact on the general population.

Examination of topics included in the second day of coverage revealed several interesting trends:

Tone   The day after his announcement, the tone of the stories in the newspapers we examined continued to be positive. The *New York Times* praised Johnson for his "courageous leadership" ("Magic Johnson as President," p. 12). The positive tone that pervaded coverage is best exemplified by the comment that Johnson's forthright announcement was the type of decisive action that one would expect of a president of the United States (p. 12).

The *Times* did print a story quoting Johnson as admitting that he had "been messing around with too many women" ("Day Later, It Remains a Shock Felt Around the World," p. 33), but such themes (which eventually would evolve into major topics) did not command the spotlight at this early stage of the Johnson story.

Mediated Image   The image of Johnson as a crusader against the spread of AIDS continued to emerge in the second day of coverage. The *Examiner* recounted Johnson's appearance on the Arsenio Hall Show with a photo and headline, "Magic Takes Crusade to the Air."

Another article further substantiated the positive impact of Johnson's leadership in the AIDS crisis, albeit in a strictly business-oriented perspective. Headlined "Magic Has Impact on Wall Street," the article outlined how stock in Trojan and Carter-Wallace, America's largest condom manufacturers, surged on Wall Street following Johnson's revelation.

In a *USA Today* story, Johnson's decision to be a spokesperson for the AIDS epidemic was addressed in a story headlined: "This Is Not Like My Life Is Over." Admiration and compassion for Johnson, major themes during this stage of the coverage, were reflected in an editorial in the *Times* ("Magic, Now and Forever"), which praised Johnson's leadership and honesty in dealing with his condition.

November 10 Daily Editions

Topic The Sunday editions of all the newspapers offered readers a synopsis of the Johnson-related events that had occurred since the Thursday announcement. The *Boston Globe* offered a historical comparison to Johnson's role as a potential advocate for AIDS education. According to the *Globe*, Johnson could do for AIDS what Lou Gehrig had done for amyotrophic lateral sclerosis (Lou Gehrig's disease) ("The Sorrow is the Same").

Offering more specificity on a related issue, the *Examiner* focused on AIDS victims of color in an article entitled "Cases by Race."

Tone There continued to be a generally positive tone in the coverage of Johnson. The *Examiner's* headline "Carrying the Suffering in His Strong Arms" suggested the larger-than-life ethos that permeated much of the weekend coverage.

Nonetheless, a tonal change was noted that began to question Johnson's protection from criticism. An example of this was evident in the *Boston Globe's* editorial ("Invisible but No Longer Denied") on the one million other victims who had not basked in the spotlight now afforded to Johnson. The *New York Times* ran a story that reflected growing recognition of Johnson's life-style, headlined "Fast Lane = AIDS Lane."

Mediated Reality Johnson was most frequently referred to as "superstar" and "hero" and as potentially America's Number 1 spokesperson for AIDS prevention.

Week of November 11th

After the first few days of intense media interest on Johnson's HIV status, coverage diminished significantly in all the newspapers we analyzed. Thus, the remainder of this chapter summarizes stories related to Johnson on a weekly basis.

Topic Johnson's condition served as rich context for other AIDS-related stories in the week following his November 7th announcement. For instance, the *New York Times* ("Johnson's Influence a Study of Class") mentioned Johnson in an article focusing on Black ministers who were urging their congregations to practice abstinence in combating the spread of AIDS.

Many articles openly identified Johnson's revelation as an impetus for such journalistic interest on AIDS: "Following Magic Johnson's announcement that he is HIV positive" ("Lakers Slowly Adjusting to Life Without Magic").

Several newspapers contained stories that actually sought to delve beyond Johnson's superstar/spokesperson status to examine his medical condition, as well as to explore the issue of sexual promiscuity in the AIDS epidemic. For example, the *New York Times* focused on Johnson's life-style in a story in which Magic admitted "having unprotected sex with a woman who has the virus. I can't specify the time, the place or the woman, it's a matter of numbers" ("Johnson Talks About Sex Life," p. 39). Another *Times* story entitled "Magic as Hero: It's Not the Most Comfortable Fit," openly questioned the positive accolades heaped on Johnson in media coverage and questioned his personal responsibility in contracting the virus. The *Times* article read, "Think of all the women Johnson may have infected. They will suffer with less support" (p. B17).

Tone   The overall tone within coverage remained upbeat. Yet, serious questions began to emerge about Johnson's character and life-style—issues that would continue to dull his superstar/spokesperson status and the degree of sympathy extended to the former Laker.

For example, the *New York Times* reported that Johnson had formed a committee to assist him in becoming "America's AIDS Ambassador" because everyone was interested in hearing from "Magic and his words of wisdom" ("Johnson Talks About Sex Life," p. B9). Emerging questions about Johnson's life-style were quieted somewhat by the superstar's announcement that he planned to compete in the Olympic games in Barcelona in 1992.

Mediated Reality   Near the end of the first week after Johnson's revelation that he was HIV positive, Johnson's positive mediated image was seriously challenged in selected stories within the examined coverage. Of those newspapers examined, *USA Today* remained the most positive in the mediated reality it offered its readers, with negative data placed well within the story and countered by positive material.

An example of the growing assault on Johnson's credibility is found in a guest columnist headline in the *Examiner*: "Promiscuity Is The Road To Hell." This mood change also was noted in another article in the *Examiner*, which read: "Two columnists Thursday joined in the nationwide praise for Magic Johnson's approach to learning that he is infected with the HIV virus, but were critical of his sexual lifestyle or the reaction by some to it" ("Magic Johnson Named to National AIDS Panel," p. A-4).

A *New York Times* column entitled "Sorry, But Magic Isn't a Hero" also attempted to debunk Johnson's positive ethos:

The dazzle of that smile seems to have blinded some people to the egotistical essence of Earvin Johnson's having tested positive. . . . He has been hailed by many as a "hero" when hedonist might be the better word. (p. B1)

Week of November 18th

USA Today and the *San Francisco Examiner* featured more press coverage of Johnson's HIV status than the other newspapers examined. Coverage dropped sharply in the *New York Times* and the *Boston Globe*, while the *Denver Post* mentioned Johnson only once during the entire week.

Topic A favorite topic of the *Examiner* continued to be Johnson as a healthy and heroic spokesperson with an abiding commitment to lead the way in AIDS prevention. *USA Today* addressed the general AIDS issue on a national level with several related articles. An elaborate discussion regarding premarital sex was featured in the paper's "Today's Debate" section on November 19, peppered with references to Johnson's revelation.

A major forum for Johnson-related stories appeared in special letters-to-the-editor sections of *USA Today* and the *Examiner*. Generally negative, readers referred to Johnson's "scandalous behavior" and pointed out that the goal was not safe sex but "safe people." There were also related stories in most of the papers on Johnson's past sexual encounters and on rumors, denied by Johnson, that he was bisexual.

Tone The second week of coverage witnessed further confirmation of a mood change regarding Johnson. As well as praise for his candor, he received criticism of his fast-paced life-style, which was covered in vivid detail.

Mediated Reality The reality of Johnson's condition and his responsibility for it emerged as factors that affected the mediated reality during this time period. Skepticism about his ability to be a national spokesperson was voiced. *USA Today* told readers, "educators dismiss Johnson's usefulness [in combating AIDS] as a knee-jerk reaction" (Magic's HIV Affects Health Educators' Game Plans," p. 8D). The reality of Johnson's long-term AIDS prognosis also emerged in discussion of his AZT treatment. On page 1 of the *Denver Post* was the following quote from a teen: "It really hurts me. If you really think about it, a part of him has died."

Week of November 25th

Coverage of the Johnson story decreased among all the newspapers examined. There were no related stories in the *Times* or *Examiner*. The *Boston Globe* featured more Johnson-related coverage than any of the other papers during this time period.

Topic   *USA Today* continued to feature stories with references to Johnson's HIV status. For example, in an article on sexual practices in the AIDS era an individual states, "Magic Johnson's announcement . . . has further chilled our sexual fervor" ("More Remote Sources of Satisfaction," p. 1).

The *Boston Globe* contained several related article placed in both the sports and health sections. Topics included memories of his basketball career, abstinence, and the Los Angeles Lakers' party scene, as told through the experiences of a Lakers' groupie.

Tone   Coverage continued to reflect an objective, yet increasingly human approach. With the exception of the *Boston Globe's* account of the Lakers' party scene, Johnson became more of a contextual part of stories on the AIDS crisis rather than the focus of the story.

Mediated Reality   References to Johnson as a hero continued to fade in the decreasing amount of coverage on the topic. One possible positive result from the media's focus on Johnson's HIV condition was that, according to a *USA Today* article, Americans have decreased their sexual fervor since his announcement ("More Remote Sources of Satisfaction").

Week of December 2nd

The downward spiral of Johnson-related stories continued among all newspapers examined.

Topic   Stories in *USA Today* and the *Denver Post* addressed the proposed meeting between Johnson and President Bush to discuss Johnson's potential as the nation's official ambassador against the AIDS epidemic. There also were related stories in which Johnson denied that he was suffering from any immediate health problems related to his AZT treatment. Other papers, including the *Boston Globe*, featured stories that referenced Johnson as part of the general AIDS context.

Tone   The objective tone continued to be evident. Focus of the coverage turned to Johnson's condition and the positive outlook rather than his persona or ethos as a superstar, themes that had once commanded the spotlight.

Mediated Reality   Johnson emerged as a credible, humane spokesperson for AIDS prevention.

DISCUSSION

This analysis of selected newspaper coverage of Magic Johnson's announcement that he was HIV positive and the subsequent stories on this topic during the following weeks reveals interesting findings, as well as possible phases of press coverage of this newsworthy event.

We detected differences in the amount of coverage as well as the tone and mediated image conveyed in Johnson-related stories. The *San Francisco Examiner*, possibly reflecting the interests and values of its large gay audience, was the most positive in tone and in the mediated image it offered its readers. All of the other newspapers except the *Denver Post* offered numerous features on the event and aftermath; the *Denver Post* carried the fewest Johnson-related stories. In addition, writers for the *Post* were more critical of Johnson in the coverage they did devote to his story. As with any topic, the *Post's* noncoverage of the Johnson story communicates a particular message regarding specific editorial policy, especially considering the amount of space devoted to the story in the other newspapers.

We also noted a general distinctive change in tone among the newspapers as the Johnson story evolved. In the immediate wake of his November 7 announcement, coverage was sympathetic, almost excessive, in portraying Johnson as a hero caught in the modern-day web of the AIDS tragedy. As the shock of the tragedy subsided, however, coverage centered on the context in which Johnson acquired the virus. Varying in the degree of interest and coverage of his purported fast-track life-style, the newspapers we examined projected a less glowing mediated image of the NBA superstar. However, through the media hype of the initial announcement, the outpouring of sympathy, and the scrutiny of the media, Johnson's ethos survived. The American public ultimately viewed Johnson as a persuasive force in combatting the spread of AIDS.

The Confirmation Paradigm

This study has revealed similar phases of press coverage of the Johnson story to those outlined in Payne et al.'s (1989) Confirmation of a Candidate paradigm, designed to assess media coverage of political figures in campaigns. Application of this perspective to the Johnson story can possibly provide a better understanding of the dynamics of such special press events.

According to Payne et al. (1989), political candidates proceed through five distinct phases in the course of a campaign. These include announcement, definition, debunking, judgment, and conversion. Specifically, the announcement phase characterizes the time period in which a candidate declares he or she is seeking office. During this period, press coverage tends to be positive, with the particular focus on reporting the actual announcement event.

In the definition phase, particular issues are associated with the candidate, as revealed in speeches and past and present actions. The tone of coverage begins to reflect an attitudinal disposition toward the candidate.

Debunking is the third phase of the confirmation paradigm. It is in this crucial period that a particular issue is contested by the public, or raised by the press, that questions the propriety of the candidate's past or present behavior, character, or stands on particular issues. The mediated image, as projected in the coverage, reflects the issue's importance to the candidate's survival. Coverage centers on this crucial topic, further defining the voting issue that ultimately will determine the candidate's viability and staying power in the campaign.

Judgment, the fourth phase, involves deliberation on the candidate's actions or inaction toward the charges or issues raised in the debunking phase. Once the judgment is rendered by the pubic or other agent, it is reflected in the tone of the newspaper coverage of the candidate. The mediated image offered during this phase generally reflects the public's decision on the candidate's performance on the contested issue. Newspapers do, however, often color such images according to their own agendas and biases. If a candidate does not meet the mediated burden of proof to the satisfaction of the public or other agent, as reflected in the coverage during the judgment phase, he or she no longer is presented as a viable candidate and quickly fades from coverage.

The final phase of the confirmation paradigm, limited to those candidates who do emerge victorious from the mediated debunking/judgment battle, is conversion. In the conversion phase, the candidate is recognized as having met the mediated test and has emerged as a viable and serious contender.

The evidence suggests that the coverage of Magic Johnson's announcement that he was HIV-positive reflects the steps of the Confirmation paradigm. Some general comments on Johnson's experience of the phases are offered below.

Application of the Confirmation Paradigm to the Magic Johnson AIDS Story

Announcement   The announcement phase of the Magic Johnson story characterized the weekend coverage of November 8th to the 10th. During this time, press coverage primarily was concerned with detailing the news that Johnson was HIV positive. The tone of the coverage and the mediated image were both extremely positive.

Definition   The definition phase occurred during the first full week of coverage and was characterized by the emergence of Johnson's mediated image as a potential superstar spokesperson for AIDS prevention. Johnson was described as a "hero" and an "idol" who, because of his high credibility and star quality, would bring the AIDS message to those who previously had ignored its danger.

Debunking   The debunking phase began almost immediately with the *Denver Post's* coverage of Johnson's announcement that he was HIV positive. Yet, analysis of the coverage reveals that the debunking was initiated by Johnson's admission that he was guilty of "messing around with too many women" and "accommodating as many women" as he could. Issues of personal responsibility and character were now raised. All coverage that we examined contained elements of debunking Johnson's credibility by pointing out the personal faults that led to his contracting the AIDS virus.

Judgment   Examination of the coverage suggests that despite the attacks on his character and reports of questionable sexual encounters, Johnson survived the debunking process with minimal damage to his ethos.

Conversion   Having been judged to be an able spokesperson in fighting the AIDS epidemic, Johnson emerged as a national symbol and spokesperson against the spread of AIDS. An abiding characteristic evident in Johnson's mediated image and the tone of coverage is Johnson's courage in going public with the news of his condition and his subsequent work in educating the public about AIDS.

SUMMARY

This analysis of selected news coverage of Magic Johnson's announcement that he was HIV positive provides provocative insights into how the press performs in such a special situation involving a national hero and a dreaded disease. Johnson's decision to go public, to personally make the announcement of his condition, initiated the flurry of press activity, the potential effect of which was the positive mediated image that continues to be associated with Johnson.

The controversy surrounding *USA Today's* report in April 1992 that tennis great Arthur Ashe is suffering from AIDS presents an interesting opportunity for a comparable study on press coverage in which the questionable issue was raised by an external agent—in this instance, the press. Such investigations provide better understanding of the role and ethics of reporting such events to a public growing more aware of the global impact of the AIDS crisis.

REFERENCES

Payne, J. G., Ratzan, S. C., & Baukus, R. B. (1989). National newspaper analysis of the press coverage of Jesse Jackson's 1984 presidential campaign: The confirmation of the candidate. *Explorations in Ethnic Studies, 12,*(2), 35–52.

TV Guide, March 21–27, 1992. "Magic, TV and Kids," Linda Ellerbee, p. 8.

TV Guide, March 21–27. "Should Sports Heroes be Role Models at all?", Ira Berkow, p. 12.

San Francisco Examiner

November 8, 1991
"A hero exits with a smile," Skip Myslenski and Jorge Casuso, p. 1.
"Johnson to sell HIV awareness," Carla Marinucci, p. 1.
"AIDS Community has a new champion," Lisa Krieger, p. 1.
"Johnson: Profile in courage," (column) Ray Ratto, p. D-1.
"It can happen to anyone, even Magic," (column) Matt Spander, p. D-1.
"Magic had a truly heroic basketball career," Associated Press, p. D-4.
"Warriors predict change in lifestyle," John Hillyer, p. D-4.
"Reeves worried about AIDS," Examiner Staff, p. D-2.
"Other notable victims of AIDS," Associated Press, p. A-18.
"News of Magic's condition stuns his young fans," Larry Maatz and Charles Handy, p. A-18.

November 9, 1991
"Magic takes crusade to the air," Ken Peters, p. 1.
"Magic has impact on wall street," Charolette-Anne Lewis, p. A-18.
"Lakers' hearts not in it," John Nadel, p. B-1.

November 10, 1991
"A message that worked its own kind of Magic," Lisa Krieger and Jane Garrison, p. 1.
"Carrying the suffering in his strong arms," (column) Joan Ryan, p. 1.
"AIDS Cases by Race" (chart), p. A-22.

November 11, 1991
"Magic a candidate for AIDS commission," Associated Press, p. A-2.
"Lakers get back to winnin' time at the forum," Associated Press, p. C-3.

November 12, 1991
"Heterosexual transmission of HIV rising," Lisa Krieger, p. 1.
"Magic creates stir in the business world," Associated Press, p. B-3.
"AIDS' deadly legacy" (inset), p. A-12.

November 14, 1991
"Promiscuity is the road to hell," (column) Patrick Buchannan, p. A-17.
"God has yet to create a better HIV teacher" (column), Christopher Matthews, p. A-17.

November 15, 1991
"Magic moment," Examiner Staff, p. 1.
"Magic will be at Olympics as guest if not participant," Examiner Staff, p. C-3.

November 16, 1991
"Magic Johnson named to national AIDS panel," Associated Press, p. A-4.
"Two guys who couldn't be more different," Steve Bisheff, p. D-1.
"Readers react to Magic Johnson's bombshell," Sports Mailbag section, p. D-3.

November 18, 1991
"Magic's presence inspires Lakers," Associated Press, p. D-2.
"Letters to the Editor," p. A-14.

November 20, 1991
"Magic exam: No sign of AIDS," Associated Press, p. D-2.
"Magic resolution opposed," Associated Press, p. D-2.

The Denver Post

November 8, 1991
"Magic: I have HIV." *New York Times* article, p. 1.
"Say it ain't so" (column), Dick Conner, p. 1.
"Celebrities who died of AIDS" (inset), p. A-20.
"A Primer on AIDS" (inset), p. A-20.
"The gift of Magic remains with us" (column), Woody Paige, p. 1D.
"The illness smear his reputation?" Mark Kisza, p. 1D.
"Knicks roll to victory after prayer for magic," *Denver Post* Wire Service, p. 3D.
"Westhead: Magic faces game of lifetime," Donna Carter, p. 4D.
"Report stunning to fans," Mike Monroe, p. 4D.
"Shock waves sent through league," *Denver Post* Wire Service, p. 4D.

November 9, 1991
"Magic: A New Chapter," *Denver Post* Wire Service, p. 1.
"AIDS shock works magic on teens," Janet Bingam and Stacey Baca, p. 1.

November 11, 1991
"Bush may add Magic to AIDS board," Marlene Cimons, p. 3A.

November 13, 1991
"Nonsense erupts as America absorbs Magic Johnson's AIDS revelation" (column),
    Patrick Buchannan, p. 11A.
"Do you believe in Magic?" (column), Cal Thomas, p. 11A.
"That Magic Johnson smile is real" (column), Anna Quindlen, p. 13A.
"Maybe Magic will get the message to us" (column), Arthur Caplan, p. 13A.

November 14, 1991
"Olympics give Johnson big welcome," Staff, p. 1D.
"Disease grabs attention of Broncos," Jim Armstrong, p. 1D.

USA Today

November 8, 1991
"HIV forces Magic to retire; 'This is not like my life is over,'" Greg Boek, p. 1.
"His was the name of the game," David DuPree, p. 1.
"Reactions mix emotion with sense of purpose," USA Staff, p. 1.

"Positive HIV test forces retirement," Michael Hurd, p. 1.

"Networks ponder future of NBA without Magic," USA Staff, p. 1C.

"Doctor says source of virus unknown," USA Staff, p. 2C.

"Children need help in coping with news," Anita Manning, p. 2C.

"AIDS education gains eloquent spokesman," Kim Painter, p. 2C.

"Teens: time to act," Karen S. Peterson, p. 2C.

"At least 1 million in USA HIV infected," USA Staff, p. 2C.

"After disbelief and discomfort, a new disposition" (column), Peter Vecsey, p. 26.

November 11, 1991

"Some questions don't deserve answers" (column), Janice Lloyd, p. 10A.

"Connie Chung draws out her 'old friend' Magic," USA Staff, p. 1B.

"Johnson ideal for AIDS panel," USA Staff, p. 1C.

"Mandatory testing by teams begs questions about motives" (column), Len Elmore, p. 10C.

"Announcement should awaken minorities" (column), Anita Taylor, p. 10C.

"Rumors fly about Magic but the motives are selfish" (column), Peter Vecsey, p. 10C.

"HIV-infected workers get little support," Julia Lawlor, p. 1D.

November 13, 1991

"Magic tells his side, denies bisexual rumors," USA Staff, p. 1C.

"Clippers set to steal some of the Lakers' thunder," USA Staff, p. 8A.

November 14, 1991

"The name of the game is sex," USA Staff, p. 1.

"Magic ads target teens," Martha T. Moore, p. 1.

"Promiscuity risky business for athletes," Greg Boek and Mike Dodd, p. 1.

"Analyses: AIDS related stocks' fall will continue," Gary Strauss, p. 13B.

"Magic still welcome," USA Staff, p. 2C.

November 15, 1991

"Magic's disclosure hits home," Kim Painter, p. 1D.

"Mail for Magic overwhelms Lakers," USA Staff, p. 9C.

"Writers contest reaction," USA Staff, p. 9C.

November 18, 1991

"Magic back to cheer Lakers on," Lisa Dillman, p. 1C.

November 19, 1991

"Condoms, schools: A civics lesson. Battle rages over safe sex versus abstinence," Mimi Hall, p. 1.

"Outrage greets Washington plan," Deanne Glamser, p. 1.

"Magic's HIV affects health educators' game plans," Marybeth Marklein and Robin DeRosa, p. 8D.

"Reaction is wide-ranging," USA Staff, p. 8D.

"How schools tackle the subject," USA Staff, p. 8D.

"Condoms make sex safer," USA Staff, p. 12A.

"Save sex for marriage," Beverly LaHaye, p. 12A.

"Magic Show" (column), USA Staff, p. 1C.

"Nascar drivers say they'd keep HIV quiet," Beth Tuschak, p. 3C.

November 21, 1991
"Women support Martina's stand," Greg Boek, p. 4C.
"Dual standard seen on sex," USA Staff, p. 4C.
"Ad agency people agree on disparity," Michael Heestand, p. 4C.
"Public attitude seems to be 'good guys' vs 'bad guys,'" Greg Boek, p. 4C.

November 26, 1991
"More remote resources of satisfaction," Elizabeth Snead, p. 1.

December 5, 1991
"Magic won't attend meeting with Bush," David Leon Moore, p. 1C.
"Agent says Magic 'fine,' blasts cancellation report," David DePree, p. 1.

December 8, 1991
"Magic courts readers: autobiography, safe-sex book," Diedre Donahue, p. 1.

New York Times

November 8, 1991
"Basketball star retires on advice of his doctors," Richard Stevenson, p. 1.
"Magic Johnson's legacy," Ira Burkow, p. B11.
"Riley fights to keep poise," Harvey Araton, p. B11.
"A career of impact, a player with heart," Clifton Brown, p. B11.
"Studies cite 10.5 years from infection to illness," Gina Kolata, p. B12.
"Magic's loud message for young black men," Michael Specter, p. B12.
"The sports world, although stunned, takes the message," Robert Thomas Jr., p. B13.
"Athletes endorsement may now be in doubt," NYT Staff, p. B13.

November 9, 1991
"Magic, now and forever" (column), Tom McMillen, p. 13.
"Magic Johnson as President," op-ed piece, Staff, p. 12.
"Believe in Magic," op-ed piece, Staff, p. 12.
"Proposal seeks to speed up federal approval of drugs," Philip J. Hilts, p. 10.
"Johnson will get drug treatment to fight virus," Lawrence K. Altman, p. 33.
"Day later, it remains a shock felt around the world," Robert Thomas Jr., p. 33.
"Leagues remain cautious on conducting HIV tests," Gerald Eskanazi, p. 33.

November 10, 1991
"Fast lane could mean AIDS lane," Harvey Araton, p. C1.
"A jarring reveille for sports" (column), Robert Lipsyte, p. C1.
"The plague finally reaches the box scores," George Vecsey, p. C4.

November 11, 1991
"Johnson souvenirs skyrocket in price," NYT Staff, p. 2C.

November 12, 1991
"After Magic, the extra mile," op-ed piece, p. 13.
"Johnson's influence a study of class," Harvey Araton, p. B12.

"Bush asks Johnson to join AIDS panel," Philip J. Hilts, p. B12.

November 13, 1991
"For anyone but Johnson," Jane Gross, p. 18.
"Keep Magic in the mainstream," Dave Anderson, p. B7.
"Lakers slowly adjusting to life without Magic," Michael Martinez, p. B7.
"Johnson talks about sex life," Associated Press, p. B9.

November 14, 1991
"Sorry, but Magic isn't a hero," Dave Anderson, p. B1.

November 15, 1991
"Magic as hero: it's just not the most comfortable fit," Robert Lipsyte, p. B17.

November 16, 1991
"Johnson agrees to join commission on AIDS," NYT Staff, p. 32.

November 17, 1991
Mailbox section of the *New York Times,* p. 21.

November 21, 1991
"Magic, Quayle and a message," Dave Anderson, p. B13.
"Lakers riding high with Magic at their side," NYT Staff, p. B19.

November 28, 1991
"Back surgery sidelines Dival 6–8 weeks," NYT Staff, p. B20.

December 4, 1991
"Warning on AIDS surprises NHL," Robert Thomas Jr., p. B18.

December 5, 1991
"Canada's time of reckoning on AIDS," John F. Burns, p. B21.

December 6, 1991
"3 Books by Magic Johnson," NYT Staff, B3.
"Montreal coach, an ex-cop, deals with AIDS threat," Joe Lapointe, B3.

December 17, 1991
"HIV tests up 60% since the disclosure from Magic Johnson," Calvin Sims, p. 1.

The Boston Globe

November 8, 1991
"Star, 'healthy now,' to speak out about illness to youth" Jackie Macmullan, p. 1.
"Young hoop players voice sorrow, disbelief," Diego Ribadeneira, p. 1.
"A lesson about vulnerability hits Americans hard," Joseph P. Cahn, p. 1.
"Text of Johnson's speech," *Globe* Staff, p. 56.
"A great star and a good guy" (column), Bob Ryan, p. 51.
"He'll never be as attractive to advertisers," Kimberly Blanton, p. 54.
"Finals chapters climaxed legendary rivalry," Peter May, p. 54.
"Some Magic moments," Staff, p. 54.

"The revelation brought the NBA to a standstill," Jackie Macmullan, p. 53.
"Grieving is unbelievable" (column), Michael Madden, p. 51.
"Auerbach expresses sadness and concern," Will Mcdonough, p. 55.

November 9, 1991
"Now AIDS shadows the pros," Mark Blaudschun, p. 1.
"Magic opens a window on AIDS," Philip Bennet, p. 1.
"Students jolted into talk of disease," Peggy Hernandez, p. 8.
"AIDS information lines swamped," *Globe* Staff, p. 8.
"Insurers rely on AIDS testing," Doug Bailey, p. 9.
"A friend's pain hits home to Bird" (column), Dan Shaughnessy, p. 29.
"Patriots mull AIDS testing" *Globe* Staff, p. 29.
"He may wait to gain fame" (column), Will Mcdonough, p. 29.
"Lakers, Magic despite the grief," Peter May, p. 29.
"Ailing star appears on Hall show," Bob Duffy, p. 29.

November 10, 1991
"Experts discuss retirement issue," Delores Kong, p. 31.
"Friends, fans express support," Robin Romano, p. 34.
"How the virus is transmitted and how to minimize the risk," Delores Kong, p. 1.
"Spaulding, Converse noncommittal on plans," Associated Press, p. 28.
"Magic Johnson gave AIDS prevention a needed jolt," Richard A. Knox, p. 28.
"The sorrow is the same" (column), Bob Ryan, p. 55.
"First impressions—and lasting impact" (column), Michael Madden, p. 55.
"Dancers raise cash for AIDS committee," *Globe* Staff, p. 37.
"Invisible but no longer denied" (column), Mike Barnicle, p. 32.
"Now, off the court, a chance for Johnson to perform some other Magic" (column),
    Derrik Z. Jackson, p. A35.
"In the AIDS fight, a Magic moment," op-ed piece, Staff, p. 34.

November 11, 1991
"Back home, LA plays on," Peter May, p. 39.
"AIDS post may go to Magic Johnson," *Globe* Staff, p. 6.

November 12, 1991
"AZT for Johnson," *Globe* Staff, p. 30.
"For heterosexuals, too, AIDS figures are grim," Associated Press, p. 20.

November 13, 1991
"Magic's impact tied to infection source," Thomas Palmer, p. 10.
"Magic Johnson invited to AIDS summit," Associated Press, p. 10.
"AIDS activists eager to answer the questions," Renee Graham, p. 15.
"Experimental drug offered for pneumonia tied to AIDS," Reuters, p. 15.
"Olympic dream remains in Magic's mind," Pete Goodwin, p. 41.
"A shattered team must cope—and hope," Peter May, p. 41.

November 14, 1991
"Divisions deep on condoms for youth," Don Aucoin, p. 1.
"Two advertisers stick with Magic," Paul Hemp, p. 1.

November 15, 1991
"Advertisers and the AIDS fight," op-ed piece, Staff, p. 20.

November 16, 1991
"Magic Johnson to join national AIDS commission," Rita Beamish, p. 30.

November 18, 1991
"Magic greeted by cheers," Associated Press, p. 37.
"Putting AIDS scourge in perspective," Judy Foreman, p. 25.

November 21, 1991
"Sex talk in the Magic era," Ellen Goodman, p. 25.

November 27, 1991
"Magic's fast lane," John Strege, Donna Wares, James V. Grimaldi, p. 45.
"This groupie wants out of the group," *Globe* Staff, p. 49.

November 28, 1991
"Poll says concern grown on AIDS," *LA Times* Wire Service, p. 10.
"Rockers reassessing fast-lane lifestyles in the age of AIDS," Steve Hochman, p. 45.

November 29, 1991
"Memories of Magic," Staff, p. 70.

November 30, 1991
"Celtics cruise as LA trips up," Peter May, p. 37.
"Magic was gone, but show went on," Dan Shaughnessy, p. 37.

December 2, 1991
"Parents worry about kinds," Patti Doten, p. 30.
"Singles turn cautious," Mark Muro, p. 30.

December 4, 1991
"NHL receives AIDS jolt," Pete Goodwin, p. 77.

December 6, 1991
"Telling kids about AIDS, sex," Barbera E. Melte, p. 37.

Part Three

AIDS: The Cutting Edge of Awareness, Action, and Policy

Chapter Nine

Freedom of the Press to Cover HIV/AIDS: A Clear and Present Danger?

John Marlier

THE PROBLEM

Whatever impact the media coverage of the first decade of the human immuno-deficiency virus (HIV)/acquired immune deficiency syndrome (AIDS) epidemic may have had, it has clearly not been sufficient to limit the spread of HIV infection, and this fact represents a grave threat to the medical and economic security of the United States and the world.

According to the National Commission on AIDS, more than 100,000 Americans had died of AIDS by 1991, more than had been killed in the Korean and Vietnam wars combined, and this figure is expected to rise to more than 350,000 by 1993, as 600,000 new HIV infections also occur (Marwick, 1991). Longer range predictions vary, but even the best-case scenario identified by Johnston and Hopkins (1990) in their analysis of the range of predictions projects 1.5 million HIV-positive cases; 200,000 active AIDS cases; and 863,000 cumulative AIDS deaths in the United States by 2002. Their worst-case scenario projects 14.5 million HIV-positive cases and 1 million active AIDS cases by that date. Their *most likely* scenario is 6 million

HIV-positive cases and 400,000 active AIDS cases by the end of the coming decade.

Johnston and Hopkins (1990) also noted that although half of the HIV infections in the United States by 1990 were in heterosexuals, the majority of heterosexuals were not modifying their sexual practices to protect themselves. They suggest that voluntary universal testing and sexual segregation based on knowledge of who is infected could be better controllers of AIDS than any medical developments in the 1990s. Yet the Centers for Disease Control estimated that 75% of the 1 to 1.5 million HIV-positive persons as of 1991 were not aware of their infection (Findlay, 1991). A majority of male and female high school students report being sexually active, yet in a recent study ("Students Polled," 1992) fewer than a quarter of them reported using a condom during their last experience of intercourse, which is consistent with data from the late 1980s documenting both adolescents' inclination to engage in high-risk sexual and drug-related behaviors and failure to adopt self-protective sexual practices (DiClemente, 1990; Kegeles, Adler, & Irwin, 1988).

These data exemplify the extensive available information that leads inexorably to the conclusion that efforts to date to limit the spread of HIV infection have been insufficient.

With regard to the goal of promoting diagnosis and treatment, the aforementioned fact that as many as 75% of HIV-infected Americans are unaware of their infections is sufficient to show the inadequacy of efforts to date; however, problems in the delivery of adequate care to those who *are* aware of their infections have also been documented (Strauss, Fagerhaugh, Suczek, & Weiner, 1991).

Many public policy issues stimulated by the spread of HIV/AIDS also remain unresolved and largely undebated after a decade of media coverage of the crisis. At the end of 1991 the *Wall Street Journal* was reporting that "people who test positive for HIV, the virus that causes the disease, are finding that their health status often brings discrimination that defies legal remedies" (Lambert, 1991, p. B1) in areas of employment, housing, health care, insurance and personal liberties associated with public health, and even criminal laws—in each case because of an ongoing lack of legislation, settled public policy and regulations, and/or consistent enforcement standards.

Meanwhile, the public policy debate related to HIV/AIDS, to the extent that it has occurred, has centered largely on such red herring questions as whether to ignore the consensus recommendation of the scientific community and spend significant resources on universal HIV testing of health care workers to avoid repetition of a unique single case of transmission (the Bergalis case).

The cumulative impact of these failures to respond effectively on either the individual or collective level to the HIV/AIDS epidemic is threat to the economic as well as the medical security of the United States and the world.

In mid-1991, the *New York Times* reported that the current annual expenditures for treatment of HIV infection in the United States had reached $5.8 billion, with projected increases to $10.4 billion by 1994 (Altman, 1991). Without effective response to limit the spread of the infection, it is only a question of more or less time until American employers recognize the possibility (which has already been recognized in such African nations as Zimbabwe) that "their work forces will be decimated by the deadly disease" ("The World Battles a Deadly Plague," 1992, p. 13), with a consequent depressing effect on economic productivity, even as the burden of financing health care grows. According to the report of the National Commission on AIDS released in the fall of 1991, by as early as the end of 1993, AIDS

> will outstrip all other diseases in years of potential life lost, . . . There is only a little time left to recognize that the threat of HIV is all around us. To have a chance of winning this battle, we must energize our nation and transform indifference into informed action. (Marwick, 1991, p. 2050)

The National Commission's report includes 30 recommendations, one of which is that a national plan for response to the HIV/AIDS epidemic immediately be developed, as has been done in all other developed nations (Marwick, 1991). The remainder of this chapter considers the requirements to be met by such a plan in terms of a public information policy, premised on the conclusion drawn from the foregoing information that nothing less than our national security is at stake if media coverage of HIV/AIDS does not soon stimulate a more effective national response than it has in the past 10 years.

The design of such an effective public information policy requires first a consideration of what types and kinds of information need to be publicly disseminated through the media in order to stimulate effective individual and collective responses to the threat of HIV/AIDS. The questions of how and why unrestricted exercise of the freedom of speech and the press with regard to HIV/AIDS in the United States has failed to elicit such a response can then be addressed. After specific areas have been identified in which media coverage of HIV/AIDS to date has arguably failed to promote, or has hindered, effective responses to HIV/AIDS, it should be possible to identify the necessary components of an effective policy to structure, limit, and/or control public information dissemination about this issue.

WHAT THE PUBLIC NEEDS TO KNOW
ABOUT HIV/AIDS

Any assessment of whether the national interest has been served by the dissemination of information about HIV/AIDS to date must begin with specification of that interest by identifying (a) the kinds of individual behavioral and collective policy/program decisions that are possible or necessary in the face of the HIV/

AIDS epidemic and (b) the types or kinds of information that reasonably could contribute to each citizen's ability to make intelligent individual behavioral choices and/or participate intelligently in the policy debates leading to collective decision making. Then it is necessary to consider whether the presentation of other types or kinds of information, which are superficially related to the HIV/ AIDS epidemic but do not fall into any of the necessary categories of information, has a harmful impact on the efficacy of response to the crisis and ought therefore to be restricted.

With regard to the question of what we can do, individually and collectively, in response to HIV/AIDS, the World Health Organization's General Program Against AIDS provides a reasonable analytic framework. According to Dr. Dorothy Blake of Jamaica, Deputy Director of the Global AIDS Program,

> We have three goals: preventing transmission of the virus, promoting and organizing care for those suffering from the disease, and coordinating international responses to it. ("The Challenge," 1992, p. 11)

On a national level, the first of these is directly applicable as a goal of public information policy and is completely uncontroversial. Nor is there much room for debate with regard to the desirability of disseminating information about diagnostic and treatment options as widely as possible, even if the terms and conditions of their availability are debatable. Furthermore, the information that fits these first two criteria is largely of an objectively factual (as opposed to evaluative or judgmental) type, and the question of just what information is relevant and useful in each of these regards is largely uncontroversial and objectively identifiable by scientific criteria.

Therefore, the arguments justifying Constitutional protection of presentations of diverse viewpoints are relevant almost exclusive to the final information need, which on a national level is to provide maximal input into the debate over a public policy that defines a collective response to the spread of HIV/ AIDS.

Given these informational needs, assessment of the failure of the public information campaign about HIV/AIDS to date to stimulate effective response requires that we examine whether this campaign has

1 Disseminated the information necessary for individuals to make self-interested behavioral decisions that would limit the spread of HIV infection, in a form that promotes such decision making;
2 made available to those at risk information about diagnosis and treatment of HIV infection, in a form that promotes both self-interested use of available treatments and modification of infection-spreading behaviors by infected but undiagnosed individuals; and
3 stimulated informed public policy debate and decision making about HIV/AIDS-related issues such as health care rationing, research priorities, na-

tional health insurance, employment discrimination, housing discrimination, insurance discrimination, etc.

In addition, it is necessary to examine what information has been disseminated that does not serve any of these needs and to consider the impact of such information on individual and collective responses to the HIV/AIDS epidemic.

EFFECTS OF MEDIA COVERAGE
OF HIV/AIDS TO DATE

The fact that large numbers of Americans continue to engage in behaviors that put them at risk of HIV infection does not appear to be the result of factual ignorance about HIV or the means by which it is transmitted. By mid-1991, "extensive research throughout the U.S. indicate(d) that public AIDS awareness among adults is virtually universal" (Brown, 1991, p. 668). Furthermore, most Americans hold accurate beliefs about how the disease is transmitted through sexual intercourse, sharing of hypodermic needles, and contaminated blood transfusion (Knox, 1991). To the extent that the general public is factually misinformed regarding transmission of HIV, that misinformation is reflected in a tendency to see themselves as being even more at risk than they really are of infection through such nonrisky transmission routes as sharing toilet seats, sneezing, sharing water glasses, etc. (KRC Communications Research, 1990). It follows that if factual belief, whether accurate or inaccurate, leads directly to behavioral risk aversion, then even individuals who are at little risk of infection would be modifying their behaviors to reduce their inaccurately perceived higher level of risk.

Unfortunately, there is abundant evidence that a high level of AIDS knowledge does not necessarily lead to safer sex practices or other risk-reducing behavior modification (Baldwin & Baldwin, 1988; Edgar, Freimuth, & Hammond, 1988), apparently because even the best informed individuals tend to consider themselves to be exceptions to the risk that they believe applies to others like themselves (McDermott, Hawkins, Moore, & Cittadino, 1987). In one study of such assessments, for example, more than 60% of college student respondents asserted a belief that heterosexuals had a moderate to high risk of contracting AIDS, but 75% of the same respondents rated their own risk as being very low (Freimuth, Edgar, & Hammond, 1987). These findings are consistent with data from the Centers for Disease Control indicating that as of mid-1991, the percentage of the American public that perceived the AIDS crisis as personally relevant to themselves was still zero (Kroger, 1991).

Thus with regard to the public information goal of disseminating information about the transmission of the HIV virus in a form that will stimulate behavior modification to limit the spread of the virus, we must conclude that the information has been disseminated, but its recipients have not yet been persuaded that it pertains to them and so have failed to respond with self-protective behavioral choices. Such a reaction is consistent with a long line of research findings on the psychology of information seeking and processing (see Mortensen, 1971, for a review of early studies in this area) in the service of what Dennett (1991) recently dubbed a "heterophenomenological" process of constantly constructing and revising views of the world that we humans all experience and to which we must each respond. As a consequence, and as suggested by numerous communication scholars (e.g., Brown, 1991), rhetorically effective information dissemination to an audience engaged in such defensively selective reception is likely to require a calculated and coordinated interplay of mediated and interpersonal communication of a type not yet widely practiced with regard to HIV/AIDS.

Accomplishment of the public information goals of both disseminating information about the diagnosis and treatment of HIV infection and promoting self-interested use of that information appears to have been similarly limited to date by the mass audience's inclination toward psychologically self-defensive selective exposure to, and interpretation of, information available through the media. On the one hand, people with newly diagnosed HIV seropositivity, who are usually asymptomatic, are imbued with a passion that comes only from seeing oneself at proximate risk, with the result that information dissemination through activist organizations and networks has proved to be very effective (Wachter, 1992). On the other hand, for the 75% of those who are infected but have not been diagnosed, this zeal is absent and, in fact, the self-awareness of their behavioral choices that led to their infection might enhance the general tendency to denial that produces the selective exposure to and interpretation of media content in others. Consequently, these people are likely to fail to find out about, let alone seek out, the early treatment that could prolong their lives. They are also likely to continue the behavioral practices that led to their own infection (and thereby put others at continued risk of infection), rather than modifying those behaviors, not because the appropriate information is unavailable, but because the form of its presentation is rhetorically ineffective in the face of their systematic resistance to effective reception, processing, and use of that information.

These same tendencies to avoidance and denial have also impeded, in a number of ways, the debate necessary for democratic participation in the development of an effective public policy in response to this massive public health crisis. In the first place, those who refuse to believe the issue has any relevance to themselves because of the realistic fear it arouses about their own HIV status are unlikely to participate in such debates because such participation would threaten the shell of avoidance that protects them from their fear. Consequently, even taxpayers with a certain and universal economic interest in the fiscal, if not the medical, consequences of the spread of HIV/AIDS might avoid discussion of pressing public issues as a means of avoiding related and implied concerns of an even more threatening personal nature. The result is that even the relatively unthreatening (for persons who are not infected with HIV) questions of public health, insurance or housing discrimination, and tax policy related to HIV/AIDS tend to drop off the end of the political agenda for the general electorate even in a presidential election year (Masterson-Allen & Brown, 1990; Wachter, 1992). Those who know themselves to be infected are frequently intimidated into silence and nonparticipation in the public policy debate by the well-documented likelihood of facing insurance discrimination, loss of necessary health benefits or employment, and/or social hostility and prejudice if their infection becomes known (Hayes & Stipp, 1991; Lambert, 1991; Mondragon, Kirkman-Liff, & Schneller, 1991). Those who are infected but do not succumb to this chilling effect in the pubic debate, meanwhile, frequently see themselves as having literally nothing to lose by resorting to the kinds of polarizing activist lobbying tactics associated with groups such as ACT UP and/or devote single-minded energy to lobbying for preferred responses to the crisis from the medical community. The cumulative results of these simultaneous influences on participation by different groups in the public policy debate are, first, a general dampening of the debate that supports the avoidance reactions of the public at large and, second, an unbalanced representation of legitimately interested points of view in the debate (to the extent that one exists) over a realistically necessary public policy on HIV/AIDS (Kong, 1991; Wachter, 1992).

The specification of a *realistically necessary* public policy response is necessary because even cursory analysis of media content related to HIV/AIDS reveals vast and voluminous coverage that only *appears* to contribute to the public information goals identified earlier and actually inhibits the realization of these goals by distracting attention and debate into areas that pander to the public's emotion-driven avoidance reaction and are logically irrelevant to the pragmatically feasible and potentially efficacious behavioral and policy choices that we face both individually and collectively.

This genre of coverage began in the 1980s with the widespread media attention devoted to hemophiliac Ryan White and arguably includes much (but not all) of the coverage of two of the biggest wire service stories of 1991—Magic Johnson's retirement after HIV infection and Kimberly Bergalis's battle with AIDS and proposal for legislation mandating universal HIV testing for health care workers—which together dominated the American media coverage of HIV/AIDS in late 1991 and early 1992 (Goodman, 1991; "The Top Ten News Stories of 1991," 1992; Weisberg, 1991). Also included in this category would be 1991's sympathetic ABC News coverage of the Ray family's support for the underage marriage of their 14-year-old HIV-positive hemophiliac son (which would put his 16-year-old fiancée at risk of infection); the *New York Times* coverage of City University of New York Professor Leonard Jeffries's genocidal conspiracy theories about the origin of the AIDS virus (Stanley,

1991); and dozens, if not hundreds, of other human-interest sidebars about atypical but emotionally evocative cases of HIV infection or AIDS.

Such coverage is counterproductive with regard to stimulating effective individual and collective responses to the HIV/AIDS epidemic because it supports the psychological avoidance defense of the viewer or reader, even as it stimulates the distraction of human and material resources into consideration of logically irrelevant issues and/or implementation of emotionally reassuring but pragmatically ineffective policies and programs.

Each of the aforementioned cases is somewhat different with regard to the means and extent of its counterproductivity, but the general problem created by such coverage is illustrated particularly well by the case of Kimberly Bergalis. As noted by Jacob Weisberg (1991) in *The New Republic*,

> In the opinion of C. Everett Koop, the former surgeon general, "the Florida case is too bizarre to be helpful in making public policy." Acer, who may have infected as many as five people in Florida, is the only proven case of a health care worker infecting a patient. . . . Yet the Bergalis bill would go to great lengths to prevent a recurrence of what may well be a freak accident. Though there is no convincing evidence that it would save a single life, Dannemeyer's bill has been estimated to cost as much as $1 billion. . . .

Coverage of Professor Jeffries's theories about the origin of the AIDS virus similarly distracted attention from the concerns that could help control the damage from HIV/AIDS, because even definite proof or disproof of his theories would not tell us what we should do *now*, no matter how emotionally satisfying it might be to have a villain to blame for our plight. Interest in the cases of hemophiliacs like White or Ray is also largely irrelevant to any viewer or reader other than the rest of the 20,000 hemophiliacs in the United States (a number that includes me but is still small enough to be minimally relevant to the public health threat posed to the nation by HIV/AIDS); but to the extent that it evokes sympathy for self-indulgent behavioral choices on the part of HIV-infected individuals that put others at risk, as in the case of the Ray boy becoming a 14-year-old bridegroom, it is actively counterproductive. As for Magic Johnson, the idea of presenting a world-class athlete and multimillionaire who has acknowledged sexual activity with hundreds of women and remains healthy enough to play in the NBA All-Star game and the Olympics after HIV infection as either a realistic role model or an object lesson would be ludicrous on its face were it not for the fact that so many of America's youth apparently identify strongly with him and are sufficiently phenomenologically self-deceptive to have responded to his disclosure of HIV seropositivity with the observation that "if Magic could catch it, then I guess anybody could" (Armstrong & Wood, 1991).

This leads to a caveat in the argument about the counterproductivity of the media's coverage of human-interest sidebars under the guise of informing the public about HIV/AIDS: that although the extent to which a particular case evokes a sense of personal identification in the mass audience may defy rational logic, such evocation, linked to pragmatically, logically, and scientifically defensible information and persuasion, must be a goal of an effective public information policy guiding coverage of HIV/AIDS. Thus, for example, if members of an at-risk demographic group such as minority youths perceive Magic Johnson's behavioral decision making to be similar to their own—however objectively irrational that perception may be—and if Magic Johnson will encourage those youths to practice responsible and pragmatically effective behavior to reduce the spread of the virus in that group, then media coverage that facilitates that persuasion is productive and should be encouraged and supported. Similarly, to the extent that coverage of Ryan White contributed to public awareness of more general issues of discrimination, then that aspect of that coverage was productive, even if coverage of the celebrities attending Ryan White's funeral was distracting from those legitimate concerns and therefore counterproductive.

By the same logic, if a similarly irrational level of audience identification with the plight of Kimberly Bergalis leads to massive distraction of deliberative energies and material resources (Congressional hearings, media space and time, etc.) into consideration (and, potentially, implementation) of pragmatically inconsequential policies, then coverage that promotes that process should be recognized as being deleterious to the public interest and should be excised from the public information environment, no matter how strong the audience interest in such stories, as evidenced by broadcast ratings or print media circulation. Media coverage that panders to the audience by giving people the content they want, because it generates a false and self-deceptive sense of security, but distracts them from focusing on the information they objectively and demonstrably need to act effectively in their own self-interest is subversive of the public interest.

DEVELOPMENT OF AN EFFECTIVE PUBLIC
INFORMATION POLICY ON HIV/AIDS

The foregoing discussion leads inexorably to the conclusion that the blessings of liberty that we the people enjoy in the United States of America are currently far less than secure for both ourselves and our posterity because of the threat to public health, economic security, and domestic tranquility posed by the spread of HIV/AIDS. Media coverage of the epidemic during its first decade has been ineffective in rallying an adequate response to this threat. Continued failure at this time to develop and implement a more effective and consistent public information policy on HIV/AIDS would be so irresponsible as to present a clear and present danger to the security of the nation.

The observations and arguments presented in the preceding section suggest a public information policy on the HIV/AIDS epidemic that offers greater hope of stimulating effective individual and collective response to the threat of HIV/AIDS than has occurred to date.

Lacking such a policy, media coverage of HIV/AIDS during the past decade has tended to pander to the mass audience's irrational and psychologically defensive demands for coverage that supports individual and collective avoidance reactions. Information related to transmission of the infection, diagnosis and treatment options, and necessary public policy issues such as insurance discrimination *has* been presented, but usually in noninvolving neutral and objective forms that a receiver could easily selectively avoid or see as irrelevant to him- or herself. Media managers, when challenged to show that they have fulfilled their social responsibilities to society in disseminating information about HIV/AIDS, cite just such coverage. Meanwhile, these same media decision makers have provided a much greater volume of coverage that at the same time it supports the public's avoidance reaction, it actually impedes effective individual and collective response to the crisis by distracting attention from issues and decisions that are pragmatically both possible and necessary. Such coverage is defended on the grounds that

1 Maximum quantities of coverage will result in the distillation of truth in a democracy, which is the rationale supporting the First Amendment rights of free speech and a free press;

2 The public has an affirmative "right to know" what it wishes to know (which assertion has no basis in law); and/or

3 Media outlets should provide the viewing/reading audience with the coverage it *wants* and have no affirmative responsibility to make informed judgments as to whether such coverage disserves the public interest by supporting a systematic avoidance of information viewers/readers *need* to make effective decisions. The fact that such counterproductive coverage may also tend to boost circulation and broadcast ratings, and therefore serve the economic self-interest of the media managers and the shareholders for whom they toil, contributes, of course, to the zeal with which this last argument, in particular, is made.

The cumulative impact of the editorial policies that have resulted from such thinking is a polity that has a reasonable grasp of the factual information but has not yet meaningfully responded to the threat to the commonwealth on either the individual or the collective level. Although information necessary for responsible individual and collective decisions about how to limit the spread of the contagion has been presented, it has not been presented in a sufficiently persuasive form to be efficacious in stimulating the individual and collective behavior changes necessary to realize that goal. Similarly, information about diagnosis and treatment has, in fact, been available through the mass media; yet 75% of HIV-infected Americans have so far been able to avoid concluding from that coverage that they should seek diagnosis and treatment (Findlay, 1991). Coverage of public policy questions has not led to either settled policy or consistent implementation, with the consequence that ongoing discrimination against HIV-infected individuals and avoidance of the issue by the general public distort the public debate about policy choices (to the extent such debate even occurs). The bulk of coverage related to the HIV/AIDS epidemic in the mass media has so far been irrelevant to the pragmatically necessary behavioral and policy decisions we must make individually and collectively to protect ourselves, and this irrelevant coverage distracts attention and resources from the coverage of information that *could* play a constructive role in stimulating an effective response.

In sum, the hypothesis that unrestricted freedom of the press and of speech with regard to the issue of HIV/AIDS would be efficacious in securing the blessings of liberty to ourselves and our posterity has been empirically tested in an ongoing, decade-long experiment and has been disconfirmed.

THE FOURTH ESTATE AS SERVANT
OF THE PUBLIC INTEREST

When the framers of the Constitution of the United States provided in the First Amendment that "Congress shall make no law . . . abridging the freedom of speech, or of the press," their stated purpose was, among other things, to "insure domestic Tranquility, provide for the common defence, promote the general Welfare, and secure the Blessings of Liberty" to themselves and to us, their "posterity" (U.S. Constitution, Preamble). They assumed that this purpose could most effectively and parsimoniously be achieved by forbidding restriction of the amounts and types of information available to the citizens of the fledgling republic.

Subsequent events in the history of the republic have, however, resulted in the recognition that some circumstances require different means to achieve the ends sought by the framers. The Supreme Court of the United States, as interpreter of the Constitution, has upheld restriction of freedoms of both speech and the press in circumstances in which the national interest might be harmed by unrestricted exercise of these rights. As formulated by Justice Oliver Wendell Holmes,

> The question in every case is whether the words used are used in such circumstances and are of such a nature as to create a clear and present danger that they will bring about the substantive evils that Congress has a right to prevent. (*Schenck v. United States*, 1919)

Furthermore, on the obverse side of the issue and in spite of legally defined limits to the right of privacy for public figures, there is no legal basis whatever for the media's claim that the public has a "right to know" that justifies disclosure of information potentially harmful to the commonwealth.

Continued media coverage of HIV/AIDS of the ineffective type that has occurred to date constitutes a clear and present danger to the republic because of the massive scale of the economic and medical consequences of continued avoidance and nonresponse to the epidemic. Furthermore, the time to act is short; if we wait for enough HIV-infected people to become sufficiently sick to stimulate personal concern in their acquaintances among the public at large, the number of others who will by then be infected but not yet ill will be unmanageably large.

What is needed is a consistent policy that governs coverage of HIV/AIDS to promote media coverage with the following characteristics:

1 Rhetorical presentation of factual information about how the infection is transmitted, in a persuasive form combining mediated and interpersonal channels and focused on promoting behavior modification to reduce the spread of HIV infection.

2 Universal dissemination through media and other channels of information on diagnosis and treatment that is strategically designed to promote use of diagnosis and early treatment by those at risk who have to date failed to recognize and effectively respond to that risk, coupled with counseling and persuasion to reduce the chances that newly diagnosed HIV-positive people will continue to practice behaviors that might further spread the disease.

3 Systematic agenda setting in the domain of politics and public discourse to break down public avoidance of the issue, promote widespread participation in public debate about its implications, and stimulate the development of settled public policy and regulatory/enforcement options related to HIV/AIDS, particularly in those areas (e.g., discrimination and access to health care) that, as long as they remain unresolved, generate a chilling effect on public discussion of relevant policy by HIV-infected citizens and others who are immediately affected, thereby distorting the public debate about policy options.

4 Deletion of media content (regardless of audience demand for such coverage) that panders to the mass audience's defensive avoidance of the issue by providing emotionally evocative human-interest sidebar stories that are logically and objectively irrelevant to any pragmatically efficacious individual or collective decisions that could or should be made.

Such a policy would result in media coverage of HIV/AIDS that would more effectively focus public attention on what we the people *need* to know to respond effectively to the threat, regardless of what we, from an uninformed and psychologically defensive perspective, think we *want* to know. It would therefore fulfill the responsibility of media outlets as social institutions to contribute to the commonwealth. Ideally, those who are collectively responsible for determining media content, through their professional organizations, will see fit sooner rather than later to promulgate such a policy in the public interest and will enforce its use by members of those professional organizations. The evidence of the past decade, however, is not encouraging with regard to the likelihood of their doing so; the economic self-interest of the media shareholders in pandering to the mass audience's self-destructive avoidance reaction while rationalizing that they are serving the public through exercise of First Amendment rights appears to dominate editorial policy regarding coverage of HIV/AIDS.

Should media decision makers fail to implement a policy like that described above in the very near future, however, the magnitude of the threat to national security represented by continuation of their current practices will justify governmental imposition of such a policy.

REFERENCES

Altman, L. K. (1991, June 20). Cost of AIDS care in the U.S. is seen at $5.8 billion in '91. *New York Times*, p. A16.

Armstrong, S., & Wood, D. (1991, November 13). Magic Johnson's situation raises awareness of AIDS. *Christian Science Monitor*, p. 7.

Baldwin, J. D., & Baldwin, J. I. (1988). Factors affecting AIDS related sexual risk-taking behavior among college students. *Journal of Sex Research, 25,* 181–196.

Brown, W. (1991). An AIDS prevention campaign: Effects on attitudes, beliefs and communication behavior. *American Behavioral Scientist, 34,* 666–678.

Dennett, D. C. (1991). *Consciousness explained.* Boston: Little, Brown.

DiClemente, R. (1990). The emergence of adolescents as a risk group for human immunodeficiency virus infection. *Journal of Adolescent Research, 5,* 7–17.

Edgar, T., Freimuth, V., & Hammond, S. (1988). Communicating the risk of AIDS to college students: The problem of motivating change. *Health Education Research, 3,* 59–65.

Findlay, S. (1991, June 17). AIDS: The Second Decade. *U.S. News and World Report,* pp. 20–23.

Freimuth, V., Edgar, T., & Hammond, S. (1987). College students' awareness and interpretation of the AIDS risk. *Science, Technology and Human Values, 12,* 37–40.

Goodman, W. (1991, November 17). The story TV can't resist. *New York Times*, p. 31.

Hayes, A., & Stipp, D. (1991, November 15). Cap on AIDS-related insurance claims is upheld by U.S. Appeals Court. *Wall Street Journal*, p. 3.

Johnston, W. B., & Hopkins, K. R. (1990). *The catastrophe ahead: AIDS and the case for a new public policy.* New York: Praeger.

Kegeles, S., Adler, N., & Irwin, C. (1988). Sexually active adolescents and condoms: Changes over one year in knowledge, attitudes, and use. *American Journal of Public Health, 78,* 460–461.

Knox, R. A. (1991, June 17). Most favor bigger U.S. role in AIDS fight. *Boston Globe,* pp. 1, 22–23.

Kong, D. (1991, October 2). AIDS group faults CDC in effort to halt disease. *Boston Globe*, p. 22.

KRC Communications Research. (1990).

Kroger, F. (1991, September). Keynote address presented at the AIDS Crisis: Effective Health Communication for the '90s conference, Emerson College, Boston, MA.

Lambert, W. (1991, November 19). Discrimination afflicts people with HIV. *Wall Street Journal,* pp. b1, b6.

Marwick, C. (1991). Congressional AIDS commission in limelight, likely to remain there for another year. *Journal of the American Medical Association, 266,* 2050.

Masterson-Allen, S., & Brown, P. (1990). Pubic reaction to toxic waste contamination: Analysis of a social movement. *International Journal of Health Services, 20,* 485–500.

McDermott, R., Hawkins, M., Moore, J., & Cittadino, S. (1987). AIDS awareness and information sources among selected university students. *Journal of American College Health, 35,* 222–226.

Mondragon, D., Kirkman-Liff, B., & Schneller, E. (1991). Hostility to people with AIDS: Risk perception and demographic factors. *Social Science Medicine, 32,* 1137–1142.

Mortensen, C. D. (1971). *Communication: The study of human interaction.* New York: McGraw-Hill.

Schenck v. United States, 249 U.S. 47. (1919).

Stanley, A. (1991, August 7). City college professor assailed for remarks on Jews. *New York Times,* pp. B1, B3.

Strauss, A., Fagerhaugh, S., Suczek, B., & Weiner, C. (1991, July/August). AIDS and health care deficiencies. *Society,* pp. 63–73.

Students polled on risky behavior. (1992, February 18). *Boston Globe,* p. 9.

The challenge facing Africa. (1992, January). *World Press Review,* p. 11.

The top ten news stories of 1991. (1992, February). *World Press Review,* p. 9.

The world battles a deadly plague. (1992, January). *World Press Review,* p. 13.

Wachter, R. M. (1992). AIDS, activism and the politics of health. *New England Journal of Medicine, 326,* 128–132.

Weisberg, J. (1991, October 21). The accuser: Kimberly Bergalis, AIDS martyr. *The New Republic,* pp. 12–14.

Chapter Ten

Communication Disorders in Adults with AIDS

Cynthia L. Bartlett

The ability to communicate is central to functioning as a human being. It allows people to make vital personal connections with others as well as to conduct the business and the pleasure of daily life. Success in these activities depends in large measure on the extent to which the myriad communicative abilities are intact. What is more, patient reports are central to medical decision making, and a patient's comprehension, insight, and recall are critical to his or her compliance with the recommendations of health care givers. Thus impairments in patients' abilities to express themselves or take in, understand, retain, and carry out instructions have the potential to interfere with both day-to-day life and the delivery of optimal health care. In general, impaired communication isolates people from those around them, whether information providers, health care givers, friends, or loved ones.

Few people with acquired immune deficiency syndrome (AIDS) are spared communicative disorders. As the human immunodeficiency virus (HIV) crosses the blood–brain barrier (Diedrich et al., 1988; Elder & Sever, 1988; Gyorkey, Melnick, & Gyorkey, 1987; Ho et al., 1985; Levy, Bredesen, & Rosenblum, 1988; Rosenblum, Levy, & Bredesen, 1988), cerebral tissue is vulnerable to direct infection. Furthermore, opportunistic infections and neoplasms may affect specific communication-critical areas of the brain, producing communicative disorders similar to those in stroke. A variety of dementing disorders are common in AIDS (Levy, Bredesen, & Rosenblum, 1985; McArthur, 1987; Navia, Jordan, & Price, 1986; Snider et al., 1983) and may be the only or first sign of the disease (Navia & Price, 1987). Dementia has been reported as well in asymptomatic seropositive individuals (Mirra, Anand, & Spira, 1986; Skoraszewski, Ball, & Mikulka, 1991), although others recommend caution in interpreting such findings (Gibbs, Andrewes, Szmukler, & Mulhall, 1990). Brain and peripheral nerve disorders can also affect the mechanics of producing speech (Dalakas & Pezeshkpour, 1988; Langford-Kuntz, Reichart, & Pohle, 1988), as can conditions that compromise the integrity of speech production structures (Marcusen & Sooy, 1985). Finally, people with AIDS (like any other group of people) may have communication disorders unrelated to their HIV-based disorders. When a person with AIDS has either preexisting or AIDS-related communication impairments, the resulting isolation compounds the isolation originating from others' fear of the disease, homophobia, social alienation, or the patient's own withdrawal. For these reasons, it is important to address communication disorders in people with AIDS.

The term "communication" is used here to encompass a variety of specific functions. These relate broadly to understanding others' messages (whether delivered by speaking, writing, gesturing, drawing, or some combination) and conveying messages to others (by the same means). A wide variety of communication disorders pervade the population of individuals with AIDS. This chapter summarizes them and offers suggestions, where applicable, for optimizing the effectiveness of communicative interactions with people with AIDS.

Ideally, the communicative function of patients with AIDS should be assessed by specialists in communication disorders (certified audiologists and speech–language pathologists) at the first hint of problems. Most hospitals, nursing homes, home health agencies, and other health care organizations have speech–language pathologists either on staff or available as consultants. What follows is not intended to substitute for the services of these professionals but rather to alert others to the prevalence of communicative disorders in persons with AIDS and to emphasize the importance of accurately identifying and adequately addressing these problems. The sections are organized into an (a) introductory segment; followed by (b) signs or symptoms to note, where applicable; and (c) suggestions for adapting communicatively to the problem being addressed.

UNDERSTANDING OTHERS' MESSAGES

For a person to understand others' messages, at least two systems must be either intact or sufficiently augmented (as with eyeglasses or hearing aids) to ensure that messages are first received and then decoded and stored. These systems are (a) the primary sensory systems related to communication (especially hearing and vision) and (b) the central nervous system supports for higher cognitive–linguistic function. These are discussed below.

Hearing Problems

Intact ability to comprehend and retain a message is of little use if the message does not first gain access to the language centers of the brain. Thus, a first communication-related consideration for health care givers interacting with a person with AIDS is how well the person hears. It is important to note that what is referred to generically as "hearing" includes more than the ability to perceive an incoming signal as being adequately loud. Hearing also relates to the extent to which the auditory system differentiates various components of that signal so that potentially similar-sounding signals are distinguished from each other. Impairment of the latter is referred to as a speech–sound discrimination problem. This type of hearing loss can exist even in the presence of the ability to perceive speech as being adequately loud. The existence of a prior hearing loss should be documented as part of the medical history.

Hearing impairment can also occur as one of the sequelae of the disease (Breda, Hammerschlag, Gigliotti, & Schinella, 1988; Flower & Sooy, 1987; Gherman, Ward, & Bassis, 1988; Hart, Cokely, Schupbach, Dal Canto, & Coppleson, 1989; Kohan, Rothstein, & Cohen, 1988; Real, Thomas, & Gerwin, 1987; Strauss & Fine, 1991). In a 1989 report, the National Institute on Deafness and Other Communication Disorders's Task Force on the National Strategic Research Plan estimated that 75% of adults with AIDS and 50% of adults with AIDS-related complex have demonstrably abnormal auditory system function. These abnormalities can affect the structure and function of the middle and external ears and eustachian tubes and can interfere with the transmission of acoustic signals virtually throughout the neural portion of the auditory system, from the hair cells of the cochlea to the primary auditory cortex of the brain. Along with many other AIDS-related disorders, hearing loss can be among the primary or secondary impairments associated with pneumocystis carinii, candidiasis, fungal infections, meningitis, toxoplasmosis, demyelinating processes, tumors, and polyps.

Impaired hearing is also among the possible side effects of ototoxic treatments for HIV infections and for AIDS-related conditions. For this reason, any patient on a medication known or suspected of ototoxicity should have his or her hearing monitored regularly. Finally, it is reasonable to assume that HIV-positive and AIDS patients will experience fluctuating hearing levels.

Signs People whose hearing is impaired may exhibit observable signs of their difficulty. Although some of these may reflect other or additional problems, the following are some of the common behavioral indicators of hearing loss.

1 Patient adjusts television or radio too loudly.

2 Patient does not note that someone has entered the room until he or she is within view.

3 Patient frequently requests repetitions.

4 Patient appears puzzled by others' words.

5 Patient appears to ignore what is being said to him or her unless speaker specifically indicates that he or she is addressing the patient.

6 Patient misunderstands what has been said by questioningly repeating or questioning the presumed message (e.g., "You want me to swallow these *bills*?").

7 Patient complains of "ringing" or "buzzing" in the ear (tinnitus).

Suggestions   If a patient is known to have a hearing loss and to have been fitted for a hearing aid, it should be available to him or her regularly. For those in inpatient facilities, insertion of the aid should become part of routine morning care and its removal routinely incorporated into bedtime evening care. It is important to stress that hearing aids are delicate high-tech equipment and therefore require special daily checking and care to function properly. Replacement batteries must also be on hand. Information on the maintenance of hearing aids, if a patient is unable to perform it, can be obtained from a partner/significant other familiar with the procedures or by requesting the information from the staff audiologist (or audiology consultant), from the distributor of that brand and model of aid, or from the office of a local otolaryngologist who has an audiologist in his or her practice.

If at all possible, the patient with AIDS who has a hearing loss (whether preexisting and unaided or of recent onset) should be evaluated by a certified audiologist who can advise on the feasibility of amplification. If a hearing aid is not recommended, the aid is rejected by the patient, or the hearing loss may be temporary, the patient can be provided with telephones having amplifiers, and, if the patient is at home, devices that alert through vibration or light can be substituted for items such as doorbells, telephones, and alarm clocks, which typically signal acoustically.

Whether the person with AIDS has aided hearing or not, there are a number of things speakers can do to optimize listening conditions and provide maximal cueing for the patient. Although these are important for health care practitioners to incorporate into their interactions with hearing-impaired patients with AIDS, it is equally important to convey them to patients' families, partners, and any others with whom the patient interacts.

1 *Directly face the person.*   Don't talk to a hearing-impaired person unless you can "see the whites of their eyes." At the same time, it is important that your face be lighted. Depending on the patient's level of alertness, it may also be necessary to turn the patient's head and direct his or her gaze to your face before speaking. Relative to this point, it is clearly important to determine at the

outset whether the patient wears eyeglasses and, if so, obtain them and be certain that they are worn consistently.

2 *Don't shout.* It is a nearly reflexive action to raise the voice when speaking to someone who appears not to understand. In the case of someone who has diminished hearing (whether aided or not), speaking too loudly tends to distort both the acoustic signal produced and the facial movements ("lip reading") that could otherwise assist comprehension. Especially in the case of people with impaired speech–sound discrimination, being spoken to very loudly is also disconcerting. For some listeners, being spoken to in a slightly louder (but not too loud) voice may be helpful. A useful guideline for speakers in this regard is to maintain a vocal volume within a range that feels natural. Once it feels unnaturally loud or forced, the voice is likely too loud.

3 *Speak at a natural rate and with natural articulatory movements.* For some speakers, talking at a faster than normal rate is typical (as it is for those who are rushed). At the same time, many speakers slow their speaking rate to an equally unnatural pace and exaggerate their speech movements when addressing someone with a hearing loss (and others who they assume have not understood). Each of these strategies tends to interfere with a listener's ability to ascertain what has been said. Thus, a conscious effort on the part of speakers is required to speak naturally in terms of both loudness level and the rate and excursion of articulatory movements.

4 *Ask for confirmation of understanding.* Especially for critical information, it may be useful to ask the listener to confirm that he or she has understood. This request could take the form of a simple "Do you understand what I said?" Alternatively, in certain situations, it may be useful to ask the listener to recount his or her understanding of the material just heard.

5 *Minimize background noise.* A noisy listening environment makes it more difficult to hear even for people with intact auditory systems. Competing stimuli (speech or others) are an even greater problem for individuals with hearing loss (whether aided or not). Thus, it is important to minimize extraneous noise when addressing a person whose hearing is impaired. Especially when it is critical for the person to understand, speakers should consider doing the following to diminish ambient noise before talking: Close windows and hall doors; turn off the television or radio; when multiple speakers are present, have only one speak at a time; and try to deliver important information to the person when roommates have no visitors.

6 *Be sure everyone who comes into contact with the person understands the preceding strategies.* The importance of this point is clear in terms of health care delivery, but it is equally critical in efforts to minimize patients' isolation from partners and others with whom they interact.

Comprehension Problems

As indicated earlier, hearing and differentiating a spoken message are the necessary precursors to understanding what the message means. Whereas hearing is a combined function of peripheral nerves and other structures of the brain, comprehending messages is supported by cerebral processes (principally in the left hemisphere of the brain). Comprehension is also more difficult to assess than is hearing acuity.

Signs   People who hear but do not understand speech may at times act like they are either confused or uncooperative. They may respond inappropriately to others' conversation (as in possible confusional states) or may fail to comply with requests (as may be the case in lack of cooperation). Because each of these potential causes (confusion, lack of cooperation, and comprehension difficulty) has its own implications medically and socially, differentiation among them is of the utmost importance to optimizing treatment and assuring appropriate interactions. Needless to say, any of these conditions can also exist simultaneously or in fluctuating combinations given the multifaceted nature of the disorder and varying forms AIDS may assume even in one person.

Suggestions   The first priority when a person with AIDS appears to have difficulty comprehending or to be confused or uncooperative is to establish the source(s) of the behaviors. The collective expertise of a variety of specialties (neurology, speech–language pathology, neuropsychology, and psychiatry, among others) is frequently needed to sort through the symptoms. Specific strategies for interacting with any person with AIDS who may not comprehend what is said depend on both the reason(s) for the problem and the specific features of any individual's difficulty. These features can vary considerably from person to person depending on the nature, severity, and combination of problem(s). General suggestions for comprehension problems related to aphasia are addressed in the Aphasia section.

CONVEYING MESSAGES TO OTHERS

For a person to convey messages to other people in ways that are considered "normal," again at least two systems must be intact. The first system comprises the speech production structures of the vocal tract (those involved in respiration, voice production, nasality control, and oral articulation). The other system encompasses the communication-critical portions of the central and peripheral nervous systems that are responsible for controlling vocal tract movement and coordination and higher linguistic and cognitive functions.

Language is the rule-governed cognitive–linguistic process required to produce the content of a message (*what* is said). Language is also responsible for the ability to understand messages that are heard or read. On the other hand, speech is *how* something is said—a mechanical process that is the principal mode of expression for language. Both speech and language can be compromised in AIDS. As with other AIDS-related communication disorders, the causes for, symptoms of, and treatments or compensations for speech and language problems are varied.

Speech Problems

The elements of vocal tract function listed earlier (respiration, phonation, resonance, and articulation) operate in concert to produce strings of speech sounds that are sufficiently differentiated and loud at a rate that allows the composite to be heard and understood. Any decrement or combination of decrements in loudness, rate, or speech–sound differentiation, or an excess of speed, can interfere with speech intelligibility.

Loudness Persons with AIDS who speak too softly may do so for any number of reasons, ranging from generalized weakness to impaired respiratory musculature to an inadequately functioning voice production mechanism.

Suggestions Perhaps the most natural response to someone who has spoken too softly is to ask the person to repeat what he or she said or to speak louder. However, a very ill patient with AIDS may be quite weak, and to comply with either of these requests requires considerable extra effort. Those who speak too softly or too rapidly may be assisted by augmentative communication devices that amplify or alter certain physical aspects of speech production.

A less physically taxing choice than asking an ill person who has low vocal volume to speak louder is to use a portable amplification system. These are frequently available in a hospital's audiovisual or conference department. They consist of a hand-held, lavaliere, or clip-on microphone; amplifier; and speaker and are plugged into a regular wall socket. Less cumbersome (but sometimes difficult to find) are small, battery-powered amplification units. These have a microphone that clips onto an eyeglass frame (or is mounted on a headband) and an amplifier–speaker that fits into a breast pocket or can lie on the person's bed.

Rate A variety of neurological disorders that occur in AIDS-associated conditions can affect the rate and rhythm of speech. Some disorders slow the speaking rate, and others quicken it; some disorders affect the rhythm with which speech is produced; and nearly all of the disorders weaken to some extent the musculature that supports speech.

Because being understood (as opposed to sounding "normal") is the central communicative concern in irreversible conditions, it should be emphasized that slowed speaking alone seldom interferes with intelligibility and consequently is addressed minimally if at all under such circumstances. When speaking rate is slowed, speeding up is extremely difficult because of the weakened condition of the speech muscles and the other constraints on muscle control imposed by both likely underlying neurological damage and generally diminished vigor due to illness.

By contrast, a too rapid speaking rate does interfere with intelligibility; however, speaking rate should be considered in relative terms. Faster than usual speech may well remain understandable if other aspects of speech muscle control and the speech structures themselves have been essentially spared. However, in many AIDS-related neurological conditions, an otherwise "normal" speaking rate is too fast given weakened speech musculature and difficulty coordinating aspects of speech production other than rate (such as the range, force, direction, and cadence of the movements). In other cases, speaking rate is increased in an absolute sense and may even accelerate within an utterance, as in Parkinson-like conditions.

Decreasing a speaking rate that is too fast (in either relative or absolute terms) seems like an easy enough expectation, but in actuality is rather difficult, especially if the slower rate must be constant. The mechanics of speech typically occur at an all but unconscious level. People concentrate more on the content of their utterances and on adjusting to changing environmental conditions and to feedback from listeners than on the production process.

Suggestions Even in light of the foregoing, a slowed speaking rate can effect a noticeable increase in intelligibility, and it is worth helping a patient to achieve or approach it when possible. The most obvious means to this end is to ask the speaker to slow down. A few individuals may be able to comply with such a request, but many need repeated reminders. Speech pacing devices are an alternative to such prompts and are of two general types: Some produce an audible "beat" at an adjustable rate (like a metronome); others can be manipulated. These vary in elaborateness, from high-tech to homemade, as well as in expense.

The general principle behind using pacing devices is that they provide external prompts for rate control besides those from other people (whose reminders inevitably begin to sound like nagging) and are a support for the control. Because not all people are able to use pacing devices, the decision to offer one to any particular person should be made only after the potential efficacy of pacing for him or her has been assessed and then the utility of any specific device evaluated. Should pacing be recommended, the patient typically also needs training and practice to use it to maximal effect.

Speech–Sound Differentiation   The mobile articulators (velum and pharynx, tongue segments, mandible, and lips) function in minutely timed sequential and simultaneous interactions with each other and with the immobile articulators (hard palate, teeth, and maxilla). These movements segment an undifferentiated buzz (produced by vibration of the vocal folds in the larynx) into strings of recognizable speech sounds. Given appropriate loudness and speaking rate, intact articulatory structures and adequate neural control over their movement, intelligible speech is generally possible.

Numerous AIDS-related conditions can interfere with the physical integrity of speech structures and the neural control of their movement. These range from oral mass lesions and oral inflammatory conditions to neurological disorders ranging from cryptococcal meningitis and toxoplasmosis to progressive multifocal leukoencephalopathy and neurosyphilis to central nervous system lymphoma.

In the case of neurological disorders, dysarthria, apraxia of speech, or a combination of the two may be evident. Either may affect the functioning of other vocal tract segments (such as those performing respiration and voice production) in addition to articulatory function. Thus the origin of the compromised speech intelligibility can range from an alteration in the size or shape of speech articulators to disorders that affect their movement, including disturbed praxis, paralysis, ataxic incoordination, the choreiform movements of hyperkinesia, the Parkinsonian hypokinetic disorders, or almost any combination of these.

Suggestions Speech–language clinicians assess speech and determine the potential for benefit from direct therapy for people with speech production problems. Other communicative choices may exist for those who may not benefit from direct treatment.

People whose speech has become difficult or impossible to understand may be assisted by alternative communication devices. Like augmentation devices, these range in complexity and cost from the alphabet and numbers written on the cardboard back of a pad of paper to multicomponent, custom-designed, computer-assisted systems.

The suitability of any particular alternative communication device for a given individual depends on the status of a number of factors, including motor skill, alertness and attention span, and the person's cognitive–linguistic system, among others. Assessing these factors, determining the potential benefit to a patient of using an alternative device, and fashioning it are the responsibilities of speech–language pathologists. These people evaluate the function of the patient's speech and language and may work with a neuropsychologist to determine cognitive and attentional levels and with the physical or occupational therapist to define the nature and extent of relevant motor skills.

Language Problems

The language problems associated with AIDS-related brain conditions are manifested in multiple ways. All affect the structure and content of language in identifiable but varying ways. Although these communication disorders are frequently called "aphasia," not all are the result of focal lesions in critical areas of the affected person's language-dominant cerebral hemisphere, the most clinically useful conception of aphasia. Rather, many apparently aphasic language disorders in AIDS are related to other central nervous system damage or to a combination of aphasic and nonaphasic language disorders. These aphasic and nonaphasic language disturbances are discussed below.

Aphasia Aphasia is the result of focal brain damage and is typically manifested by some degree of naming difficulty and auditory comprehension problems (the latter can be minimal, but are demonstrable). These two problems may be combined with varying degrees of speech fluency and of ability to repeat material spoken by another person. The resulting combinations of relatively spared or diminished fluency, comprehension, repetition, and naming produce the classic types of aphasia (Broca, Wernicke, conduction, global, and the like).

In most discussions of aphasia, reference is made principally to spoken language and its comprehension by way of the auditory system. Except in relatively rare instances, aphasic people's written language and reading comprehension are compromised in ways similar to their oral-auditory problems. As a consequence, for people who are aphasic, reading and writing (including typing and pointing to letter boards) do not generally provide satisfactory alternatives to heard and spoken language.

In addition, spoken language in aphasia may be characterized by a number of other features. The frequency with which any of the other features is observed depends on the type and severity of the aphasic disorder. These output errors include substituting one or more speech sounds in a word ("ked" for "bed") or substitution of related words ("yes" and "no," proper names, "chair" for "table," and the like). People may use nonsense words, perseveration (continued use of an utterance after it is no longer appropriate), or uncharacteristic swearing. They may omit small "grammatical" words, causing the result to sound like the language used in telegrams (telegraphic speech) or may seem to be using normal grammatical strings of real words but the whole lacks content (empty paragrammatic speech).

Suggestions Communicating with an aphasic person is often frustrating for all parties in an interaction. Specific strategies for interacting with any given aphasic individual depend on that person's constellation of problems and preserved abilities. These are best defined by someone experienced with aphasic language and its assessment (usually the speech–language pathologist or neuropsychologist). Nonetheless, the following are general guidelines that are appropriate for most people with aphasia.

1 *Assume that the person comprehends.* Even though the person has demonstrable auditory comprehension problems, most aphasic people understand some of the language they hear. Thus it is especially important to exercise

COMMUNICATION DISORDERS AND AIDS

caution when holding discussions with other people within the hearing range of an aphasic person, whether he or she is the subject of the discussion or not.

2 *Talk to the person.* For health care givers, this provides a humanizing element to care and can involve simply speaking directly but soothingly about the procedure being carried out (bathing, feeding, administration of mediations, and the like).

3 *Give the person time to talk.* When aphasic people are able to speak to some extent, most need extra time to do so.

4 *Help the person with his or her message.* Many people hesitate to fill in the blanks when someone with aphasia has word-finding difficulty. Because this is done when nonaphasic individuals encounter the problem, it is thus a normal repair strategy and there is little need to hesitate engaging it with aphasic people. The only real caution is that it is best not to jump in too quickly, but to allow the person sufficient time to retrieve the word him- or herself.

Dementia   The result of diffuse brain damage, dementia results in global decline in cognitive function. According to Cummings and Benson (1983),

> Dementia can be defined as an acquired persistent impairment of intellectual function with compromise in at least three of the following spheres of mental activity: language, memory, visuospatial skills, emotion or personality, and cognition (abstraction, calculation, judgment, etc.). (p. 1)

Published accounts of the epidemiology of dementing disorders in the population of persons with AIDS have reported its prevalence to range from 30% to 70% (McArthur, 1987; Navia et al., 1986), and some writers have estimated that the cognitive decline of dementia is the most frequently occurring manifestation of both HIV infection and AIDS (Levy et al., 1985; McArthur, 1987; Navia et al., 1986).

Suggestions   As with aphasia, the constellation of symptoms in dementia varies in nature and severity, making a list of recommendations for communicating with dementing individuals difficult to compile. Again, however, general principles may prove to be useful until the successful communicative strategies for a particular person have been defined in light of speech–language and neuropsychological assessments.

1 *A number of publications are available that have been written for lay persons caring for dementing people* (Heston & White, 1983; Mace & Rabins, 1981; Ostuni & Santo Pietro, 1986; Powell & Courtice, 1985). They are also instructive for professional health care providers.

2 *The nature of the decline in dementia renders specific aspects of language difficult for cognitively impaired people to handle and thus these aspects are better avoided.* Among these are verbal analogies; sarcasm and irony; open-ended questions; conversations with more than one person; long, grammatically complex sentences; multiple bits of information presented at the same time;

introduction of a new topic without warning; and conversations about abstract material. Bayles and Kazniak (1987) have provided a superb elaboration of language and communication in dementing disorders.

3 *Avoid attempts to persuade.* To be persuaded requires that a person be able to take in information contrary to a current belief, compare and analyze the two, and alter the held belief in light of the presented evidence or argument. Accomplishing this requires thinking and reasoning. Because these are impaired in dementia, attempts to argue with patients (regardless of the topic) typically result in agitation for them and frustration for yourself.

4 *Approach and speak to dementing individuals calmly.* It is frequently useful to place a hand gently on the person's arm to alert the person to the fact that he or she will be addressed. For people whose dementia is more severe, it may be necessary to turn their head gently so that they are facing you and making eye contact before you initiate any interchange.

5 *For those whose symptoms include prosopagnosia (inability to recognize faces), it may be helpful to have people who enter the room identify themselves by name.* This should include individuals who might be expected to be recognized, such as partners, close friends, and family.

Other Problems

It is important to emphasize that persons with AIDS may be deprived of the ability to express themselves in the absence of any communication disorder. Endotracheal intubation and tracheotomy often interfere with speaking, and individuals with such devices need special consideration communicatively. A simple communication board may be very helpful for such people assuming that their language and cognitive status allows them to use it.

CONCLUSION

Communication disorders are widespread in the population of people with AIDS. Attending to the communication needs of these individuals has the potential to assist in ensuring quality health care, is crucial in helping them to maintain as much contact as possible with partners and other loved ones, and is central to the preservation of dignity.

REFERENCES

Bayles, K. A., & Kazniak, A. W. (1987). *Communication and cognition in normal aging and dementia.* Austin, TX: PRO-ED.

Breda, S., Hammerschlag, P., Gigliotti, F., & Schinella, R. (1988). *Pneumocystis carinii* in the temporal bone as a primary manifestation of the acquired immunodeficiency syndrome. *Annals of Otology, Rhinology, and Laryngology, 97,* 427–431.

Cummings, J. L., & Benson, D. F. (1983). *Dementia: A clinical approach.* Boston: Butterworths.

Dalakas, M. C., & Pezeshkpour, G. H. (1988). Neuromuscular diseases associated with human immunodeficiency virus infection. *Annals of Neurology, 23*(Suppl.), S38–S48.

Diedrich, N., Ackermann, R., Jurgens, R., Ortseifeu, M., Thun, F., Schneider, M., & Vukadinovic, I. (1988). Early involvement of the nervous system by human immunodeficiency virus (HIV). *European Neurology, 28,* 93–103.

Elder, G., & Sever, J. (1988). AIDS and neurological disorders: An overview. *Annals of Neurology, 23*(Suppl.), S4–S6.

Flower, W., & Sooy, C. D. (1987). AIDS: An introduction for speech-language pathologists and audiologists. *Asha, 11,* 25–30.

Gherman, C. R., Ward, R. R., & Bassis, M. L. (1988). *Pneumocystis carinii* otitis media and mastoiditis as the initial manifestation of the acquired immunodeficiency syndrome. *American Journal of Medicine, 85,* 250–252.

Gibbs, A., Andrewes, D. G., Szmukler, G., & Mulhall, B. (1990). Early HIV-related neuropsychological impairment: Relationship to stage of viral infection. *Journal of Clinical and Experimental Neuropsychology, 12,* 766–780.

Gyorkey, F., Melnick, J., & Gyorkey, J. (1987). Human immunodeficiency virus in brain biopsies of patients with AIDS and progressive encephalopathy. *Journal of Infectious Diseases, 155,* 870–876.

Hart, C. W., Cokely, C. G., Schupbach, J., Dal Canto, M. C., & Coppleson, L. W. (1989). Neurotologic findings of a patient with acquired immune deficiency syndrome. *Ear and Hearing, 10,* 68–76.

Heston, L. L., & White, J. A. (1983). *Dementia: A practical guide to Alzheimer's disease and related illnesses.* New York: W. H. Freeman.

Ho, D., Rota, T., Schoaley, R., Kaplan, J., Allan, J., Groopman, J., Resnik, L., Felsenstein, D., Andrews, C., & Hirsch, M. (1985). Isolation of HTLV-III from cerebrospinal fluid and neural tissues of patients with neurologic syndromes related to the acquired immunodeficiency syndrome. *New England Journal of Medicine, 313,* 1493–1497.

Kohan, D., Rothstein, S. G., & Cohen, N. L. (1988). Otologic disease in patients with acquired immunodeficiency syndrome. *Annals of Otology, Rhinology, and Laryngology, 97,* 636–640.

Langford-Kuntz, A., Reichart, P., & Pohle, H. D. (1988). Impairment of cranio-facial nerves due to AIDS. Report of 2 cases. *International Journal of Oral and Maxillofacial Surgery, 17,* 227–229.

Levy, R. M., Bredesen, D. E., & Rosenblum, M. D. (1985). Neurological manifestations of the acquired immunodeficiency syndrome (AIDS): Experience at UCSF and review of the literature. *Journal of Neurosurgery, 42,* 475–495.

Levy, R., Bredesen, D., & Rosenblum, L. (1988). Opportunistic central nervous system pathology in patients with AIDS. *Annals of Neurology, 23*(Suppl.), S7–S12.

McArthur, J. C. (1987). Neurologic manifestations of AIDS. *Medicine, 13,* 255–260.

Mace, N. L., & Rabins, P. V. (1981). *The 36-hour day: A family guide to caring for persons with Alzheimer's disease, related dementing illnesses, and memory loss in later life.* Baltimore: Johns Hopkins University Press.

Marcusen, D. C., & Sooy, C. D. (1985). Otolaryngologic and head and neck manifestations of acquired immunodeficiency syndrome (AIDS). *Laryngoscope, 95,* 401–405.

Mirra, S. S., Anand, R., & Spira, T. J. (1986). HTLV-III/LAV infection of the central nervous system in a 57-year-old man with progressive dementia of unknown cause [letter to the editor]. *New England Journal of Medicine, 314,* 1191–1192.

National Institute on Deafness and Other Communication Disorders. (1989). *A report of the Task Force on the National Strategic Research Plan.* Bethesda, MD: Author.

Navia, B. A., Jordan, B. D., & Price, R. W. (1986). The AIDS dementia complex: I. Clinical features. *Annals of Neurology, 19,* 517–524.

Navia, B. A., & Price, R. W. (1987). The acquired immunodeficiency syndrome dementia complex as the presenting or sole manifestation of human immunodeficiency virus infection. *Archives of Neurology, 44,* 65–69.

Ostuni, E., & Santo Pietro, M. J. (1986). *Getting through: Communicating when someone you care for has Alzheimer's disease.* Plainsboro, NJ: The Speech Bin.

Powell, L. S., & Courtice, K. (1985). *Alzheimer's disease: A guide for families.* Reading, MA: Addison-Wesley.

Real, R., Thomas, M., & Gerwin, J. (1987). Sudden hearing loss and acquired immunodeficiency syndrome. *Otolaryngology, Head and Neck Surgery, 97,* 409–412.

Rosenblum, M., Levy, R., & Bredesen, D. (Eds.). (1988). *AIDS and the nervous system.* New York: Raven Press.

Skoraszewski, M. J., Ball, J. D., & Mikulka, P. (1991). *Journal of Clinical and Experimental Neuropsychology, 13,* 278–290.

Snider, W. D., Simpson, D. M., Nielson, S., Gold, J. W. M., Metroka, C. E., & Posner, J. B. (1983). Neurological complications of acquired immunodeficiency syndrome: Analysis of 50 patients. *Annals of Neurology, 14,* 403–418.

Strauss, M., & Fine, E. (1991). Aspergillus otomastoiditis in acquired immunodeficiency syndrome. *American Journal of Otology, 12,* 49–53.

Chapter Eleven

Neurosurgical Professionalism and Care in the Treatment of Patients with Symptomatic AIDS

Michael L. Levy
Joseph P. Van Der Meulen
Michael L. J. Apuzzo

The current epidemic of acquired immune deficiency syndrome (AIDS) not only is causing the deaths of young, viable individuals but also is creating doubt about the traditional roles of the physician in the care of their patients. In this chapter, we explore this issue by initially discussing the response of societies in the past to progressive and ostensibly irreversible epidemics and then analyzing the currently changing perceptions of and loss of trust in the traditional patient–physician relationship.

As long as the potential cure for AIDS continues to avoid us, it is essential that physician and patient education be maximized. Health care professionals and educators should be made aware of stigmatizing, negative attitudes on the part of physicians and medical students toward patients with AIDS and develop programs to educate themselves about their prejudices in an effort to promote knowledge and understanding. This will allow physicians to understand their own perceptions of the disease and potentiate effective treatment of those with symptomatic disease. Patients should be made aware of risk factors for becoming contaminated and of their rights as an individual and a patient should they become infected. Such education can result in a reappraisal of the role of the physician in the care of AIDS patients and return the decision-making process to the understanding and trust on which medical care is based.

We conclude our discussion with an overview of the disease processes that commonly afflict the central nervous system (CNS) in AIDS patients and detail the options for diagnosis and treatment.

HISTORICAL SUBSTRATE

To understand the political and medical implications of caring for patients with AIDS, we must first evaluate historical responses of society to progressive and devastating epidemics. The perception of any disease is based on the moral and social preoccupations of a society, in addition to the perceived specificity of the disease for certain minority groups, ethnic or otherwise. Historically, reactions to epidemics have included punishment of the afflicted community, belief that the origin of the disease is foreign to the community, and belief that the disease is specific to a foreign minority. These beliefs eventually become more generalized to include fear of those with the disease and the assumption that societal members who become afflicted with the disease are innocent victims of the contagion. Finally, the fear can lead to the belief that the disease will result in an end to society.

It has been stated that whereas death is the great equalizer of people, illness is the great differentiator. A society's reaction to an epidemic thus results in stereotypical characterizations of the disease and its victims (McCullum, 1992). Perceptions of individuals who have the disease as unclean and immoral may determine how aggressively the origins and potential treatment of the disease are researched and the patients managed. In a recent essay, McCullum (1992) identified the origins of social-disorder-based response to epidemics. Specifically, a society initially responds to an epidemic or disease as being foreign or specific to a stereotypical race, culture, or group. A forced response to the disease occurs either when the society must take responsibility for its own involvement in the progression and perpetuation of the disease or when the disease begins to involve members of the community who themselves have relegated the stereotype to a minority group and believe themselves to be immune to the disease. Eventually widespread progression of the epidemic throughout the community and the resultant chaos can result in social acceptance of the disease in addition to justification of research on its origin and cure.

The most obvious example of societal maladaption to a disease is the response to the spread of sexually transmitted diseases. Venereal diseases by nature define uncleanliness and a breach of morality. Historical support for this tenet is evident in the response of American society to the syphilis epidemic in the late 18th century. Prostitutes were said to be responsible for the origin and perpetuation of the disease. They were subsequently socially and/or legally isolated. Misinformation regarding the disease led the public to believe that syphilis resulted from excessive sexual intercourse or routine nonsexual contact with infected individuals. Further sequestration of the disease to specific groups became evident in the perception that prostitutes were usually immigrants or poor. Thus, immigration itself was cognitively linked to the nurturing and spread of the disease. In addition, it was promoted that the disease could be controlled by abstinence from sexual contact and adherence to the societal virtues of family life.

McCullum (1992) concluded that despite the progression of knowledge regarding the origin and spread of disease in modern society, our response to the AIDS epidemic is not unlike responses to past epidemics. The chaos resulting from the AIDS epidemic has also compromised our ability to evaluate inadequacies of our perceptions of disease in the past and benefit from such an evaluation. AIDS continues to be treated as a sociopolitical issue as opposed to a public health issue in America.

PERCEPTIONS OF AIDS
IN THE MEDICAL COMMUNITY

Kelly, St. Lawrence, Smith, Hood, and Cook (1987b), in a randomly selected sample of 157 physicians, were able to document that physicians manifested harsh attitude judgments toward patients with AIDS and were less willing to interact with patients with AIDS than with patients with other illnesses. Evaluation of 119 medical students revealed that they also held negative and prejudiced attitudes toward both AIDS and homosexual patients. Kelly et al. reported that the students believed that AIDS patients were more deserving of their diseases than patients with leukemia, in addition to being more deserving to die, lose their jobs, and be quarantined. Finally, the students were less willing to interact on a casual basis with AIDS patients than with patients with leukemia even in the absence of the potential for contracting the disease.

It has been suggested that health care professionals and educators should be made aware of these stigmatizing, negative attitudes on the part of physicians and medical students and develop programs to educate them about their prejudices toward patients with AIDS in an effort to promote knowledge and understanding (Kelly, St. Lawrence, Hood, Smith, & Cook, 1988; Kelly, St. Lawrence, Smith, Hood, & Cook, 1987a; Kelly et al., 1987b). Education should also be directed at a better understanding of the psychosocial implications of the disease as well as potential risk avoidance and management for health professionals. One would hope, in fact, that such an atypical response on the part of the physician is based more on a fear of the politicization of the disease than of the potential to become contaminated by patient contact (Fumento, 1990).

The question of whether to provide or withhold medical treatment is not an issue, regardless of whether a patient has AIDS or any other manifest disease. The proper care of any patient is based on the interaction of the potential benefits and complications that the physician may provide for the patient and the patient's disease, and the understanding and trust between the patient and physician. The refusal by a physician or health care worker to treat a patient with AIDS, when such treatment represents the standard of care, is a violation of the Americans With Disabilities Act of July 1980 and will likely result in prosecution. In addition, various organizations such as the AIDS Legal Task Force and American Medical Association specialize in civil litigations and the possibility of license revocation for those physicians who refuse to treat AIDS patients (Clarke & Conley, 1991).

LAWS RELATING TO HUMAN IMMUNODEFICIENCY VIRUS

Legislation regarding human immunodeficiency virus (HIV) infection is designed to protect the population against contamination (and to protect certain rights of the infected individual in the state of California). Patients who test positive for HIV should be aware of the laws. Blood tests to determine HIV status cannot be used to determine health insurability or employability. The results of these tests can be recorded in the patient's medical record by the ordering physician and released to other physicians for the purpose of diagnosis, care, or treatment of the patient without the patient's written consent.

Physicians may notify potential contacts (sexual or otherwise) of an infected individual but may not identify the individual in so doing. The physician should first notify the patient of his or her HIV status and provide counseling. If the patient is unwilling or unable to consent to the notification of potential contacts, the physician may proceed without consent. HIV testing of inmates, suspects, or parolees is permitted under limited circumstances. The obligation rests with the prison medical authorities. Persons with AIDS or who are HIV positive and knowingly donate blood, semen, or body organs are committing a felony. Federal law prohibits discrimination against persons with HIV infection with regard to their employment and/or medical treatment.

RESPONSIBILITIES OF PHYSICIANS

A recent commentary by Faria (1992) provides a concise summary of the difficulties physicians face in their care for patients with AIDS:

> The physician is no longer the venerated, respected healer in our society, but instead, a vulnerable provider fighting tooth and nail for his/her survival against an ever more intrusive government in an adversarial litigious society. We as physicians are on the defensive and in a state of siege. We are under attack and assailed on all fronts by insurance company bureaucrats, malpractice attorneys, workers compensation carriers, Medicare sanctioning authorities, and a sundry of agencies.

Frankly, [physicians] are in no position to refuse to treat anybody, especially a patient with AIDS. In fact, with the new AMA proclamation, the physician is now both legally and "ethically" compelled to treat any patient with AIDS who walks into the office despite the physician's expertise or experience in this field. The AMA has thus effectively added the element of force to intimidate further its already beleaguered members, out of political expediency rather than historical wisdom. We should treat our patients with AIDS always with sensitivity, compassion, and tolerance; yet we must also as physicians have the courage to state the truth, even when it is not "politically correct." (p. 39)

THE CONCEPT OF TRUST

Fear and distrust are the progeny of any life-threatening epidemic. With the progression of the AIDS epidemic over the last decade and the public's increasing awareness of the presence of the disease in physicians and health care workers, the issue of trust is becoming tantamount. The concept of trust in the physician–patient relationship has become tattered and strained given the combustive publicity surrounding the infection of Kimberly Bergalis following a routine dental procedure performed by a dentist who was HIV positive. Public and legislative response ranged from desire for mandatory HIV testing of all health care professionals to the desire for identification of high-risk procedures by hospitals, the performance of which would be banned to HIV-positive health care professionals (Miller, 1992).

Ironically, hospitals make widespread use of policies that regulate infection control and epidemiology. Modification of existing policies concerning health care workers infected with transmissible pathogens has become the mainstay of response to recent public outcry. Official policy of the University of California, San Francisco (UCSF), School of Medicine AIDS Coordinating Council is that patient and physician protection can be maximized through teaching, monitoring, and enforcement of infection control. Recommendations for health care workers caring for HIV-positive patients made by the UCSF Task Force on AIDS were initially published in the *New England Journal of Medicine* in 1983 (Cone, Hadley, & Sande, 1983).

Miller (1992) reported that in more than 10,000 cases in which a patient was treated by an HIV-infected physician, none have become infected. In contrast, of the more than 1 million cases of HIV infection to date, approximately 50 cases represent health care workers who have become infected through occupational exposure. Current policy regarding physicians is that patients are not eligible to become aware of a physician's HIV status. In addition, there is no mandatory testing for physicians or health care professionals. All patients are made aware of this policy. Patients undergoing invasive procedures with exposure to potential hematologic contamination are informed of the physician's HIV status either immediately or following testing and are subsequently counseled.

In August 1987, the Centers for Disease Control published their "Recommendations for Prevention of HIV Transmission in Health-Care Settings," which recommended that blood and body fluids precautions be consistently used for all patients, regardless of their blood-borne infectious status. These are referred to as the Universal Precautions. The Universal Precautions apply to blood and other body fluids containing blood. They do not apply to saliva, feces, nasal secretions, sputum, sweat, tears, urine, breast milk, or vomitus unless these contain visible blood. Appropriate barrier techniques should be used to prevent skin and mucous membrane exposure when contact with the blood or other body fluids of any patient is anticipated. This includes the use of masks, protective eyewear, gowns, aprons, and mouthpieces to minimize the need for mouth-to-mouth resuscitation. If a health care worker's hands or skin becomes contaminated, the area should be washed immediately. Care should be taken in the disposal of needles, scalpels, and other sharp instruments, and they should be disposed of in puncture-resistant containers. Precautions are also detailed for office housekeeping and the sterilization of surgical instruments in physicians' offices.

The risk to health care workers of contracting HIV infection following exposure to blood known to be HIV infected is approximately 1 in 250. The majority of such exposure results from needle sticks ("Centers for Disease Control Update," 1987). At the University of Southern California Medical Center, after exposure both the exposed health care worker and the infected patient undergo serum electrolyte panels, complete blood counts, HIV, hepatitis, and Venereal Disease Research Laboratories determinations. For low-risk exposure, the contact presents for evaluation and has serial HIV serum evaluations at 3, 6, 12, and 24 months. For high-risk exposure, the contact is placed on a 6-week course of ziduvodine (AZT).

In the operative suite, contamination control and the requirement for absolute sterility during surgical procedures continue to protect both the surgeon and patient from the transmission of disease. A number of modifications in both surgical technique and protective equipment have been developed to prevent contamination. Clear plastic visors and protective goggles are now routinely worn intraoperatively to prevent blood and tissue debris from splashing into the eyes or drenching the facemask. The practice of wearing two sets of gloves on each hand, versus the use of stronger monofilament or metallic gloves, can reduce the incidence of laceration of the hands by scalpel blades or puncture wounds from needles, jagged bone edges, or foreign objects. Water-repellent surgical gowns and drapes reduce the incidence of blood or fluid soaking through to the abdomen, groin, or lower extremities of the physician. Even in the presence of these additions to the operating room, nothing can replace the use of rigorous and technically sound surgical techniques, the control of bleeding, and a controlled approach to complication avoidance and management.

RESPONSIBILITIES OF PHYSICIANS TO PATIENTS WITH REGARD TO INFORMATION

Guidelines have been established to determine which patients are at high risk for contracting HIV and thus should have antibody testing. Physicians not only should be aware of these guidelines but also should be able to easily communicate this information to their patients. It should be noted that despite current statements to the contrary, 88% of AIDS in the United States is transmitted by intravenous drug abuse or high-risk sexual behavior (Centers for Disease Control, 1990). Patients who fall into high-risk categories include men who have sex with men (notably anal intercourse), patients who have a large number of sexual partners, prostitutes, hemophiliacs, patients who present for treatment of sexually transmitted diseases, patients with a history of intravenous drug abuse, patients whose sexual partners have identifiable risks, patients who received blood transfusions from 1978 to 1985, and women of childbearing age with any identifiable risk factors.

HIV TESTING

There are a number of assays to detect infection of a patient by HIV, and a basic understanding of these tests is essential for physicians to optimize the care of their patients. These include enzyme-linked immunosorbent assay, which detects host-produced antibody to HIV via spectrophotometric analysis; Western blot, which detects host-produced antibody to HIV via electrophoretic analysis; immunofluorescence assay; radioimmunoprecipitation assay; P24 viral core antigen assay; viral culture for HIV; and the polymerase chain reaction. Seroconversion with the production of detectable levels of antibody by one of the foregoing tests usually occurs within 12 weeks of exposure, although the presence of viral genome has been detected by polymerase chain reaction 42 months prior to antibody tests' becoming positive.

NEUROLOGICAL MANIFESTATIONS OF AIDS

There are a multitude of disease states that can affect an immunocompromised individual. Our focus here is on those manifestations that are associated with the CNS given our experience in the Department of Neurological Surgery at the University of Southern California School of Medicine.

Disease Entities

Patients may present in the acute stages of HIV infection with an aseptic (i.e., of undetermined etiology) meningitis. The presentation of the patient is notable for headache, fever, cranial nerve palsies, stiff neck, and changes in the number of white blood cells in the cerebral spinal fluid. This may occur in up to 10% of patients. AIDS dementia is notable for a progressive dementia, behavioral changes, and psychomotor retardation. This may occur in up to 66% of patients and is present in 90% of patients at autopsy. Peripheral neuropathies, which are usually sensory, present with symmetric radiating pain and numbness. Up to 90% of patients may present with neuropsychiatric disturbances including impaired cognition, memory loss, and sleep disturbances. Vacuolar changes in the spinal cord can result in progressive weakness, loss of function, and incontinence in afflicted patients.

Other disease entities include CNS involvement by cryptococcus, toxoplasma, herpes encephalitis, papovavirus, cytomegalovirus, Kaposi's sarcoma, and lymphoma.

Given the myriad of pathogens that can afflict the CNS in patients with AIDS, effective treatment depends on accurate diagnostic capabilities. Various CNS diseases and their potential treatments are identified in Table 1 (Levy, Bredesen, & Rosenblum, 1985).

Surgical Management

The development of methodologies of medical imaging over the past decade has expanded the clinician's comprehension of the nature and extent of structural disease processes in many areas. Our appreciation of structural alteration and certain elements of physiological disease in the brain has been refined by computed tomography (CT), magnetic resonance imaging (MRI), digital subtraction venous angiography, and positron emission tomographic scanning. The combination of these imaging capabilities and stereotactic instrumentation has initi-

Table 1 Neurological Manifestations of AIDS and Their Treatment

Disease	Treatment
Viral syndromes	
Aseptic meningitis	None
Herpes simplex encephalitis	Acyclovir or Arabinose-A (ARA-A)
AIDS dementia	None
Progressive multifocal leukoencephalopathy	ARA-A
Nonviral syndromes	
Toxoplasma gondii	Pyrimethamine and sulfadazine
Cryptococcus neoformans	Amphotericin B and 5-fluorocytosine
Candida albicans	Amphotericin B and 5-fluorocytosine
Atypical mycobacteria	Ethambutol and rifampin
Tumors	
Central nervous system (CNS) lymphoma	Radiation therapy
Kaposi's sarcoma	Radiation therapy and chemotherapy
CNS and systemic lymphoma	Radiation therapy and chemotherapy

ated reappraisal of the indication for larger, more invasive procedures involving the biopsy and excision of lesions in the brain.

Stereotactic biopsy refers to the identification of a lesion within the brain in three dimensions or in X, Y, and Z coordinates. The lesion is identified using CT or MRI following the placement of a localizing frame onto the patient's head. The various coordinates required to perform a biopsy are determined by the CT or MRI coordinates made at the level of the lesion. The coordinates are then processed by computer and a biopsy performed based on the calculated anteroposterior, lateral, and vertical points. Stereotactic biopsy is less invasive and associated with less morbidity/mortality than craniotomy and has expanded the neurological surgeon's options for patient management, many of which are threatening to the patient. Currently, images, although providing significant structural information, do not present a reliable assessment of the tissue type or infectious origins of the lesion. Our experience is based on methods and applications of imaging-directed stereotactic biopsy employed by the neurosurgical services of the University of Southern California Medical Center, where approximately 1,000 such procedures have been undertaken since 1981.

During the past decade, neurosurgery has seen the evolution of increasingly sophisticated imaging devices that allow unusual refinements in the radiological appreciation of normal and abnormal intracranial structures. During the past 5 years, stereotactic devices that allow a wedding of imaging techniques and stereotactic neurosurgical concepts have become available. Being privileged to have had available a prototype instrument (Brown-Roberts-Wells imaging-directed stereotactic system) during the early stages of this evolving discipline (Heilbrun, Roberts, Apuzzo, Wells, & Sabshin, 1983) we have elsewhere reported our initial experiences and application of these techniques in the evaluation and management of intracranial mass lesions (Apuzzo, Chandrasoma, Zelman, Giannotta, & Wells, 1984; Apuzzo & Sabshin, 1983). Stereotaxis offers multiple options to the neurological surgeon. Specifically in relation to structural alteration, applications that may be considered include (a) precise point tissue retrieval for biopsy and tissue assay (Fulling & Nelson, 1984; Ostertag, Mennel, & Kiessling, 1980), (b) cystic structure or abscess cavity aspiration (Rivas & Lobato, 1985), (c) installation of permanent or temporary drainage conduits (Apuzzo et al., 1984; Apuzzo & Sabshin, 1983), (d) installation of single or multiple catheter arrays for point source or colloid-based radiation therapy (brachytherapy) (Apuzzo, Chandrasoma, Zelman, & von Hanwehr, 1987; Gutin et al., 1984), (e) precise direction of cerebroscopic instrumentation with concurrent biopsy aspiration or excision (Iizuka, 1975), and (f) point localization of abnormal tissue and guidance during surgery (Kelly, Kall, & Goerss, 1984). We are reporting our experience and the neurosurgical perspectives gained from over 1,000 cases in which imaging-directed stereotaxy was used in the evaluation and management of intracranial structural abnormalities.

General Methodology

Because the goal of biopsy technique is rapid and safe point access, with retrieval of tissue from the target point with minimization of risk but maximization of accuracy of assay, our perspective led us to adopt methods that permitted

1 Rapid translation of accurate imaging data to an operating-room setting;
2 Compacted time use of imaging areas during the procedure;
3 Performance of all aspects of the procedure with local anesthesia with neuroanesthesiologists standing by (this approach was adopted to ensure full cooperation of the patient, rapid recognition of complications, and optimization of the period of patient recovery);
4 Minimization of tissue trauma and handling;
5 Close interaction with surgical pathologists, cytopathologists, neuropathologists, and microbiologists during the biopsy procedure and tissue processing.

These goals were achieved employing the Brown-Roberts-Wells system (Apuzzo et al., 1984; Apuzzo & Sabshin, 1983; Heilbrun, 1983; Heilbrun et al., 1983) and by developing a close amalgam with the neuroanesthesiology, neuroradiology, and surgical pathology departments as a composite involved and interested stereotactic team (Apuzzo, Chandrasoma, Cohen, et al., 1987; Apuzzo, Chandrasoma, Zelman, & von Hanwehr, 1987). Without adequate support in these ancillary areas, the capabilities of imaging-directed stereotactic biopsy or instrumentation cannot be fully or satisfactorily exploited.

Diagnosis

The use of stereotactic biopsy in AIDS is controversial. In our experience, the occurrence of any mass lesion in the brain is associated with short survival in HIV-positive patients. We use stereotactic biopsy in our institution only for mass lesions for which a strong suspicion of malignant lymphoma exists after a trial of antitoxoplasma drugs.

The expectations of stereotactic biopsy are less for nonneoplastic lesions than for tumors. Infections we have encountered include tuberculosis, coccidioidomycosis, mucormycosis, cryptococcosis, cysticercosis, herpes simplex, cytomegalovirus encephalitis, progressive multifocul leukoencephalopathy, and toxoplasmosis. Recently Levy et al. (1992) reported performing stereotactic biopsy in 50 neurologically symptomatic patients with AIDS. Patients were diagnosed with HIV encephalitis (3 patients), infarction (2 patients), cryptococcosis (1 patient), atypical mycobacterial infection (1 patient), progressive multifocal leukoencephalopathy (14 patients), lymphoma (14 patients), toxoplasmosis (13 patients), and metastatic tumors (2 patients). They reported a definitive diagnostic efficacy of 96%.

Stereotactic biopsy requires a piece of tissue for permanent sections from which multiple slides are cut for immunoperoxidase studies for viruses (herpes simplex, cytomegalovirus, and progressive multifocal leukoencephalopathy) and toxoplasma. The next priority for tissue is for electron microscopy. If tissue remains, a sample for mycobacterial, fungal, and viral culture is taken before the rest is submitted for routine sections.

CONCLUSION

Innovation in neurosurgical imaging, techniques, and methodology have allowed neurosurgeons to markedly enhance the diagnostic potential while decreasing the morbidity and mortality of classic surgical approaches. It is of concern that such progression in our knowledge and technique is countered by bias that exists in some physicians' perception of patients with AIDS. The fear of both the disease and its political ramifications has compromised physicians' ability to provide care. A similar fear, based on a lack of understanding, exists in the general population and has further compromised any potential bond that can be formed between a physician and patient. Much as technical innovation has increased the potential benefits to patients with AIDS, education of the physician and general population is essential to return AIDS to its categorization as an infectious disease and to return patient care to the level of the patient–physician relationship.

REFERENCES

Apuzzo, M. L. J., Chandrasoma, P. T., Cohen, D., Zee, C. S., & Zelman, V. (1987). Computed imaging stereotaxy: Experience and perspective related to 500 procedures applies to brain masses. *Neurosurgery, 20,* 930–937.

Apuzzo, M. L. J., Chandrasoma, P. T., Zelman, V., Giannotta, S. L., & Weiss, M. H. (1984).Computed tomographic guidance stereotaxis in the management of lesions of the third ventricular region. *Neurosurgery, 15,* 502–508.

Apuzzo, M. L. J., Chandrasoma, P. T., Zelman, V., & von Hanwehr, R. I. (1987). Applications of stereotaxis. In M. L. J. Apuzzo (Ed.), *Surgery of the third ventricle* (pp. 751–792). Baltimore: Williams & Wilkins.

Apuzzo, M. L. J., & Sabshin, J. K. (1983). Computed tomographic guidance stereotaxis in the management of intracranial mass lesions. *Neurosurgery, 12,* 277–285.

Centers for Disease Control. (1990). *HIV/AIDS surveillance report.* Atlanta, GA: Author.

Centers for Disease Control update: Human immunodeficiency virus infections in health-care workers exposed to blood of infected patients. (1987). *Morbidity and Mortality Weekly Report, 36,* 285–289.

Clarke, O. W., & Conley, R. B. (1991). The duty to "attend upon the sick" [editorial]. *Journal of the American Medical Association, 266,* 2876–2877.

Conte, J. E., Hadley, W. K., & Sande, M. Special Report: Infection control guidelines for patients with the acquired immunodeficiency syndrome (AIDS). *New England Journal of Medicine, 309,* 740–744.

Faria, M. A. (1992). To treat or not—can a physician choose? A commentary. *The Pharos, 55,* 39–40.

Fulling, K. H., & Nelson, J. S. (1984). Cerebral astrocytic neoplasms in the adult: Contribution of histologic examination to the assessment of prognosis. *Seminars in Diagnostic Pathology, 1,* 152–163.

Fumento, M. (1990). *The myth of heterosexual AIDS.* New York: Basic Books.

Gutin, P. H., Phillips, T. L., Wara, W. M., Liebel, S. A., Hosobuchi, Y., Levin, V. A., Weaver, K. A., & Lamb, S. (1984). Brachytherapy of recurrent malignant brain tumors with removable high activity iodine-125 sources. *Journal of Neurosurgery, 60,* 61–68.

Heilbrun, M. P. (1983). Computed tomography-guided stereotactic systems. *Clinical Neurosurgery, 31,* 564–580.

Heilbrun, M. P., Roberts, T. S., Apuzzo, M. L. J., Wells, T. H., & Sabshin, J. K. (1983). Preliminary experience with Brown-Roberts-Wells computerized tomographic stereotaxic guidance system. *Journal of Neurosurgery, 59,* 217–222.

Iizuka, J. (1975). Development of a stereotaxic endoscopy of the ventricular system. *Confinia Neurologica 37,* 141–149.

Kelly, J. A., St. Lawrence, J. S., Hood, H. V., Smith, S., Jr., & Cook, D. J. (1988). Nurses' attitudes towards AIDS. *Journal of Continuing Education in Nursing, 19,* 78–83.

Kelly, J. A., St. Lawrence, J. S., Smith, S., Jr., Hood, H. V., & Cook, D. J. (1987a). Medical students' attitudes towards AIDS and homosexual patients. *Journal of Medical Education, 62,* 549–556.

Kelly, J. A., St. Lawrence, J. S., Smith, S., Jr., Hood, H. V., & Cook, D. J. (1987b). Stigmatization of AIDS patients by physicians. *American Journal of Public Health, 77,* 789–791.

Kelly, P. J., Kall, B. A., & Goerss, S. G. (1984). Computer-assisted stereotactic biopsies utilizing CT and digitized arteriographic control. *Acta Neurochirurgica (Wien), 33*(Suppl.), 233–235.

Levy, R. M., Bredesen, D. E., & Rosenblum, M. L. (1985). Neurological manifestations of AIDS. *Journal of Neurosurgery, 62,* 475–495.

Levy, R. M., Russell, E., Yungbluth, M., Frias Hidvegi, D., Brody, B. A., & Dal Canto, M. C. (1992). The efficacy of image-guided stereotactic brain biopsy in neurologically symptomatic acquired immunodeficiency syndrome patients. *Neurosurgery, 30,* 186–190.

McCullum, C. (1992). Disease and dirt: Social dimensions of influenza, cholera, and syphilis. *The Pharos, 55,* 22–29.

Miller, J. (1992). HIV: Infection control and your health. *UCSF Magazine, 13,* 24–27.

Ostertag, C. B., Mennel, H. D., & Kiessling, M. (1980). Stereotactic biopsy of brain tumors. *Surgical Neurology, 14,* 275–283.

Rivas, J. J., & Lobato, R. D. (1985). CT-assisted stereotaxic aspiration of colloid cysts of the third ventricle. *Journal of Neurosurgery, 62,* 238–242.

Chapter Twelve

Adolescents and HIV: Two Decades of Denial

Karen K. Hein
Jill F. Blair
Scott C. Ratzan
Denise E. Dyson

As we enter the second decade of the human immunodeficiency virus (HIV) epidemic, many challenges arise; one of the foremost centers on the adolescent community. The sexual and drug activities associated with increased prevalence of HIV infection often begin during adolescence. Hence the epidemic of acquired immune deficiency syndrome (AIDS) poses a significant threat to this population. However, HIV research, prevention, and service programs frequently fail to address the unique needs of this critical group (Hein, 1991a). With educational attention principally directed to children or adults, adolescents, who are neither big children nor small adults, often are not reached through traditional venues.

The lack of sufficient programs that address adolescents' needs stems from the fact that HIV among adolescents is largely an invisible epidemic. Because adolescents do not flock into emergency rooms, clinics, or private offices dying of AIDS, it is easier to overlook their needs when those who are dying present such obvious, pressing concern (Kipke, Futterman, & Hein, 1990). However, if there is to be any potential control of the AIDS epidemic, the acknowledgment that adolescents are susceptible to the disease must be registered through programs designed to meet this group's particular needs (Hein, 1991c).

The focus of this chapter is to analyze the scope and magnitude of adolescents' concerns during this era of AIDS; to look at the ways in which those needs have been neglected; and to make suggestions for improvement within the health care system and educational, social service, and media sectors. As a recommendation for the future, we discuss comprehensive services and technical assistance on the local, regional, and national levels, based on the New York City Adolescent AIDS Program. By applying the results of recent program research on medical, psychosocial, and risk assessment issues, we hope to provide a better understanding of the problems of the adolescent during this epidemic. Chancellor Joseph Fernandez and his staff's contribution to AIDS activism in the New York City school system is examined, along with the power waged by the formation of coalitions of educators, health care workers, parents, and students in the battle for control of this pandemic disease.

STEREOTYPES, FEAR, AND DENIAL

In the late 1980s, AIDS was the sixth leading cause of death in young people ages 15 through 24 (Des Jarlais et al., 1990); now it approaches the rank of fifth place (Novello, 1988). Because there is often a delay of a decade from HIV infection to AIDS, the fact that numerous adolescent AIDS cases presently exist indicates that these adolescents were infected years ago.

The story of Ryan White, a hemophiliac adolescent who acquired HIV through blood transfusions, helped Americans comprehend that adolescents with HIV can die of AIDS. Ryan White helped Americans to break through stereotypes, fear, and denial as he moved from exclusion from one community to inclusion in another.

The media characterization of adolescents with HIV has been and still is highly stereotypical. Teenagers, especially adolescents, with HIV are stereotyped in newspapers and magazines as either innocent victims or rebellious juveniles guilty of unacceptable behavior (see Chapter 6). Many magazines, including *Psychology Today* (Hersch, 1988), have carried excellent articles dealing with the issues of HIV in the adolescent world, while accompanying these articles with photographs portraying infected adolescent girls as prostitutes or infected adolescent boys as delinquents. There is little representation of the thousands of adolescents who are in school and have jobs, partners, friends, and loving and supportive families.

The example of Henry Nichols, the Eagle Scout who was commended by Norman Schwartzkof, demonstrates the stereotypical view portrayed by the media. Henry acquired HIV through blood transfusion as a young person with hemophilia, not through sexual transmission. For this reason, newspapers praised him for his achievements.

Other examples abound, including the *New York Newsday* (Nov. 6, 1991) article entitled, "Poor Kids Spreading AIDS." The use of the word *spreading*, instead of *contracting*, as well as other sensational language, reinforces stereotypical views. The separation of adolescents with HIV into "bad kids" and "good kids" creates judgmental images that hamper the promotion of education, awareness, and prevention of the epidemic.

FUEL FOR THE FUTURE:
THE ADOLESCENT AIDS PROGRAM

Although both the media and the majority of HIV programs have not addressed the needs of the adolescent during the last decade of the AIDS crisis, some organizations and groups have rallied to this cause. One example is New York City's Adolescent AIDS Program, which is part of the Montefiore Medical Center and the Albert Einstein College of Medicine in the Bronx. In July 1987, the doors were opened to a center that had no patients. Five years later, the program has cared for 65 adolescents with HIV, only 4 of whom have developed AIDS and died (Hein, 1987).

Although the New York City Adolescent AIDS Program is hospital based, it nonetheless is structured to accommodate a variety of adolescent needs. At the heart of the program are the clinical services, which operate under the title of Risk Evaluation Program (REP). The term "AIDS" was purposely excluded from the title because of the stigma that still exists in coming to a program that specializes in this disease. The REP staff includes a physician's assistant, adolescent medicine specialist, social worker, and psychologist. In addition to this core team, professionals such as a lawyer, an ethicist, a priest, and a group of outreach workers and health educators help to connect the program with the community-based agencies that serve youth (Futterman & Hein, 1990). Many concerned adolescents do not know how to approach such a system, so the Adolescent AIDS Program is part of the AIDS and Adolescent Network of New York City. The network, also founded in 1987, operates with more than 750 members in an effective partnership that links medical centers, youth care agencies, educators, and social service organizations (Hein, 1990b).

The three principal goals of the Adolescent AIDS Program are clinical care, clinical research, and advocacy for youth. The unique aspects of HIV infection in adolescents are explained to help other health providers through the U.S. adapt successful elements of this program to their setting. The research compares the different modes of HIV transmission among adolescents, young children, and adults. An additional goal of the program is to bring attention on the local, state, and national levels to the fact that adolescents embody the next wave of the HIV epidemic. As an example, until 1991, teenagers between the ages of 13 and 17 could not participate in the national clinical trials as there were no established protocols for their age group. Finally, in the fall of 1991, seven adolescent units were funded to help adolescents have access to clinical trials designed specifically for them. Nevertheless, in most areas of HIV/AIDS research, adolescents continue to be a forgotten segment of the population during this epidemic.

In the Adolescent AIDS Program, HIV testing is conducted confidentially, and counseling sessions continue for as long as it takes an individual to understand the risks and benefits of being tested. Sometimes, pretest counseling can take 6 months. Parental consent or knowledge is not required for counseling and testing, although an adolescent always is encouraged to discuss the situation with a parent or guardian if possible (Hein, 1991b).

Central to the Adolescent AIDS Program's philosophy is the belief that one cannot take care of adolescents unless one attends to the existing barriers of consent, confidentiality, and payment. If adolescents are going to visit the center confidentially, without the knowledge or consent of their parents or guardians, they probably will be unable to pay. As a solution, a free first visit is offered, at which time a payment schedule is worked out. If adolescents are included under their parents' or guardians' insurance plans but wish their visits to remain confidential, they are asked to pay an amount as low as 50 cents or a dollar per session, or an amount they can afford.

Medical, Psychosocial, and Risk Assessment Issues

In 1990, the Adolescent AIDS Program reviewed the experiences of its 65 young clients with HIV. Although most of them appeared to be healthy, a surprising discovery was made that half of them had immune systems that were severely impaired, with CD4 counts under $500/mm^3$ when they walked in the door (Futterman & Hein, 1990). Most of these young people had no clinical symptoms.

At present, the exact natural history of HIV in adolescents is unclear. What is known is that infected adolescents get many of the ailments that adolescents without HIV commonly get (Futterman, Hein, Legg, Dell, & Shaffer, 1991). Skin conditions, including acne and seborrhea; sinus infections; as well as vaginal infections for females are the common manifestations among adolescents. Therefore, having an active primary care focus in the HIV clinic becomes extremely important. In the REP, immunizations, flu vaccine, measles-mumps-rubella, and pneumococcal vaccine are provided so adolescents can be kept as healthy as possible. In addition to primary care activities, the program also provides secondary and tertiary care, including backup hospitalization (Hein, 1990a). In addition to linking adolescents to counseling and testing opportunities, it is essential that a hospital is located nearby, ready and willing to take an adolescent when an HIV-related illness or complication requires hospitalization.

Although the psychosocial issues are varied, many are related to the time period directly following the adolescents' discovery that they are HIV positive and before they have learned to integrate the implications into their lives. Often the 14-day waiting period between having the blood test and learning the results is an extremely tense time for adolescents. It is essential that staff are available to answer any questions and provide support in case anxiety levels get exceedingly high.

Once adolescents are informed, the main concern for those who test HIV positive is suicidal ideation or attempt. Research conducted in the program indicates that the circumstances of counseling and testing are fundamental factors in determining the response of an infected adolescent (Hein, 1991b). If adolescents find out through programs that require HIV testing as a prerequisite for training or employment, such as in the military or Job Corps, where follow-up services may not be offered, they are prone to reacting much more negatively than if they find out through comprehensive care facilities, where staff are prepared to provide support, as well as psychological and medical services (Futterman, Hein, Kipke, et al., 1990).

Issues of disclosure create the next traumatic turning point. What is a 15-year-old supposed to tell his or her friends, community, school teachers, employer, or parents, and how? Many young people in the Adolescent AIDS Program have chosen not to disclose to anybody but the staff in the program for many months after learning they are HIV infected. The staff then are placed in a position of acting as family for adolescents during those first few months while they come to grips with the implications of the disease and determine how they can inform their inner and outer circles.

Another difficult time is when an adolescent's CD4 blood cell count changes from one of the arbitrary markers of more than 500 to less than 500/mm^3. Studies have shown that when the immune system declines to this level, treatments with specific medications such as zidovudine (AZT) can help keep recipients healthy by either buffering the faulty immune system or helping to prevent or treat specific infections. When the marker falls between 200 and 500, discussion of the possibility of taking AZT is instigated. When the marker falls under 200, the idea of prophylaxis against *Pneumocystis carinii* pneumonia is introduced.

Risk Reduction Strategies

In the major national strategies, the messages to adolescents are

- Be abstinent,
- Be monogamous,
- Limit the number of partners, and
- Use condoms.

It is educational to examine each of these messages (Hein, 1991c). The declaration "Be abstinent," although the safest lifestyle, is not an attractive alternative to many adolescents. The message "Be monogamous" is confusing to adolescents, because most consider themselves to be so. If they have had intercourse, they have had it with one person for a while, and then perhaps with another person for a while. This pattern is a kind of monogamy. The message should be that it only takes one infected partner to become infected, and one's risk of being infected from just one partner is increasing rapidly (Emans, Brown, Davis, Felice, & Hein, 1991).

Regarding the message to "Limit the number of partners," again, a person has a much higher risk of getting HIV if his or her one partner is infected than if the person had a hundred partners who are not infected. The notion of limiting one's number of partners has an epidemiological truth, but it is not helpful in securing the protection of individual adolescents.

The third message, "Use condoms," ignores the fact that it is a difficult challenge for most female adolescents to convince male partners to use condoms; thus, the preventive message is lost. Female adolescents cannot use male condoms because condoms are not designed for the female body. (The recently approved female condom is expensive and not yet readily available.) Specific communication of appropriate images through the word choices that ultimately affect societal behavior will take time.

Unfortunately, many of the adolescents with HIV in the Adolescent AIDS Program do not practice safer sex because they are afraid that by either using a condom or asking for a condom to be used, they might imply that they have a reason to need one. Until condom use is more widely accepted, adolescents will continue to think that they would be suspect if they used or requested one. One 16-year-old girl was able to get her partner to use condoms by saying that she had an ovarian cyst and that condoms were essential in her condition. Her story made no medical sense, but the alternative of telling him that she had HIV was unacceptable to her.

A young man in the program refused to use condoms because, he said, "if I do my partner will somehow know or suspect that I have HIV." Another young woman sat in her AIDS education class at school and wanted to correct the teacher's misinformation. But she did not dare; so great was her fear of disclosure that she could not take the risk of sharing the information she knew to be true.

Another patient in the REP, a 20-year-old, is afraid to lose the independence that is so important to him. He has continued to work, but when he is forced to miss work for treatment purposes, he tells his employer that he has diabetes and that he needs to receive injections at the hospital. Because of this fear of losing his job, he is not able to have his medical care covered by employee insurance.

Adolescents are concerned not only about disclosure about their HIV condition but also of the behavior that may have caused the infection. Whether it be sexual abuse, living on the streets and being engaged in "survival sex," or same-sex activities, often adolescents do not feel comfortable disclosing the secrets of their past or present lives unless a bond of trust is established (see Chapter 1 for a discussion of trust). Over time, they usually recount their stories to a counselor at the center, although often they never reveal their experiences to the people with whom they are sharing their lives. One young man has arrived with his girlfriend for every clinic visit. She now is knowledgeable about safer sex, as is he. They are both very bright and have memorized the guidebook for young people, *AIDS: Trading Fears for Facts* (Hein & Di-Geronimo, 1992). They can quote it chapter and verse. However, the young man has perianal warts. This is an indication that at some point, he has been the recipient of anal intercourse, but this is not something he is willing to discuss with his program counselors even after a year of being in their care.

In addition, it is important to consider the extreme vulnerability of adolescent gay males and heterosexual females (Brooks-Gunn, Duke-Duncan, Ehrhardt, Hein, & Shafer, 1989). Adolescent gay males, certainly if they cannot talk about HIV, often cannot talk about being gay, and these communicative barriers increase the feeling of isolation. Often gay male adolescents have sexual relationships with older men, who they believe will not judge their sexuality. However, in their search to be accepted, these adolescents may increase their risk by having unprotected sex with men who have a greater prevalence of the HIV virus. For those gay male adolescents who have been kicked out of their homes or have run away and are trying to survive on the streets, it is important to realize that people who buy sex often will pay an adolescent more if he does not insist that a condom be used.

Heterosexual females also are an extremely vulnerable group if they have unprotected sexual intercourse. Half of the young woman in the Adolescent AIDS Program with HIV had fewer than five lifetime partners before they contracted the disease. They had no way of knowing that they or their partners were at risk of contracting HIV. In this case, it is a myth about risk reduction that an adolescent girl should "know her partner," when 90% of people with the virus do not know they have it. Many young heterosexual females are discovering almost inadvertently that they are HIV positive, when they donate blood in college, when they are pregnant, or when they are tested for other sexually transmitted diseases and find out that HIV counseling and testing are available.

It takes very sensitive antennae to learn how to approach adolescents who are frightened of disclosure (Kipke, Futterman, & Hein, 1990). If words like "boyfriend" and "girlfriend" are used, it is very unlikely that adolescents will disclose information about same-sex activities. In the program, the staff use words like "partners." No assumptions are made about the partners' genders. It is presumed that sexual abuse has been an issue for many young people who have sexually transmitted diseases or HIV; a nonjudgmental approach provides the opportunity for disclosing that kind of experience. Open-ended questions are asked, such as "Has anything ever happened to you sexually that has made you uncomfortable?" Often, adolescents who come to the center will answer that question no and then 6 months or a year later, when they feel safe, will reveal that the answer is in fact yes.

OPTIMISM AND ACTIVISM IN NEW YORK CITY[1]

New York City is Number 1 in the list of American cities with diagnosed AIDS cases. The city has 20% of the country's cases in the age group of 13 to 21, although it holds only 3% of the nation's youth population (Vermund, Hein, Gayle, Cary, & Thomas, 1989). In addition, New York City provides schooling for 956,616 children from kindergarten to high school.[2] Because the AIDS epidemic has hit New York City first and hardest, this city can act as a "crystal ball," lighting the way for the rest of the nation.

On February 27th, 1991, the New York City Board of Education, in a four to three vote, broke new ground in its adoption of the most far-reaching HIV/AIDS education initiative in the country—a program that includes the availability of condoms at the high school level, without parental notification or consent, for all students enrolled in school. This bold and challenging program is not only unique because of its component parts; it speaks to the need to raise consciousness and demands that controversial issues be discussed in public, that the opposition reveal itself, and that the community at large take responsibility.

What makes the New York City Public Schools HIV/AIDS Education Program including condom availability special is that it required a public debate and a public vote. It demanded accountability from all sectors of the community, from the Mayor to the Commissioner of Health.

In the spring of 1990, a subcommittee of the HIV/AIDS Advisory Council wrote a letter to Chancellor Joseph A. Fernandez requesting a meeting. The Chancellor scheduled a meeting to discuss their concerns. The subcommittee presented evidence of neglect by the school system and a lack of commitment by the administration on this issue, and presented the Chancellor with a call for a high-quality curriculum, an upgraded Advisory Council with broad representation, and condoms in the schools. They presented statistics. They spoke of children with whom they had worked, whose lives had been decimated by the HIV virus, and of adolescents who reported being HIV positive. They spoke of

---

[1]Portions of this section originally appeared in "Politics and Practice: HIV/AIDS Education Including Condom Availability in New York City Public Schools" by J. F. Blair, December 1991/January 1992, SIECUS Report, 20(2). Reprinted with permission. Copyright © Education Council of the U.S., Inc. 130 West 42nd Street, Suite 2500, New York, NY 10036. (212)819-9770, fax (212)819-9776.

[2]Statistic taken from Facts & Figures 1991–92, published by the New York City Public Schools (Joseph A. Fernandez, Chancellor); produced by the Division of Public Affairs.

young people who were not educated about their own risk of infection, and who had no access to information about HIV/AIDS prevention.

On August 30, 1990, the AIDS Advisory Council met with the Chancellor. This was the first time in its history that the Chancellor had met with the Council, and as a result, there was a record turnout, with representatives from the Catholic Church, as well as advocates and activists. The Chancellor discussed their recommendations and stated his intention to adopt every recommendation with the exception of condom availability, which he would have to investigate and present to the members of the Board. Staff members, with assistance from the New York City Department of Health, collected materials and reviewed the statistics on adolescent sexuality. In September, the Chancellor expressed his personal support of the availability of condoms, and on September 26, 1990, the headline in *New York Newsday* read, "Chancellor: Schools Should Hand Out Condoms. Fernandez Pushes AIDS Education Plan."

Members of the New York City Board of Education requested that the Chancellor present them with a comprehensive plan for K–12 on HIV/AIDS education. The plan was developed over several months, beginning in early October 1990, when an extraordinary advocacy coalition came together from a broad spectrum of educators, health professionals, and HIV/AIDS activists to organize an education initiative with the goal of helping to protect New York City's youth from a deadly epidemic.

By November 15th, a draft plan had been written. Meetings were scheduled with labor unions, the Federation of Parent Associations, district and high school superintendents and principals, members of locally elected community school boards, clerical leaders, and advocacy organizations. The consultation process for an issue of this kind requires affirmative outreach. The development of the Chancellor's plan included a range of actions and activities, from updating and developing a K–12 HIV/AIDS curriculum to organizing HIV/AIDS Education Teams comprised of parents, students, and faculty at every high school in the city. The plan was revised a half dozen times, as a result of the consultation process, prior to its presentation to the Board of Education. Although the changes were relatively minor, the process proved helpful both in generating support for the Chancellor's initiative and in broadly disseminating the content of the plan.

In early December, a memo was issued to more than 1,000 individuals and institutions inviting written comment on the plan. Four public sessions were scheduled on Saturdays and weekday evenings, with the Chancellor's staff available for comments and questions. At the same time, there were other forums for public debate. To demonstrate the interest generated by this issue, when the Board of Education presented its budget proposal for the school system, a $6.5 billion plan for school expenditures, only a handful of citizens came to comment on the proposed budget. Yet, from October to February, more than 500 people signed up to speak on HIV/AIDS education in the schools. One session lasted 6 hr. Eventually the Board of Education scheduled a 12-hr public hearing to allow all parties to be heard. The hall of the Board was crowded with spectators and speakers, with television cameras from as far away as Australia.

Citizens spoke about adolescent sexuality and family morals, about religious conviction and the risk of disease, about the breakdown of society and the crime of ignorance. Some speakers asserted that children were dying, and others called people who are infected deviants. There were protests and prayer vigils. The newspapers and television news reported the sometimes hysterical and chaotic atmosphere that pervaded the public sessions of the Board. But beyond the anger and the outrage, there were moments of gripping emotion.

One 17-year-old described the tragedy of her best friend, who committed suicide after discovering she was HIV positive because she could not find the help she needed. Joey DiPaolo, a student who attends a New York City elementary school and is HIV positive, stood on a chair to reach the microphone and spoke of his own illness, his friends' ignorance about the infection, the lack of information, and the importance of the program. Joey's voice cracked as he pleaded with those present to "please educate the children."

Since Chancellor Fernandez launched the campaign to promote comprehensive HIV/AIDS education including condom availability, many school districts across the country have begun to discuss the issue and examine the need for new pedagogic strategies to affect adolescent knowledge and behavior. The public debate of the New York City program has been critical to its success, not only in New York, where significant dialogue has been generated among young people and adults about HIV, but across the nation where New York City's program has been the subject of heated debate. It is, in fact, these discussions, which can raise public awareness of the issues of HIV/AIDS education and prevention, that will have an impact on the HIV/AIDS epidemic.

In addition to public awareness, there are other critical program components, and very important distinctions must be made as this issue is further discussed and new program designs are developed. Not all condom availability initiatives are alike, and in order to assess the objectives and effectiveness of different models, it is important to cite the differences:

• *Clinic based versus school based.* Clinic-based programs usually require some form of parental consent, either affirmative or passive, and are designed as a medical intervention model, not as a component of education and counseling about HIV/AIDS for adolescents.
• *Parental consent versus nonconsent.* The New York City program is the only school-based program using faculty volunteers that has no consent requirement of any kind. A parental consent requirement, by definition, inhibits open communication between the young person and the adult school professional in discussing issues of adolescent sexuality and HIV/AIDS.
• *Comprehensive versus compartmentalized.* This distinction, again, ties

into a clinic-based program versus a school-based program. The New York City model is a comprehensive HIV/AIDS education program for K–12. The program includes a curriculum that is designed in collaboration with health professionals, staff development for curriculum implementation, and training—specific to the implementation of condom availability—for parents, students, and faculty who volunteer to participate on the HIV/AIDS Education Teams.

- *Levels of training.* This is the only program where training is provided to all members of the school community—parents, students, and faculty—in the same environment. The response to this strategy has been overwhelmingly positive. The training includes three sections:

Orientation (1 half day, for all HIV/AIDS Education Team members): An informational and motivational seminar.

Tier I (1 full day, for all HIV/AIDS Education Team members): Team building, understanding adolescence, and basic factual overview of HIV infection and related health topics via small group exercises.

Tier II (2 full days, for faculty only): Learning to reinforce abstinence as the most effective method of prevention of sexual transmission of HIV and other sexually transmitted diseases, emphasizing resistance to peer pressure; understanding the risks of use and misuse of condoms; understanding adolescent sexuality within the context of broader developmental issues; clarifying roles and responsibilities; using referrals effectively; and communication skills building.

After schools successfully complete all three training components, they are visited by a health educator and a licensed school supervisor. This team observes a lesson in HIV, visits the health resource sites identified by the school as condom availability sites, and meets with faculty members who have volunteered to make condoms available. This site visit represents the last step in the review process prior to implementation.

- *Community organizing initiative versus school-based initiative:* Some school districts pride themselves on being able to implement HIV/AIDS education programs without controversy. In truth, one of the most effective aspects of any HIV/AIDS education initiative is the degree to which it raises community consciousness and generates public debate. Whether people agree or disagree, it is critical that the community at large become engaged in a dialogue to address this issue.

Since February 27, 1991, when the New York City program was adopted by the Board of Education, the following have occurred:

- Implementation guidelines were developed.
- High schools were offered technical assistance in developing their condom availability plans.
- A training committee of outside experts was established to design the HIV and condom availability training for the high schools.

- A K–6 curriculum was written and shared with national readers, and was submitted to the Board for adoption.
- $195,000 was donated by private corporations and foundations to establish a small grants program for high school students on student-developed HIV/AIDS education projects.
- $510,000 was provided privately to hire staff to assist with the implementation of condom availability in the high schools.
- 500,000 condoms were donated by Carter-Wallace and London International, leading condom manufacturers.
- 16 high schools began their training in June 1991.
- 2 of those 16 schools began condom availability on November 26.
- More than 100 of the city's high schools are in the process of completing or have completed their training.
- By June 1992, 112 of the 120 high schools were making condoms available.

This chronology gives the impression that things have gone smoothly since February 27, 1991. However, a lawsuit has been filed by a member of the Board and four parents against the Chancellor and the Board of Education for violating parental rights, and charges are pending before the State Education Commissioner against the Chancellor. In addition, letters still are received from people who oppose the program, many on religious and moral grounds.

However, strong signs exist that the program is beginning to take effect. At John Dewey High School, one of the first of the two schools that launched the New York City initiative, the program began with frenzied activity as students converged on the health resource sites in large numbers for the first day or so. However, after the program had been in place for a week, students were quietly lining up their chairs and waiting outside the health resource sites to meet with the faculty volunteer to talk about issues of concern. Students were asking to see a condom, many for the first time, and to learn about HIV, sexually transmitted diseases, and pregnancy prevention. The health resource sites were being used, as planned, as sources of information, support, and guidance.

The New York City school system plan offers a powerful weapon, fighting the epidemic on three levels, through the insistence of factual awareness, the development of necessary communication skills, and the expansion of available services. The plan will provide not only the students but also teachers and parents with the facts. It will help individual young people to learn how to think, talk, and act toward their friends about the epidemic and to practice safer sex. It will provide referral services to health centers in each community for the purposes of counseling and HIV testing. In addition to learning about risk and safety, the young adults of tomorrow also are learning how they will be able to do an effective job in dealing with a pandemic that clearly will be a devastating part of their adult lives.

Ongoing HIV/AIDS education in public schools is absolutely critical if a dent is to be made in the spread of HIV infection among adolescents. For too long, administrators of some schools have neglected or ignored this issue, hoping it would go away. And in other cases, their approach has been so timid that their programs merely reflect society's self-consciousness about human sexuality, failing to present a well-developed instructional program on HIV/AIDS. The central initiative of the New York City high school program is to permeate the schools with AIDS educational messages, in all classes, not just health classes. But most importantly, it is the tenor that is being changed so the "c" word can be said without inhibitions by teachers and students alike. But the fight has only just begun. Public schools need to work in tandem with local health departments and community-based organizations to provide services and information about HIV/AIDS. Parents also must be educated, and the political battles must be public.

CONCLUSION

Babies who were born when the virus was starting to spread in the mid 1970s are now adolescents. Many cannot remember a time before the epidemic. Now the responsibility has fallen on the adolescents of this generation to do more than just protect themselves from contracting HIV. Because of a newfound awareness, it is hoped they will foster a compassionate, more involved response to this epidemic. The challenge of the 1990s is to help all Americans realize that the AIDS epidemic is not a problem that will go away on its own, that it is one that will touch the lives of each person in this country and around the world well into the next century (Hein, 1992b). The words of a pamphleteer in 1926 aptly apply to the threat of AIDS in this decade: "When ignorance, superstition, and prejudice prevail, preventable disease will be allowed to slay right and left, especially among children. . . . With the practical knowledge already at our command, every case . . . and every death therefrom is a direct challenge to our intelligence" (American Association for Medical Progress, 1926). By taking a realistic step toward effective communication about AIDS, through the elimination of stereotypes about adolescents via the repetition of HIV transmission and prevention messages, society will be better prepared to deal efficiently with the next wave of the HIV epidemic.

REFERENCES

American Association for Medical Progress. (1926). *Diphtheria—curable and preventable*. New York: Author.
Brooks-Gunn, J., Duke-Duncan, P., Ehrhardt, A., Hein, K., & Shafer, M. A. (1989). Adolescent HIV Infection. *Pediatrics, 83,* 299–301.
Des Jarlais, D., Ehrhardt, A., Fullilove, M., Hein, K., Menken, J., Mensch, B., Miller, H., Turner, C. (1990). AIDS: The second decade. In H. Miller, C. Turner,

& L. Moses (Eds.), *AIDS and adolescents* (pp. 147–252). Washington, DC: National Academy Press.

Emans, S. J., Brown, R., Davis, A., Felice, M., & Hein, K. (1991). Position paper on reproductive health. Society for Adolescent Medicine. *Journal of Health Care, 12,* 649–661.

Futterman, D., & Hein, K. (1990). Medical management of adolescents. In P. Pizzo & C. Wilfert (Eds.), *Pediatrics AIDS: The challenge of HIV infection in infants, children and adolescents* (pp. 546–560). Baltimore: William & Wilkins.

Futterman, D. C., Hein, K., Kipke, M., Reulbach, W., Clare, G., Nelson, J., Orane, A., & Gayle, H. (1990, June.) *HIV+ adolescents: HIV testing experiences and changes in risk related sexual and drug use behavior.* Presented at the 6th International Conference on AIDS, San Francisco, California.

Futterman, D. C., Hein, K., Legg, N., Dell, R., & Shaffer, N. (1991, June). *Comparison of HIV+ and HIV− high risk adolescents in a NYC HIV clinic.* Presented at the 7th International Conference on AIDS, Florence, Italy.

Hein, K. (1987, June 18). *Aids and teenagers: Emerging issues.* Testimony before the Select Committee on Children, Youths and Families, United States House of Representatives. *Congressional Record,* pp. 93–141.

Hein, K. (1990a). Adolescent AIDS: A paradigm for training in early intervention and care. *American Journal of Diseases of Children, 144,* 46–48.

Hein, K. (1990b). Lessons from NYC on HIV/AIDS in adolescents. *New York State Journal of Medicine, 90,* 143–146.

Hein, K. (1991a). Fighting AIDS in adolescents. *Issues in Science and Technology, 7,* 67–72.

Hein, K. (1991b). Mandatory HIV testing for youth: A lose-lose proposition. *Journal of the American Medical Association, 266,* 2430–2431.

Hein, K. (1991c). Risky business: Adolescents and human immunodeficiency virus. *Pedriatics, 88,* 1052–1054.

Hein, K. (1992a). Adolescents at risk for HIV acquisition. In R. DiClemente (Ed.), *Adolescents: A Generation in Jeopardy* (pp. 3–16). Menlo Park, CA: Sage.

Hein, K. (1992b). Magic Johnson and the great American pendulum. *Society for Adolescent Medicine Newsletter, 2,* 1.

Hein, K., & DiGeronimo, T. (1992). *AIDS: Trading fear for facts. A guide for young people.* New York: Consumer Reports Books.

Hersch, P. (January, 1988). Coming of age on city streets. *Psychology Today,* pp. 28–39.

Kipke, M., Futterman, D., & Hein, K. (1990). HIV infection and AIDS during adolescence. *Medical Clinics of North America, 74,* 1149–1167.

Novello, A. (chair). (1988). *Report of the secretary's work group on pediatric HIV infection and disease.* Washington, D.C.: U.S. Department of Health and Human Services.

Poor kids spreading AIDS. (1991, November 6). *New York Newday.*

Vermund, S. V., Hein, K., Gaye, H., Cary, J., & Thomas, P. (1989). AIDS among adolescents in NYC: Case surveillance profiles compared with the rest of the U.S. *American Journal of Diseases of Children, 143,* 1220–1225.

APPENDIX I: STRAIGHT TO THE SOURCE

The following case study is reported by Sarah Dubitsky, who is trained in psychology and human sexuality and designed and implemented a sexuality education and HIV/AIDS prevention curriculum.

From January to May 1991, I taught 160 students, Grades 9 through 12, at a Connecticut high school. The students were primarily Caucasian, upper middle-class youths. Surveys of the students' sexual experiences and behaviors exposed the high rate of sexual activity within their school, particularly in the 12th grade; yet a pretest showed that the majority of students lacked basic knowledge about sexuality, reproduction, and contraception. Furthermore, the majority of students did not believe that they were at risk for pregnancy, sexually transmitted diseases, rape, or HIV/AIDS infection, or that these risks affected students in their school. Many students believed that this perception of invulnerability was the reason most students do not protect themselves with condom usage, practice other safer sex activities, or abstain from sexual activity.

The goal of the course I designed was to help students identify, communicate, explore, and become comfortable with their sexuality and the issues, dangers, and concerns that center on sexual activities. Material was not excluded because it might be considered inappropriate or provocative. In order to address specific needs, the students were placed as the subject of the course and were required to design the curriculum content. In this way, issues were personalized, and a logical and realistic element of threat and danger was maintained. As the educator, I provided the material, information, and knowledge of resources, while the students created educational activities that helped them to obtain a working knowledge of the social, scientific, and emotional aspects of sex in the 1990s and the threat of HIV/AIDS.

The following are examples of successful approaches through which the adolescents explored, evaluated, and commented on the sexual behaviors, risks, and beliefs of their peers and themselves. By doing so, each adolescent was involved actively as both student and educator.

Video

The video medium was used as an educational tool by both the students and myself. The camera was set up on a tripod in the classroom so it was possible to move the camera around as well as easily detach it in case the students wanted to use it outside of the classroom. The students were never specifically instructed to use the video camera, rather it was suggested as a possible medium for research projects.

Throughout the semester, the students were shown several educational videos that were produced by a variety of sources, such as ABC Afterschool Specials. After the video ended, the class would discuss the material as well as explore what was successful about the way the video was produced, whether or not the material was realistic, and if it was presented in a way conducive to furthering an adolescent's understanding of the issue. Also explored was how the students would produce the videos differently so their peers would enjoy and learn from them. Students were challenged to create videos that would be more successful, realistic, entertaining, and educational.

The topics were inspired by class discussions; television shows; newspaper articles; and personal experiences, concerns, and interests. To help the students become comfortable using the camera, I had them interview each other in class in a manner similar to talk shows, whereby students would take on certain characteristics and personalities, discussing and debating current issues. For example, on one "show," the topic was parenting. Students played the roles of principle, teacher, mother, father, sex educator, etc. These in-class activities helped the students prepare for their own activities outside the classroom. The students' own videos were shown in class and evaluated and critiqued by peers.

Business Lunches

Students formed groups of three. Each group invented, on the basis of factual knowledge of how the reproductive system works, new types of birth control. The students were allowed time during class as well as being required to work on the projects outside of class. The students brainstormed on how to present their projects to each other in an innovative forum. They came up with the idea of a business lunch. The lunch was to be taken seriously and approached as a professional sales meeting. Students dressed up, brought food, created charts. The mock seriousness of the presentation evoked great interest. After each group's presentation, questions were asked and the realistic success of the contraceptives was debated on the basis of the students' knowledge of sexual behavior, especially among adolescents. The team with the most effective and marketable product was rewarded.

Music

The motivation to create and perform songs was inspired by discussion in class about the performer Madonna and rap music. The power of MTV in the students' lives was discussed. Consequently, the students produced rap songs or catchy lyrics that would help them learn, for example, contraceptive practices or protection from HIV/AIDS.

Teach-a-Day

The students were required to teach a class on any particular subject covered in the course, give a solo presentation on a topic, or write an in-depth research paper on an individual unit. There was a great deal of concern from the older students for their younger peers. "Peer Education" thus became a critical part of this process.

Conclusion

All activities were designed to stress the elements of respect, challenge, partici-pation, and communication.

Self-exploration is an extremely important step in educating adolescents about sexual responsibility and the fight against AIDS. By involving the target adolescent group directly in the course, information becomes applicable to the adolescents' actual lives. Allowing personal response and contribution to the curriculum provides an opportunity to explore values, behaviors, and attitudes toward sexuality, which helps adolescents to understand themselves. The advantage of a curricular format in which the adolescents become the primary educational material is that the curriculum is automatically transferrable to almost any population.

APPENDIX 2: WHO'S WHO AMONG AMERICAN HIGH SCHOOL STUDENTS. AIDS SURVEY OF HIGH ACHIEVERS, 1992

Sample Size: 1,150
(Note: Where percentages do not add up to 100%, the difference indicates "No Answer." Percentages rounded to nearest whole number.)

PROFILE

Males	30%
Females	70%
16 years old	3%
17 years old	80%
18 years or older	17%
Caucasian	83%
African-American	4%
Asian-American	6%
Hispanic	5%
Other	2%
Protestant	34%
Catholic	32%
Jewish	1%
Other	23%
None	9%
Attend public school	82%
Private school	10%
Parochial school	8%
East/Northeast	20%
Midwest	28%
Southwest	7%
South	26%
Pacific/West	17%
Urban	16%
Suburban	42%
Rural/small town	39%

QUESTIONS

BEFORE MAGIC JOHNSON ANNOUNCED HE HAD CONTRACTED THE HIV VIRUS, TEENS DISCUSSED AIDS WITH:

Family	66%
Friends	83%
Teachers	74%

AFTER MAGIC JOHNSON ANNOUNCED HE HAD CONTRACTED THE HIV VIRUS, TEENS DISCUSSED AIDS WITH:

Family	73%
Friends	89%
Teachers	76%

TEENS REPORTED THAT AIDS CAN BE CONTRACTED BY:

Sharing needles	100%
Sexual intercourse	99%
Homosexual sex	97%
Blood transfusions	95%
Being near an infected person while they are coughing or sneezing	3%
Open mouth kissing	18%

BEFORE MAGIC JOHNSON'S ANNOUNCEMENT, TEENS BELIEVED THEIR RISK OF GETTING AIDS WAS:

Impossible-- it could never happen to me	19%
Slight chance but probably not	68%
Worried	11%
Very worried	1%

AFTER MAGIC JOHNSON'S ANNOUNCEMENT, TEENS BELIEVE THEIR RISK OF GETTING AIDS IS:

Impossible-- it could never happen to me	11%
Slight chance but probably not	68%
Worried	18%
Very worried	4%

TEENS REPORTING THEY HAVE HAD SEXUAL INTERCOURSE: 28%

TEENS REASONS FOR ABSTAINING FROM SEXUAL INTERCOURSE:

Want to wait for marriage	65%
Not ready	63%
Religion discourages it	46%
Parents would not approve	54%
Not in a relationship	50%
Concerned about reputation	31%
Fear of pregnancy	53%
Fear of contracting the HIV virus	54%
Fear of contracting STDs	51%
The only safe sex is no sex	51%

TEENS WHO SAY THEY WILL ENGAGE IN SEXUAL INTERCOURSE EVEN IF A CONDOM IS NOT AVAILABLE: .. 42%

BEFORE JOHNSON'S ANNOUNCEMENT, TEEN OR THEIR PARTNER(S):

Used condoms:
Always	44%
Frequently	28%
Infrequently	15%
Never	8%

Used birth control pills:
Always	26%
Frequently	4%
Infrequently	5%
Never	47%

Used nothing:
Always	2%
Frequently	8%
Infrequently	10%
Never	51%

AFTER JOHNSON'S ANNOUNCEMENT, TEENS OR THEIR PARTNER(S) ARE NOW ABSTAINING FROM INTERCOURSE: 8%

AFTER JOHNSON'S ANNOUNCEMENT, TEEN OR THEIR PARTNER(S):

Use condoms:
Always	45%
Frequently	17%
Infrequently	9%
Never	12%

Use birth control pills:
Always	27%
Frequently	4%
Infrequently	3%
Never	42%

Use nothing:
Always	2%
Frequently	4%
Infrequently	8%
Never	50%

RESPONSES BY TEENS WHEN ASKED IF THEY HAD BEEN TESTED FOR THE HIV VIRUS:

Yes, before Johnson's announcement	5%
Yes, after Johnson's announcement	0.8%
No	84%
No, but plan to	8%

Educational Communications, Inc.
721 N. McKinley Road • Lake Forest, IL 60045 • (708) 295-6650 • Fax (708) 295-3972
Also publishers of The National Dean's List and Who's Who Among America's Teachers

Chapter Thirteen

Thinking Globally, Acting Locally: AIDS Action 2000 Plan

Scott C. Ratzan
J. Gregory Payne

AIDS is the greatest communication challenge this country has faced since World War II. On the face of it, and deep down, this challenge is essentially one of education and motivation. Neither alone will suffice.
  (Reardon, 1990)

$$AIDS = HIV + CD4 < 200$$

In 1992, the U. S. Centers for Disease Control (CDC) considered a new medical definition of acquired immune deficiency syndrome (AIDS)—a positive HIV test with a CD4 lymphocyte count of less than $200/mm^3$. This expanded definition would make AIDS essentially a laboratory diagnosis, widening the population now infected with the AIDS virus. As of January 31, 1992, 206,932 cases of AIDS were reported in the United States. The federal government predicts the number of cases in the United States (the country with the most AIDS cases) to increase more than 50% nationwide, with a 300% increase in dense urban areas. Presently in the United States, more than 200 new cases of AIDS are diagnosed each day. An AIDS victim dies every 10 min, as the global picture grows even more bleak with each passing day. The Global AIDS Policy Coalition based at Harvard University estimates that more than six million people will have developed AIDS by the year 1995, with the projection of about 20 million new diagnoses of HIV by 1995, leading to 30 to 40 million infections worldwide (Critical Moment 1992). In the last 9 months of 1991, one million people were infected with HIV worldwide by the end of the century. This amount equals the total number of people infected in the United States since the epidemic began more than a decade ago ("HIV Hit 1 Million," 1992). In addition, a United Nations (1989) report projected that if the virus were to increase in urban areas and to spread extensively in selective rural areas, there could actually be a negative population growth in certain countries worldwide. This translates into an annual cost of over $2 billion per year, with the individual cost for treatment estimated at $50,000–60,000 annually.

The quest for an answer to meet the medical challenge of our lifetime continues. Last year, 88 medicines were under study for treatment of AIDS (Mossinghoff, 1991). Yet, despite the technological and biological advancements of the era, experts candidly admit that a vaccine or cure is still merely a faint hope as we approach the next century.

Barring a major medical breakthrough in the immediate future, our concerted efforts must focus on the only means available in helping thwart the deadly spread of AIDS. The National Commission on AIDS (1991) reported that "until a cure or vaccine is found, education and prevention are the only hope for altering the course of the HIV epidemic" (p. 19). Furthermore, the Commission echoed the historical findings of other sexually transmitted diseases in its recommendations for steps to be taken regarding AIDS: "It can be said with certainty that medical science alone will not be able to vanquish AIDS, even with a magic bullet" (p. 19).

Given that the new CDC definition for AIDS will double the estimate of infected individuals, the major focus must be on educational prevention among the population. A major component of the health communication equation on AIDS is health care delivery, currently a topic of debate because of the ever-changing political agenda and crippling costs. Furthermore, the health care industry, and its proclivity to address chronic degenerative diseases and institute highly specialized diagnostic and surgical interventions, is driven principally by its profit motive (Bronberg, 1981; Ginzberg, 1992; Gray, 1991; Vogel, 1980).

Aggravating rather than alleviating the situation, the popular press frequently contributes to "disinformation" by sensationalizing AIDS through features on high-profile stars such as Rock Hudson, Magic Johnson, or Arthur Ashe, or focusing on the raw numbers of lives lost to the disease. A major message of the educational prevention program that must be communicated to the public is that by 1993 within the United States, AIDS will overcome cancer, heart disease, and stroke victims as the greatest disease of potential years of life lost. All too often, the AIDS epidemic tragically illustrates the failure of the popular press to serve the public good. Without the proper context and ethical development of a storyline, journalists choose to describe AIDS with raw data that have limited impact to shape public opinion, attitudes, or behavior.

The goal of this analysis and subsequent recommendations is to begin to remove the attitudinal and behavioral constraints inherent in the public's inability to adequately address the AIDS crisis and its ramifications. What is called for is a concerted, grass roots campaign, the AIDS Action 2000 Plan, complete with international dimensions. The common goal of such an effort is to enhance the quality of life; the major focus is educational prevention. For those who are presently infected, the educational message is two pronged: (a) to advocate comfort and support in a professional setting with the best treatment possible and (b) to outline specific information on inhibiting further spread of the disease. Of course, a major requirement of such an extensive effort is financial capital, which is in short supply because of the current state of the economy as well as the competing medical interests in findings cures and treatment. What is needed is a persuasive worldwide effort to recognize that waiting for a cure or treatment without a plan for today translates into even more staggering statistics brought on by ignorance of the facts of this deadly virus.

It must be recognized that the AIDS Action 2000 Plan will use the traditional venues now available to the public. However, education about the human immunodeficiency virus (HIV) must move beyond these channels of communication. Intravenous drug users, prostitutes, and other high-risk groups are neither traditional nor accepted members of our society. Therefore, development of creative strategies, potentially carried out by social workers and law enforcement officers, health care professionals, religious groups, or private or governmental organizations, is paramount in seeking a comprehensive plan.

In targeting specific audiences defined as those at risk by the scientific community, efforts must be made to encode the message in a manner that will be noticed and decoded effectively by individuals in the target group. Similar past campaigns have been ineffective, as witnessed by the 12 million new cases of sexually transmitted diseases reported annually in the United States.

THE COAST MODEL—HEALTH COMMUNICATION AS NEGOTIATION

The COAST model of the health communication encounter as negotiation incorporates essential elements of traditional communication models. A synopsis of such theories and their respective components applicable to this unique model can help further understanding of COAST. In the traditional information-giving model widely used in health education, facts and information are provided to the patient by the health care professional. As discussed in Chapter 2, the COAST model posits a dialectical approach, characterized by a replacement of the unidirectional flow of information and the power relationship between the patient and physician with a co-active encounter based on trust and a free flow of information.

The self-empowerment model of health education/communication also can contribute to our educational prevention campaign. Through participatory learning, individuals are instructed on how to lower their respective individual risk of contracting and spreading the disease. For instance, safe sex messages would stress using condoms, limiting partners, and outline other safer sex individual responsibilities. The key element of this strategy is the selection of various alternatives through the application of objective standards; logic over emotion and individual responsibility for one's actions are essential components of this perspective.

Within an interpersonal context, the community-oriented COAST model stresses shared experiences of individuals in addressing common needs, along with the goal of addressing such issues through collective action. Agreed-on alternatives and enhanced levels of trust among the group members are common traits of the COAST perspective. Special-interest groups in the community can provide the means for such collective action.

Expanding on agreed alternatives and enhancing trust while advocating and implementing specific actions to improve the public good defines the abiding ethical goal of communication in the COAST model. In addition, such traits are essential components of the social transformatory approach to health communication. Through participatory learning and shared experiences, group members can develop a heightened critical awareness of the social, psychological, political, and economic constraints that affect specific health issues and the overall public good. These same techniques subsequently are used to motivate groups to remove rhetorical roadblocks. The overall goal of this model is to enhance health issues and the quality of society through concerted action.

In summary, the COAST model of health communication as negotiation is rooted in an ethical and effective co-active *communication* process between the patient and the provider. The definition of health communication offered in the Introduction—the process and effect of employing ethical persuasive means in human health care decision-making—mandates that during the initial health communication encounter, both parties in the dyad address a particular medical exigence, an imperfection that initiated the communication act. Subsequently, the brainstorming of all available *options* should be explored, regardless of their viability and effectiveness. Following this important phase and through intensive communication acts, the focus of the dyadic encounter is to identify *alternatives*, agreed on by both parties, that should be employed in reaching a common goal. Such alternatives are selected on the basis of application and analysis of the options to specific *standards*, objective criteria often defined by a third party, group, or organization that has credibility among those involved in the encounter. The essential element of the COAST model, and an element that should be pervasive throughout its various phases, is *trust*, the transactional product of open and honest sharing of information and credible, expected feedback among the interested parties. The degree to which trust exists within the health encounter is a positive prediction of the degree of compliance and overall satisfaction of the parties involved.

AIDS ACTION 2000 PLAN

Echoing the sentiments expressed by Reardon (1990) in her research on AIDS, the successful application of a communication based campaign of educational prevention is the greatest challenge we face, in addition to finding a cure or vaccine. Reardon wrote, "What we need is a multichannel multimethod research that reaches out into the communities of those at risk for AIDS, research that teaches us how to effectively persuade people at risk to protect themselves and others from AIDS" (p. 269–270). Reardon and others have warned that the increasing scope of the crisis demands more than what traditionally has been marshalled together to meet past health issues.

It is our hope that the COAST model of health communication as negotiation will provoke discussion of this deadly disease far beyond the confines of the traditional academic setting. To accomplish this task, the model must permeate the general milieu of our society both as a strategy of prevention as well as a dominant approach in treatment of the AIDS patient. The AIDS Action 2000 Plan, outlined below, provides a blueprint for such a strategy. (Figure 1 illustrates the various components of the AIDS Action 2000 Plan.)

Individual/Life Partner/Family/Friends

As shown in Figure 1, there are various spheres of the society that have an impact on the individual, in terms of both educational prevention and treatment after diagnosis of AIDS. The individual is at both ends of the continuum as (a) the focal point of the informational effort to educate and prevent AIDS and (b) the patient infected with the disease. It is within the various spheres of society, comprising these two areas, that the AIDS Action 2000 Plan is applied.

In the prevention education sphere, the individual is the target receiver, dependent on the highly credible agents that make up his or her primary familial group (parents, sibling, and relatives) for important cues on appropriate behavior. The COAST model is rooted firmly in this relationship, with specific and candid information exchanged between the parties on such issues as sex and AIDS. A secondary yet important objective is for the receivers of such information to become sources in the transactional process themselves.

Developing the Message

Constraints that inhibit the development of trusting relationships characterized by open, frank communication include the following: overreaction by partner/

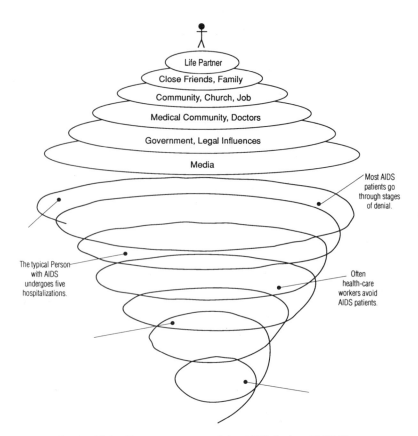

Figure 13-1   The components of the AIDS Action 2000 Plan.

familial group; fear of losing job; isolation/quarantine/insurance/health care restrictions; and fear of becoming a victim of general public hysteria, which permeates much of the discussion and the media's coverage of AIDS. The results of such ineptitude have been inadequate response and planning on all levels of society, continued sexual spread of the disease, uncoordinated health care delivery, and denial of an educational focus and the preventive role of condoms and sterile needles in meeting the challenge. Instead, attention has turned to medicine for a miracle cure or improved treatment measures. And yet, the major weapons of the AIDS 2000 Plan, and the only legitimate means we now have available for our efforts, are increased awareness and knowledge, the products of educational prevention.

The operable behavioral stimuli from groups, society, and government should arouse the basic survival instinct and further the recognition that changes in behavior must occur if one is to be AIDS free. Yet, Ostrow (1987) found that traditional motivational appeals—fear, force, pleasure, and altruism—are insufficient to induce such desired change, and should be supported by a variety of psychological, educational and institutional supports and resources.

Of specific interest to communication professionals are the type of appeals to be used in successfully conveying the finalized campaign message, that is, the use of logical versus emotional appeals. According to Edgar, Hammond, and Freimuth (1989), "The logical appeal assumes that the audience perceives a need and the message will provide the solution" (p. 7). Furthermore, logical appeals are more effective "when audiences are sophisticated, when using print media, when the competence of the source is highlighted, and when the goal of the appeal is stimulating cognitive change" (Edgar et al., p. 7). In contrast, emotional appeals "intensify motivation by creating a need where none existed" (Edgar et al., p. 7). Research favors the use of emotional appeals "when the audience is indifferent, when using broadcast channels, when the dynamism of the source is highlighted, and when the goal of the appeal is producing affective change" (Edgar et al., p. 7).

Reflecting an appreciation of pertinent factors such as race, age, sex, education, income, religion, ethnicity, and cultural perspectives, campaign messages must include facts about AIDS and how it is transmitted, realization of individual risk ratio, ability and proclivity to change behavior, and the handicap that hope for a vaccine or cure presents to particular individuals. As illustrated above, the intrinsic strategies—the types of evidence and proofs used in the message—are dependent on the target group(s).

A more intrinsic AIDS-specific agenda for the message includes appreciation of

- sexual orientation,
- sexual identity,
- economic status,
- social self-esteem,
- housing arrangements,
- sexual practices/number of sexual partners,
- intravenous drug use,
- alcohol and other drug use (average and greatest amount consumed per day),
- depression,
- family/medical/mental history, and
- number of partners who have practiced unsafe sex and/or anal intercourse.

Suffice to say, honest responses to questions about these issues are highly dependent on the degree of trust, a major component of COAST, evident in the relationship. Drs. Willard Cates and Alan Hinsman (1991) of the CDC stated in their essay on AIDS, "The data [from a *Journal of the American Medical*

Association study of adolescents] show that in populations at high risk, short-term counseling alone is not enough to effect long-term changes to safer sex behavior" (p. 1370).

To reach as many members of the public as possible, the AIDS Action 2000 Plan should consider the following contexts for message development and dissemination: job related (military, foreign service, teaching, other), premarital, prehospital (pregnancy), preimmigration, preinsurance, pre-drivers-license-registration, preschool, preblood donations, etc. If this is accomplished across the board with confidentiality, the myths of easy contagion can be dispelled and understanding and knowledge advanced.

Groups

Primary groups in the school, work, and religious realms can further the importance of the message received on the individual level or be the initial medium for such information for those who lack the familial setting. A common characteristic of these shared work, religious, or educational contexts is their collective action orientation. Agreed on alternatives (in this instance, how to approach the AIDS crisis) and enhanced levels of trust among the group members are common traits of the COAST approach.

Of critical importance is the early realization that educational prevention is only one of two goals for this sphere. The real challenge is to devise strategies that reach beyond the confines of the traditional group boundaries to high-risk groups and adolescents commonly lacking such group affiliations. A major challenge is to make initial contact with these estranged groups and individuals and begin to develop trusting relationships, the requisite for COAST and health communication as a negotiation encounter.

For instance, in a survey of college students, Reardon (1990) found that 40% desired a communication encounter with their intimate partner about AIDS but failed to follow up. Reardon concluded, "when college students find it difficult to talk about protection from AIDS with their intimate partner, there should be little wonder why less educated youngsters have such difficulty" (Reardon, p. 269). On the junior high and high school levels, Reardon cited "growing evidence that these young people are uninformed about the spread of AIDS, and many are uncomfortable with the use of condoms or with asking partners about their sexual histories" (p. 268).

A more specialized segment of this sphere involves special-interest groups, which share some of the characteristics of the primary group yet are more focused and devoted to a specific course of action designed to improve the public good. The heightened critical awareness of the societal, political, and economic exigencies is recognized within such groups. Furthermore, it serves to motivate the groups toward a concerted effort to change the status quo, thereby advancing specific health issues. The particular interests of this sphere, an important educational prevention network in the AIDS Action 2000 Plan, include

- condom distribution,
- distribution of sterile needles and education on cleanliness to avoid transmission,
- media watchdog and advocacy,
- education of health professionals,
- community-based programs,
- appropriate media emphasis with facts and repetition of effective behavioral change, and
- focus on educational prevention in various publics.

As stated earlier, a major challenge in disseminating pertinent information is that many high-risk individuals are not easily accessible, given varying degrees of estrangement from society and the absence of familial and group infrastructure. What is lacking is the social connectedness so important in communicating and reinforcing the message. Reardon (1990) highlighted the communication problem in educating those at risk:

> Communication scholars have always argued that one must know one's audience. People at greatest risk for AIDS, however, are often from backgrounds far different from those of most researchers. It is not enough to stay in our offices developing questionnaires to be distributed only to college students. Our task is a much more difficult one. It requires getting out into those workplaces, neighborhoods and schools described by Michal-Johnson and Bowen. It requires learning to persuade doctors and nurses to educate their patients about AIDS. It requires a realization that we do not know what life is like out there for young people whose peers and families do not actively advocate health protection. (p. 269)

To address this issue, the AIDS Action 2000 Plan is a safety net including comprehensive outreach programs in clinics, schools, hospitals, community centers, churches/temples, clubs, and theaters. A successful effort must reach beyond the traditional social strata and media to reach the "dropouts" of society. Reardon (1990) highlighted the problem in reaching adolescents in the formative years: "Those students most at high risk for the disease typically drop out of school or attend on a less than regular basis" (p. 268). Given this constraint, as well as other handicaps in reaching this target audience, the campaign message must be clear and, given its divergent audiences, should be specifically designed to attract attention and be assimilated into a daily regimen.

Presently, there have been few community-based special-interest organizations devoted to reaching such target groups. The Los Angeles "L.A. Cares . . . like a Mother" campaign and the San Francisco "Stop AIDS" campaign are two broad-based and focused groups that promote AIDS education messages through informal community networks designed to reach the target audience (Aggleton, 1989).

Today health care in the United States is a potential benefit of employment rather than citizenship. Because of this, HIV/AIDS education in the workplace must play a significant role in educating citizens beyond the messages provided in the primary and secondary schools' educational prevention campaigns.

A potential alternative is to link AIDS education with federal changes in health care insurance and delivery. One could apply the popular concept of "play or pay" with AIDS. By "playing," a company could provide employees health care insurance that includes HIV education/prevention. "Paying" would require the employer to pay into a pool of health insurance funds with such monies made available to the government for community AIDS prevention messages or condom distribution/needle exchange programs.

According to a *Taft Report* in 1991, fewer than 1 in 5 companies are educating employees about managing AIDS in the workplace, and only approximately 1 in 10 companies have a formal written policy on AIDS. This finding represents a failure to reach the public in one of its most common contexts—the workplace. Providing comprehensive information on treatment and referral in the workplace must be a major objective of the AIDS Action 2000 Plan.

A potential prototype for this effort is the Drug-Free Workplace Act (a federal act; also a state act in California and proposed in Massachusetts), which requires all contractors/grantees to provide a drug-free workplace with referral to professional counseling and treatment. This requirement applies to all employers who are eligible to receive federal- or state-funded contracts and grants (see potential AIDS legislation in Appendix).

Although not a highly dense community of target publics, today's college community provides a good setting for employment of the COAST model of health communication as negotiation in addressing the AIDS issue. Peterson's (1992) research suggests that various professionals/specialists/workers within the college environment, especially counseling centers and the residential staff community, are perceived by students as credible sources for information on educational prevention. The major thrust of such efforts according to Peterson, should be "to encourage the students themselves to become AIDS educators, to encourage a changing of norms through peer pressure" (p. 130). Identified as potential advocates in this effort were residence hall advisers, student government leaders, and those involved in health-related areas of study. Peterson cited successful specific programs at Ithaca College, Cornell University, and Dartmouth College.

In addition, special events that invigorate such preventative programs and further highlight the issue include special speaker series, awareness weeks, or national conferences featuring prominent leaders on the issues. One such example is the "Effective Health Communication in the 90s: The AIDS Crisis" conference held at Emerson College. The audience of the conference, held in downtown Boston, included college students and inner city youth who heard CDC AIDS Director Fred Kroger, among others, outline the latest government efforts to combat the disease. The Emerson conference on AIDS also provides an example of the COAST model in action. Members of the audience and speakers on the panels engaged in spirited discussion and debate on various issues connected with the epidemic, including the virus's origin, ethics of media coverage, and effectiveness of a national television drama in communicating the message to adolescents. A survey of those in attendance at the Emerson conference mirrored data from throughout the country on college students' uncertainty regarding and susceptibility to the virus.

The potential spiraling effect of such synergistic activities in helping further to convey the preventive message is exemplified by examining in detail the events in 1991 at Emerson College. In response to the college being the site of the production of the ABC–PBS drama on AIDS, efforts were made to host a national conference on the topic, featuring a national premiere of the made-for-television movie, "In the Shadow of Love," controversial because of its candid language regarding use of condoms. Following the conference, articles on AIDS appeared in the campus newspaper and college magazine, and the topic was a subject of debate and discussion among various constituencies within the college. In addition, the inclusion of staff from the *Boston Globe* and the *Boston Herald* furthered the agenda-setting function of the academic discussion on AIDS. Two months after the spirited criticism of the dearth of substantive media coverage on AIDS at the conference, the *Globe* featured two major educational sections devoted to AIDS.

Reflecting on using colleges as laboratories for creating and implementing important strategies on educational prevention, Peterson (1992) wrote, "If colleges and universities are truly to fulfill their ultimate purpose—that of education—they surely must address the issue of HIV now, not when it becomes convenient, or becomes perhaps too much of an unwanted burden" (p. 137).

Health Polity

The AIDS Action 2000 Plan focuses on education of the health polity on preventive measures regarding the disease and its excessive and specious demands. Cassell (1989) highlighted the crisis of confidence in effective communication, "the technological imperative appears to obliterate patients' personal needs— their individual concerns are brushed aside by the anxiety to support the function of their organs" (p. 13). Given the grim statistics of AIDS, professionals involved in the health communication encounter must develop skills to meet the emotional crush of those affected.

Highlighting this need, Jonathan Mann, chair of the 1992 International Conference on AIDS in Amsterdam, stated (Critical Moment, 1992)

When we take into account everything we've learned scientifically, in attempts at prevention, and in the experience of fighting this epidemic for 10 years, we realize that the
earlier view—which of necessity focused on the virus and on individual behavior that
transmits the virus—is too limited. In fact, it's too limited to succeed. (p. 445)

In fact, studies by Rowland-Morin and Carroll (1990) suggest that more than
one fourth of the variance affecting patient satisfaction could be explained by
ineffective verbal communication. Of particular importance given the fatal
prognosis facing AIDS patients is that health professionals become more skilled
in helping patients cope with their illness and that they be resources rather than
barriers in patients' attempt to deal with the terminal outcome. As more and
more AIDS patients enter this final phase of their lives, health communication
professionals will experience increasing demands for not only medical care, but
moral and ethical familial support and assistance. Because of the increased
number of hospices catering to the AIDS patient and the tragic, yet true reality
of many victims facing death alone, this final sector of the AIDS Action 2000
Plan will emerge as one of the larger spheres.

What are called for are not only education and development of empathic
skills among the existing health professional corps, but also an infusion of
individuals with expertise in consolation and death therapy into this sector for
the important encounters of the victim and his/her familial group. The unique
interpersonal promise inherent in COAST makes this approach to health communication an important tool in the development of personal skills among
health professionals as we prepare to meet the rising number of AIDS cases.

More than 13% of the Gross National Product is devoted to the health care
sector—health maintenance organizations, insurance companies, physicians, dentists, nurses, social workers, physician assistants, emergency medical technicians, public health workers, and the pharmaceutical industry, among others,
make up this burgeoning public. Through in-house and continuing education programs required to maintain licensure for many members of the health polity,
succinct curricular updates employing COAST concepts could reach target
providers/patients. The overall effect would be to facilitate the development of
communication skills and techniques among those deficient in formal training in
the art of effective communication. An important key theme to be emphasized at
all sectors of the campaign is an approach based on communication rather than
biology or hard sciences. The AIDS Action 2000 Plan centers on educational
prevention, a necessary strategy that must be adopted immediately, barring medical science's finding a cure, vaccine, or acceptable treatment for AIDS.

Media

Concurrent with the dyadic and intrapersonal communication strategies previously outlined, the AIDS Action 2000 Plan mandates a concerted effort by the

mass media. While sharing the skepticism of past research on the effect of mass media on long-term behavior modification, we maintain that media purveyors should intensify awareness of the AIDS issue, especially within the context of the comprehensive plan involving the numerous sectors outlined here (Brown & Einsiedel, 1990). Evidence suggests increased overall campaign effectiveness "if media messages are supplemented with interpersonal and community structures that support such changes" (Brown & Einsiedel, p. 153). Of critical importance to the campaign, according to Brown and Einsiedel, is that "effective use of the mass media requires planning, research, and consideration of the environment in which the media are used" (p. 154).

COAST's approach to health communication as negotiation and its emphasis on the individual in all sectors, as outlined in Figure 1, posit the major objective of mass media: to increase public awareness. According to Aristotle's (Cooper, 1960) appreciation of audience and McLuhan's (1967) views of communication channels/media, the message should be disseminated through a variety of appropriate means. The aim is to attract the attention of as many members of the audience as possible. One potential, but controversial, public policy step would be for the federal government to mandate that each television and radio station, in order to maintain its license, must demonstrate that it is engaged in broadcasting an AIDS prevention public service announcement/ commercial that complements the community effort. The compelling rationales for such a requirement are grim statistics and the pandemic threat of AIDS to our public good.

In addition, commercial television should address the AIDS epidemic in its regular programming in an effort to reach the wider viewing audience. As the primary source of information for most Americans, television programming must strive to break down statistics to humanistic perspectives on the AIDS epidemic. Because of the stigma associated with the disease, commercial networks were initially reluctant to include references to AIDS in scripts accepted for production. Nonetheless, the commercial success of the shows "Longtime Companion" and "The Killing Frost" ushered in a new appreciation of how audiences would accept AIDS-related dramatic productions. Joint projects such as the ABC–WGBH after-school special entitled "In the Shadow of Love" demonstrate that the mass media can play an active role in the educational prevention campaign without compromising the profit motive. In fact, such dramatic representations have greater persuasive appeal for potential modeling behavior among particular target groups than news stories of heroic figures stricken with the disease.

Concurrent with the media messages, a focus of the AIDS Action 2000 Plan is for a more personalized and coordinated effort to be adopted in each sphere by one's partner/family, support/peer group, government, and health polity groups. Without such support, messages tend to be discarded. Wallack (1981) and Milio (1986) pointed out that "mass media campaigns aimed only at affecting individual health habits may be misdirected and certainly will not have long-term effects unless they are conducted in environments that encourage and support healthy behavior'' (cited by Brown & Einsiedel, 1990, p. 158).

Effective targeting of groups and development of definitions and clear campaign objectives are crucial steps in organizing the mass media effort, as is the existence of a current infrastructure to further support the campaign effort. In a study of a particular campaign effort, Perrow and Guillén (1990) found that a past AIDS campaign in New York, aimed at intravenous drug users, focused on communicating how AIDS was spread and the dangers of the disease. Community leaders soon realized that the campaign's message was wrong; addicts knew the deadly details of the virus. The real need, or campaign objective, should have been to persuade the target audience not to share needles, a controversial topic for the mass media effort because of existing laws against needle distribution. Responding to this situation, community leaders and single-interest groups rallied behind the efforts to persuade those in power to change laws on distribution of clean needles (Brown & Einsiedel, 1990).

Government

On a larger level, the government commands an important position and responsibility to protect and inform the citizenry. The ethical issue concerning the AIDS epidemic, which has prompted discussion and heated debate in a variety of contexts, is the government's proper role in fighting the spread of AIDS. Complicating the issue is that we face the tremendous challenges of this disease with a backdrop of recession, in which fewer and fewer dollars are available to perform various public service safety net functions. Critics have faulted the government for not launching a more comprehensive and active assault on the disease, while others have faulted the government for spending too much money on a disease whose impact on society they argue has been grossly exaggerated.

Various governmental proposals and plans were implemented during the 1980s—America Responds to AIDS and the National Commission on AIDS, among others. Unfortunately, as outlined throughout this treatise, such programs alone did not or by design could not adequately halt the spread of AIDS. The sobering statistics speak to the disjointed effort: the number of deaths due to AIDS in the first three years of this decade will equal the total number of deaths to the disease in the 1980s.

The government's principal public service role concerning the disease is presently evident in examining its health communication infrastructure: the national AIDS phone information hotline, a national AIDS information clearinghouse, demographic mortality and morbidity reports, public service announcement development, and other national minority and coalition building. Yet, beyond these efforts, the evidence suggests that the government's response has been minimal, because of the lack of funding as well as heated debate on the nature of the disease and various approaches to meeting its challenge.

Summary

With the focus of the AIDS Action 2000 Plan being to reach as many individuals as possible throughout the educational, prevention, and treatment phases, it is paramount that the federal government support state, local, and municipal entities in joining with the private sector in providing community-based organizations and realistic campaign strategies. What is called for is a comprehensive national assault, a partnership of government and business, to help protect our national interests as well as the promise of countries worldwide from being ravaged by this deadly disease. Similar types of cooperative efforts have occurred in Los Angeles when business leaders joined with the government officials in 1984 to stage one of the most successful Olympics to date. The olympic challenge posed by the AIDS epidemic is another national call to arms. In previous decades, the federal government would have considered a program of grants (block, community, etc.) for community action to combat AIDS. However, with the economic, moral, and political issues endemic in the Reagan–Bush years, the federal government has shown only a token response. According to the National Commission on AIDS (1991),

> Our nation's leaders have not done well. In the past decade, the White House has rarely broken its silence on the topic of AIDS. Congress has shown leadership in developing critical legislation, but has often failed to provide adequate funding for AIDS programs. Articulate leadership guiding Americans toward a proper response to AIDS has been notably absent. (p. 3)

The federal government should approach AIDS as it did the Gulf War, in which 42 billion dollars was spent on Operation Desert Storm. The threat of AIDS is as ominous as any foreign power we have fought in terms of our national security. One could argue that capital investment in ridding society of this AIDS menace would actually achieve more long-term rewards for humanity than armaments. The perfidious use of federal funds in a variety of political arenas and our proclivity to be nearsighted and motivated by 4-year election cycles further our dilemma.

Nonetheless, even a full-fledged effort by the government necessitates an inherent complementary AIDS Action 2000 Plan and coordinated infrastructure to help combat the disease. Dr. William Roper of the CDC told the National Commission on AIDS,

> Most of the key transactions that affect the health of people take place in households, in neighborhoods, in communities. So finally, those of us at the federal level

are two steps removed, and even state health officials are one step removed from where things really happen at the community level. I believe that the most important thing I can do as a federal official is to work to strengthen local public health agencies throughout the country. (National Commission on AIDS, 1991, p. 117)

The government must spearhead the way, joining with other interest groups, not only in the educational prevention campaign (education and counseling to reduce transmission) but in the treatment of those infected with HIV. Leadership at the federal level can help guarantee AIDS patients freedom from discrimination, access to quality health care and new therapies, therapeutic interventions, funding for drugs and other treatment, confidential HIV antibody testing (for high-risk partners and other citizens), mental health counseling, and drug abuse treatment, as well as training, assistance, and support for those who serve as the caretakers of those infected with HIV.

Complementing the valiant efforts in the medical arena to find a vaccine, the federal government should take action now to explore the ethical, liability, and distribution issues inherent in the discovery of a vaccine and its testing. Furthermore, selection of subjects for drug/vaccine trial should be voluntary and conducted in a more timely fashion than the traditional model of the Food and Drug Administration.

CONCLUSION

Given the spiraling dimensions of the AIDS issue, it is crucial that any campaign be comprehensive and multipronged in its approach to educate the public. The AIDS Action 2000 Plan is rooted in the effective employment of the COAST model of health communication as negotiation. The AIDS Action 2000 Plan begins at the individual level, proceeds through various spheres of society in the educational prevention phase, and culminates with the AIDS victim throughout the treatment phase. Reaching different groups mandates many different messengers of preventive education—hence a six-pronged approach is proposed to help defeat this insidious threat to our national security and the future of humankind.

REFERENCES

Aggleton, P. (1989). Evaluating health education about AIDS. In P. Aggleton, G. Hart, & P. Davies (Eds.), *AIDS: Social, representations, social practices* (pp. 220–236). Philadelphia, PA: Falmer Press.

Bronberg, M. D. (1981). The new medical-industrial complex. *New England Journal of Medicine, 304*, 233–236.

Brown, J. D., & Einsiedel, E. F. (1990). Public health campaigns: Mass media strategies. In E. B. Ray & L. Donohew (Eds.), *Communication and health: Systems and applications* (pp. 153–170). Hillsdale, NJ: Erlbaum.

Cassell, E. J. (1989). Foreword: Making the subjective objective. In M. Stewart & D. Roter (Eds.), *Communicating with medical patients* (pp. 13-15). Newbury Park, CA: Sage.

Cates, W., Jr., & Hinsman, A. (1991). Editorial. *New England Journal of Medicine, 325,* 1369-1370.

Cooper, L. (1960). *The rhetoric of Aristotle.* Englewood Cliffs, NJ: Prentice-Hall.

Critical moment at hand in HIV/AIDS pandemic, new global strategy to arrest its spread proposed. (1992). *Journal of the American Medical Association, 268*(4), 445-446.

Edgar, T., Hammond, S. L., & Freimuth, V. S. (1989). The role of the mass media and interpersonal communication in promoting AIDS-related behavior change. *AIDS and Public Policy Journal, 4*(1), 3-9.

Ginzberg, E. (1992). The future of medicine. *New England Journal of Medicine, 326,* 73-75.

Gray, B. H. (1991). *The profit motive and health care: The changing accountability of doctors and hospitals.* Cambridge, MA: Harvard University Press.

HIV hit 1 million in 9 months—UN. (1992, February 16). *Boston Globe,* p. 8.

McLuhan, M. (1967). *The medium is the message.* New York: McGraw-Hill.

Milio, N. (1986). *Promoting health through public policy.* Ottawa: Canadian Public Health Association.

Mossinghoff, G. J. (1991). 1991 survey report: 88 medicines in testing; 3 approved in past 12 months, bringing total to 14. In *AIDS medicines: Drugs and vaccines* (pp. 1-4). Washington, DC: Pharmaceutical Manufacturers Association.

National Commission on Acquired Immune Deficiency Syndrome. (1991). *America living with AIDS: Transforming anger, fear, and indifference into action.* Washington, DC: Author.

Ostrow, D. G. (1987). Psychiatric consequences of AIDS: An overview. *International Journal of Neuroscience, 32,* 647-659.

Perrow, C., & Guillén, M. F. (1990). *The AIDS disaster: The failure of organizations in New York and the nation.* New Haven, CT: Yale University Press.

Peterson, K. E. (1992). AIDS education and prevention at colleges and universities. In M. R. Seligson & K. E. Peterson (Eds.), *AIDS prevention and treatment: Hope, humor, and healing* (pp. 121-141). New York: Hemisphere Publishing Corporation.

Reardon, K. K. (1990). Meeting the communication/persuasion challenge of AIDS in workplaces, neighborhoods, and schools: A comment on *AIDS and Public Policy, 4*(1), *Health Communication 2,* 267-270.

Rowland-Morin, P. A., & Carroll, J. G. (1990). Verbal communication skills and patient satisfaction: A study of doctor-patient interview. *Evaluation and the Health Professionals, 13,* 168-185.

Taft Report: AIDS—a special report. (1991, May). *The Taft Nonprofit Executive,* p. 1-4.

United Nations. (1989). *The AIDS epidemic and its demographic consequences: Proceedings of the United Nations/World Health Organization Workshop on Modeling the Demographic Impact of the AIDS Epidemic in Pattern II Countries.* New York: United Nations Publications.

United Nations. (1990). *Global outlook 2000: An economic, social, and environmental perspective.* New York: United Nations Publications.

Vogel, M. (1980). *The invention of the modern hospital.* Illinois: University of Chicago Press.

Wallack, L. M. (1981). Mass media campaigns: The odds against finding behavior change. *Health Education Quarterly, 8,* 209–260.

APPENDIX

Emerson College Political News Study Group:
An AIDS Educated Workforce Act

for the Commonwealth of Massachusetts

Be it enacted by the Senate and the House of Representatives assembled, and by the authority of the same, as follows:

An **AIDS** Educated Workforce Act

WHEREAS, one out of every 100 adult men and one in every 600 women in the United States are now HIV/AIDS infected; and

WHEREAS, over 100,000 Americans have already died of AIDS in the first decade since its discovery; and

WHEREAS, over 200,000 more will die of AIDS in the United States in the next two years; and

WHEREAS, the Centers for Disease Control spends less than 2% of its total budget to combat AIDS, and only a small percentage is designated to funding prevention programs.

WHEREAS, the National Commission on AIDS estimates that by 1992 the years of potential life lost to AIDS will grow to between 1.5 and 2.1 million. By 1993 AIDS will clearly overcome cancer, heart disease and stroke victims as the greatest disease of "years of life lost."

WHEREAS, despite current efforts to educate Americans on the hazards and risks of AIDS, the majority of Americans remain ill-informed and believe they are not at risk; now therefore, be it resolved that the AIDS EDUCATED WORKFORCE ACT be enacted to educate the American workforce about the hazards and risks of HIV/AIDS.

Table of Contents

Section 1. Purpose

Section 2. Definitions

Section 3. Contracts

Section 4. Violations by a Contractor

Section 5. Federal Grant Recipients

This proposed legislation was drafted by Dr. Scott S. Ratzan and David Calusdian of the Emerson College Political News Study Group for introduction into the 1992–93 session of the Massachusetts House of Representatives.

Section 6. Violations by a Federal Grant Recipient
Section 7. Effective Date

Section 1. **Purpose**

The goal of this Act is to educate the American workforce on the risks, hazards and developments of HIV/AIDS to ensure better health, productivity, and safety of working people in the United States of America. The cost of AIDS to business is great—ignorance of health issues not only reduces productivity, and increases illness, ultimately raising health costs to American citizens, but also increases the economic costs of the escalating premiums of health insurance for both workers and family members. As most Americans spend more time at the workplace during their life-span than any other educational institution, the work site is an ideal location for repetition of important health messages.

Section 2. **Definitions**

(a) "Workplace" means a place for the performance of work done in connection with a specific grant or contract.

(b) "Employee" means the employee of a grantee or contractor directly or indirectly engaged in the performance of work pursuant to the grant or contract.

(c) "HIV" means the Human Immunodeficiency Virus, that which has been implicated as the cause of AIDS—the Acquired Immune Deficiency Syndrome.

(d) "Grantee" means the department, division, or other unit of a person or organization (consisting of at least 25 employees) responsible for the performance directly or indirectly under the grant.

(e) "Contractor" means the department, division, or other unit including sub-contractors, of a person or organization (consisting of at least 25 employees) responsible for the performance directly or indirectly under the contract.

Section 3. **Contracts**

No person or organization shall be considered a responsible source for the purposes of being awarded a contract for the procurement of any property or services from any state agency unless the person or organization has certified to the contracting agency that it will provide an AIDS educated workforce by doing all of the following:

(a) Publishing a statement notifying employees of an AIDS policy and any available AIDS counseling, rehabilitation, or testing programs.

(b) Establishing a quarterly special innovative health communication educational program which will utilize different audience-specific media developed or recommended by an accredited institution of higher learning. This AIDS education package will include individual communication (through newsletters/ pamphlets/magazines), audio and video tapes, posters, etc. which will be validated with the latest health communication information on prevention, education, treatment, modes of transmission, counseling, etc.

These materials could be recommended/developed by an advisory board of communication experts which will be initially established at Emerson College, a fully accredited 501(c)3 undergraduate and graduate institution devoted to the study of communication arts and sciences.

The information above would include:

(1) The hazards of AIDS, and preventative measures to avoid HIV transmission in and out of the workplace.

(2) The person's or organization's policy of maintaining an AIDS educated workforce.

(3) The penalties that may be imposed upon employees for not attending educational/informational sessions on the hazards and consequences of HIV/ AIDS.

(c) Requiring that each employee engaged in the performance of the contract be given and sign a copy of the statement required by subdivision (a) and that, as a condition of employment on the contract, the employee agrees to:

(1) Abide by the terms of the contract and fill out an annual questionnaire on the knowledge of AIDS transmission.

(d) Making a good faith effort each month to continue to maintain an AIDS educated workforce through implementation of subdivisions (a) to (d), inclusive.

Section 4. Violations by a Contractor

(a) Each contract awarded by a state agency shall be subject to suspension of payments under the contract or termination of the contract, or both, and the contractor thereunder shall be subject to debarment, in accordance with the requirements of this article, if the head of the contracting agency or his or her official designee determines, in writing, that any of the following has occurred:

(1) The contractor has made a false certification under Section 3.

(2) The contractor violates the certification by failing to carry out the requirements of subdivisions (a) through (d), inclusive, of Section 3.

(3) The number and type of educational sessions by the grantee indicate that the grantee has failed to make a good faith effort to provide an AIDS educated workforce as required by Section 3.

(b) If a contracting officer determines that cause for suspension, termination, or debarment exists, a suspension, termination, or debarment proceeding subject to this subdivision shall, on application in writing by a contracting officer of an agency, be conducted by the agency which conducts the procurement. The agency shall, based upon a preponderance of the evidence presented, resolve all the issues of fact, determine whether a basis exists for the suspension or termination of the contract or debarment of the contractor, and issue a final decision in favor of or against suspension or termination or of the contract or debarment of the contractor. A proceeding, decision, or order of the agency pursuant to this subdivision shall be subject to appeal or review by the courts. Determinations and final decisions of the agency shall be final unless appealed by the contractor within sixty (60) days after the receipt by the contractor of a copy of a final decision of the agency.

(c) Upon issuance of any final decision under this section requiring debarment of a contractor, the contractor shall be ineligible for award of a contract by any state agency for a period specified in the decision, not to exceed five years. Upon issuance of any final decision recommending against debarment of the contractor, the contractor shall be compensated as provided by law or regulations.

Section 5. **Federal Grant Recipients**

No person or organization shall receive a grant from any state agency unless the person or organization has certified to the granting agency that it will provide a AIDS educated workforce by doing all of the following:

(a) Publishing a statement notifying employees of an AIDS policy and any available AIDS counseling, rehabilitation, or testing programs.

(b) Establishing a quarterly special innovative health communication educational program which will utilize different audience-specific media developed or recommended by an accredited institution of higher learning. This AIDS education package will include individual communication (through newsletters/pamphlets/magazines), audio and video tapes, posters, etc. which will be validated with the latest health communication information on prevention, education, treatment, modes of transmission, counseling, etc.

These materials could be recommended/developed by an advisory board of communication experts which will be initially established at Emerson College, a fully Accredited 501(c)3 undergraduate and graduate institution developed to the study of communication arts and sciences.

The information above would include:

(1) The hazards of AIDS, and preventative measures to avoid HIV transmission in and out of the workplace.

(2) The person's or organization's policy of maintaining an AIDS educated workforce.

(3) The penalties that may be imposed upon employees for not attending informational sessions on the hazards and consequences of HIV/AIDS.

(c) Requiring that each employee engaged in the performance of the contract be given and sign a copy of the statement required by subdivision (a) and that, as a condition of employment on the contract, the employee agrees to:

(1) Sign and abide by the terms of the contract and fill out an annual questionnaire on the knowledge of AIDS transmission.

(d) Making a good faith effort each month to continue to maintain an AIDS educated workforce through implementation of subdivisions (a) to (d), inclusive.

Section 6. **Violations by a Federal Grant Recipient**

Each grant awarded by a state agency shall be subject to suspension of payments under the grant or termination of the grant, or both, and the grantee thereunder shall be subject to debarment, in accordance with the requirements of this article, if the head of the granting agency or his or her official designee determines, in writing, that any of the following has occurred:

(1) The grantee has made a false certification under Section 5.

(2) The grantee violates the certification by failing to carry out the requirements of subdivisions (a) through (d), inclusive, of Section 5.

(3) The number and type of educational sessions by the grantee indicate that the grantee has failed to make a good faith effort to provide an AIDS educated workforce as required by Section 5.

(b) If a granting agency officer determines that cause for suspension, termination, or debarment exists, a suspension, termination, or debarment proceeding subject to this subdivision shall, on application in writing by a granting officer of an agency, be conducted by the agency which conducts the procurement. The agency shall, based upon a preponderance of the evidence presented, resolve all the issues of fact, determine whether a basis exists for the suspension or termination of the contract or debarment of the contractor, and issue a final decision in favor of or against suspension or termination of the grant or debarment of the grantee. A proceeding, decision, or order of the agency pursuant to this subdivision shall be subject to appeal or review by the courts. Determinations and final decisions of the agency shall be final unless appealed by the contractor within sixty (60) days after the receipt by the contractor of a copy of a final decision of the agency.

(c) Upon issuance of any final decision under this section requiring debarment of a grantee, the grantee shall be ineligible for award of any grant from any state agency and for participation in any future grant from any state agency for a period specified in the decision, not to exceed five years. Upon issuance of any final decision recommending against debarment of the grantee, the grantee shall be compensated as provided by law or regulations.

Section 7. **Effective Date**

The provisions of this Act shall become effective 120 days after the date of enactment.

Communication and Prevention—They Are All We Have

Scott C. Ratzan

It is much more difficult to be convincing about ignorance concerning disease mecha-nisms than it is to make claims for full comprehension, especially when the comprehen-sion leads, logically or not, to some sort of action. When it comes to serious illness, the public tends, understandably, to be more skeptical about the skeptics, more willing to believe the true believers. It is medicine's oldest dilemma, not to be settled by candor or any kind of rhetoric: what it needs is a lot of patience, waiting for science to come in, as it has in the past, with the solid facts.
(Lewis Thomas, "On Magic in Medicine," cited by Goldbloom & Lawrence, 1990, p. xv).

The passage above appeared in the preface by Goldbloom and Lawrence (1990), editors of *Preventing Disease: Beyond the Rhetoric*, a collaboration of the Canadian Task Force on the Periodic Health Exam and the U.S. Preventa-tive Services Task Force. In the preface of the 488-page volume, Goldbloom and Lawrence cite the suggestion of Thomas that science is the answer to many of the diseases facing humankind in the 1990s. What is disturbing is that this volume on preventing disease for medical professionals—years in the making—

had only one page dedicated to any discussion of HIV or AIDS. The medical establishment's neglect of the necessity of HIV prevention is reminiscent of Ronald Reagan's quote on the federal deficit: "Facts are stubborn things."

Perhaps the marketplace of capitalism has been the driving force behind the lack of commitment on prevention of disease. Only recently, with cost-cutting measures and other realizations of the long-term consequences of the lack of primary health care prevention, has the American public begun to recognize health care as part of the national agenda. (Presently, the United States and South Africa are the only two industrialized countries without a universal health care system.) Despite the market-oriented, profit-driven medical complex, many in the media, government, and medical community are arguing for increased federal governmental funding for AIDS beyond the 1989 level. Some, however, believe this would be disproportionate to the prevalence of diseases in the American population at large (Krauthhammer, 1990; Winkenwerder, Kessler, & Stolec, 1989).

As we examine the various criticisms and suggestions offered by the contributors to this book, examples of unethical, ineffective behavior by the media and medical establishment continue to be exposed. The coerced admission by former tennis star Arthur Ashe in April 1992 that he has AIDS presents yet another example of the inconsistencies of the modern-day media in their reporting of a disease that has killed more than 135,000 people in the United States. The concern extends beyond the important factor of informing the public about AIDS, its modes of transmission, its consequences, and possible measures of prevention. More important, it also raises questions about responsible journalism regarding the public's right to know versus an individual's right to privacy in the age of AIDS discrimination.

Because journalists tend to focus on reporting celebrity AIDS cases, often skimping on coverage of more prevalent cases, the customary questioning of the etiological mode of how the celebrity contracted AIDS becomes a highlight of the story while facts and educational messages about HIV are omitted. In Ashe's case, journalists have already raised the question in front-page articles by saying that he had become a "'legitimate' victim for whom to mourn . . . that he got AIDS the 'good way.'" (1992). As we know, HIV enters the bloodstream indiscriminately, often leading to AIDS irrespective of the mode of entry (whether it be unprotected sex, sharing of needles, exchange of bodily fluids, or blood transfusion). The American media continues to be infatuated with inquiries on the acquisition of AIDS, further raising the question of discrimination against the victims.

Despite Ashe's claim that he is 95% certain that he contracted HIV from a blood transfusion in 1983, journalists immediately raised the question of the certainty of the claim. Dr. John Hutchinson, who performed the open heart surgery on Ashe at St. Luke's Hospital in New York, called a press conference to say that he is uncertain how Ashe contracted AIDS. "There are many other ways to acquire [AIDS] than through cardiac surgery," he said in *USA Today* (Finn, 1992, p. C1).

Although journalists are trained to inquire, the ethical dimension of what to report is often more important than what not to report. The curiosity and questioning to create future stories on possible modes of transmission raise doubt, rather than ethically communicating to the public the harms associated with HIV. Just because journalists have a right to ask a question and print its response does not mean that it is the right thing to do.

Despite the fact that since 1985, only 20 people have contracted HIV from blood transfusions, the *Wall Street Journal* (Newman & Petit, 1992), reflecting the "wisdom" of the stockmarket, cited Arthur Ashe's announcement that he contracted AIDS from a blood transfusion as the reason why the companies that develop blood substitutes had strong gains during that session.

The continued perfidious media coverage of the AIDS pandemic vitiates the importance of the journalist as an educator and informant for the public. Such ethical responsibility to advocate and educate should be inherent in the case of AIDS, because it extends beyond the health, religious, and moral issues of both the journalist and society.

Abraham Lincoln said, "With public sentiment nothing can fail; without it nothing can succeed. Consequently, he who molds public opinion goes deeper than he who enacts statutes or pronounces decisions." The relevance of Lincoln's pronouncement endures today and should empower the media, the educational and health communities, and the government to prevent AIDS by informing various publics to enact change effectively.

Effective health communication is our primary and most potent weapon in preventing the spread of AIDS. Until a vaccine or cure for HIV infection is discovered, communication is all we have.

REFERENCES

Finn, R. (1992, April 9). Ashe reveals AIDS infection: Unscreened transfusion likely cause. *USA Today,* p. C1.

Goldbloom, R. B., & Lawrence, R. S. (Eds.). (1990). *Preventing disease: Beyond the rhetoric.* New York: Springer-Verlag.

Greene, L. (1992, April 9). Virus doesn't discriminate in choosing its tragic victims. *Boston Herald,* pp. 1–6.

Krauthammer, C. (1990, June 25). AIDS getting more than its share? *Time,* p. 90.

Newman, A., & Petit, D. (1992, April C6). Index jumps 2.3%; aided by Fed move, AIDS, medical stocks post strong gains. *Wall Street Journal,* p. C6.

Winkenwerder, W., Kessler, A R., & Stolec, R. M. (1989). Federal spending for illness caused by the human immunodeficiency virus. *New England Journal of Medicine, 320,* 1598–1603.

Index

Abbott Laboratories, 81
ABC-PBS AIDS drama, "In the Shadow of
     Love," 243
Acer, David, 145
ACT UP, 8, 92, 95
     baseball stadium demonstration, 96, 99,
          104
     boycotts, 97
     chapters, 93
     demonstrations, public, 93–97, 99, 100,
          104, 106
     internal conflict, 95–97, 104–105, 107
     promoting safer sex and safer drug use,
          93, 97–103
     social reform agenda, 93, 97, 103–108,
          181
     Stop the Church demonstration, 94–96,
          104
     successes of, 106–107, 180
     treatments and support of people with
          AIDS, 93, 97, 103

ACT UP/Women and AIDS Book Group, 93,
     95, 97–104
Adolescents, 10, 16, 74
     AIDS death rate, 216–217
     AIDS impact on, 10
     AIDS intervention approaches, 17
     counseling, 83, 218–219, 224
     education, 83
     indicated behavioral change, 17
     lack of HIV/AIDS prevention programs
          for, 215
     public failure to address risk, 215
     selective behavioral change, 17,
          215
     sexual and drug activities, 215
     universal behavior change, 17
Adolescent AIDS Program (NYC), 10,
     216–226
Advocacy, 92–97, 102, 222–225
Advocate, 95, 96
Africa, 1, 125, 177

AIDS:
   (*See also* Strategic Prevention
      Communication Campaigns)
   activism, 8, 28–29, 91–108, 157–158,
      181, 216, 222
     empowerment, 107
     impact of, 107
   acquisition risk of infection, 16, 18, 20,
      75–78, 80, 141, 145, 148, 152, 256
   art and, 2, 93
   attitudes toward, 120–121, 133, 235
   awareness of, 9, 26–27, 29, 151–152, 166,
      218–219, 224, 226
   behavioral modification, 124
   beliefs about, 115, 120, 123, 126,
      157–158, 179–180, 182, 217, 256
     (*See also* Health Threat
       Communication)
   case studies, 77, 78
     (*See also* Media coverage of AIDS)
   communication strategies, 3
   communicative barriers and, 221
     control (self) issues, 97–101, 103, 108,
      113–115, 123, 129, 132–136
   counseling, 83, 218, 219
     parental consent/knowledge of, 218,
      224
   crisis
     class oppression, 105
     discrimination, 104–105
     global, 175–176, 234
     heterosexism, 105, 122
     homophobia, 79, 105
     medical-economic problem in U.S.,
      175–177, 180, 183, 186, 234
     racism, 104–105
     sexism, 104–105
     socioeconomic problem, 104–105, 113,
      126, 130, 175, 180–183, 205,
      235, 241
     tax policy/implications, 180–181
   definition of, new CDC, 76, 233
   denial, 64, 122, 180
     (*See also* FRAIDS, fear of aids)
   diagnosed cases of AIDS in U.S., 56, 222,
      233–234
     of HIV, 143, 149, 175–176
     projected, 233–244
   education prevention, 234
     training in teaching prevention,
      224–227

   epidemic, 126, 176, 179, 203–205, 215,
      233–234, 243
     control of, 233
     epicenter, 1
     estimated cases of, 1, 76, 233–244
     expenditures, U.S., 176–177
     individual/collective response to, 179,
      184
   facts, 75–78, 127, 141, 239
   family/friends' involvement, 56, 237,
      243
   fear of, 7–8, 71–75, 80–81, 84, 123, 132
     cataloguing/categorizing, 123
     diagnostic debate/controversy, 72–73,
      80–81
     labeling, 71–72
     irrational reaction, types of, 82
     and psychiatric disorder, 72, 73, 113
     and psychology of denial, 122
   financial constraints, 26–27
   funding, 3, 218
     program, 225–226, 256
     research, 107
   global impact, 177, 234
     prevention, 235
   groups at risk, 120, 126, 183
     highest risk, 16, 20, 241
   guilt and, 78
   health care system response, 55
   hysteria, 145, 147, 149, 223
   individual risk, 16, 18, 20, 120, 126, 128,
      134, 176, 179, 203, 209
     high risk, 209, 241
     low risk, 145
   information, 177–180
     accessibility, 102, 255
     accuracy, 75, 102, 122, 123, 126–127,
      142
     availability, 73, 74–75, 102, 128, 144,
      176, 255
     disinformation, 8, 126, 234
     hotlines, 79
     inaccuracy, 75, 122, 124, 126–127
     misinformation, 84, 98, 122, 133,
      141–142, 148, 179, 220
     misunderstanding/confusion, 123–124,
      134, 142, 219
     omission, 123, 142, 256
   issues, 129
     quality of life, 113–115, 121–123,
      132–136, 189

leadership crisis, 91–92, 126, 159,
    247–248
managing the illness, 55, 176, 186,
    209–213
    neurological manifestations, 209–213
        (illus), 210
    neurosurgical management, 210–213
media coverage, 141–149, 256–257
mortality rate, 75
Names Project, 2
1980s view of, 1, 122
perception of AIDS
    adolescents and college students, 120
    medical community, 205–206
phobia, 71–73, 79
prevention, 152, 155, 160, 176, 256
    information, 113–115, 125
public health communication campaigns, 5,
    98, 176–177
    public prevention campaigns, 5
    strategies, 84, 98, 127, 129, 216–227,
        240–242
origin, 181, 182, 243
solution to, 8, 255–257
spread of, 106, 123–124, 126, 128, 141,
    148, 175, 177, 183
stereotypical constructs of, 2, 74, 126,
    130, 216–217, 227, 256
threat, 130–131
    perceived (see Health Threat
        Communication)
transmission of, 145, 147, 152
    health care professional statistics, 124,
        145, 147, 217
treatment and support, 93, 97–98, 103,
    105, 108, 176, 178, 191, 203–213,
    234, 237
    preventive treatment and support,
        103
    therapies, 98
U.S. diagnosed AIDS cases, 56, 222,
    233–234
    projected, 233–234
U.S. diagnosed HIV cases, 143, 149,
    175–176
U.S. deaths, 123, 143, 149, 175–176, 216,
    237, 256
    adolescent, 216
    projected deaths, 1, 76
U.S. prevention of, 3, 9, 15, 84
    failure to act, 104

    strategies to overcome, 26, 135,
        255–257
    vaccine/cure, 203, 234, 248
    victims, 144
        classification, 106
    and women, 99, 104–105, 129
    workforces, impact of, 177
AIDS Action Council, 146
AIDS Action 2000 Plan, 10–11, 233,
    237–248, (illus.) 238
AIDS and Adolescent Network, 217
The AIDS Caregiver Handbook, 56
AIDS Coalition to Network, Organize and
    Win (ACT NOW), 93
AIDS Coalition to Unleash Power, (see ACT
    UP)
AIDS decade (1981–1991), 142, 174, 235
AIDS education, 94, 102
    of adolescents, 10, 74, 83, 102, 107, 117,
        135–136, 216–226
    of children, 135–136, 151, 216–226
    of college students, 73–74, 82–83, 102,
        131, 135–136, 240
    of groups, 16, 106, 183, 235, 240
    of people of color, 107, 160, 183
    of prisoners, 106–107
    preventive, 233–248
    of prostitutes, 106–107, 235
    of the public, 2, 94, 114, 165–166
    of women, 106–107
    (See also Adolescent AIDS Program)
AIDS antibody testing, 141
    universal testing, 176
    (See also (HIV/AIDS antibody testing)
"AIDS is everybody's business" leaflet, 94
    (See also ACT UP, FDA)
AIDS Legal Task Force, 206
AIDS-related complex (ARC), 2, 191
Albert Einstein College of Medicine, 217
Alzheimer's disease, 108
AMA (see American Medical Association)
American Responds to AIDS, 29
American Medical Association (AMA) 147,
    206–207
Americans With Disabilities Act, 206
Anal intercourse, 221, 256
ARC (see AIDS related complex)
Ashe, Arthur, 165, 234, 256–257
Atlantic Monthly, 121–123
Audiologists, 190, 192
AZT (zidovudine), 107, 161, 219

Behavior modification, 115–117, 121–123,
    134–135, 176–177, 179–180, 182–183,
    220, 235, 239, 245
Behavioral theory (see Theory)
Bergalis, Kimberly, 134, 142, 145, 147, 176,
    181, 182
Bisexuality, 123, 125, 148, 152, 157
Blake, Dorothy, 178
Blood screening, 125
Blood testing, 206
Blood transfusions, 147, 179, 209, 216,
    256–257
Bodily fluids, 25
Bush, George, 148

Campaigns, AIDS, 6, 18, 23–30, 131, 178,
    179, 217, 239–240, 242, 248
    agenda, 239–240
    AIDS Action 2000 Plan, 233–248
    appeals, 239
    Global AIDS Program, 178–179
    goals of, 178
    Grim Reaper campaign, 114
    L.A. cares . . . like a Mother campaign,
        211
    Sex Respect, 131
    "Stop AIDS" campaign, 141
Campaign: evaluation and reorientation, 23,
    25, 26, 28, 29–32, 178–179, 235
    implementation, 27
    objectives, 30, 179
    success, 29
    (See also Strategic HIV/AIDS Prevention
        Communication Campaigns)
Canadian Task Force on the Periodic Health
    Exam, 255
Cancer, 108
Capitalism, 256
Care Partners, 55–58
    normative standard per AIDS care
        management, 56, 192
    relations with medical personnel,
        57
    stress, strain, burnout, 56
    support groups for, 56
    triadic model in quality health care
        delivery, 56
    (See also COAST Model of Health
        Communication as Negotiation)

Case, Patricia, 103
Catholic policy/position on AIDS, 92, 94–99,
    222
Centers for Disease Control, U.S. (CDC), 29,
    124, 142, 147, 149, 176, 179, 207,
    209, 233–234, 239–240, 242
    CDC health care worker infection
        statistics, 79–80
    CDC "Recommendations for Prevention of
        HIV Transmission in Health-Care
        Settings," 207
    CDC Universal Guidelines for infection
        control, 78
Center for Population Options, 131
Channel Analysis and Selection, 26, 235
    interpersonal, 26
    marketing mix, 27
    mass media, 27
    maximization of, 26
    mediated, 26
    types of, 26
    (See also Strategic HIV/AIDS Prevention
        Communication Campaigns)
Chris, Cynthia, 100
Civil litigation, AIDS-related, 206, 226
    study, 81
COAST Model of Health Communication as
    Negotiation, 10, 235–237, 242,
    244–245
    (See also trust)
College students, 73–74
    HIV seroprevalence, 74
    sexual practices, 82–83
Communication, 190–191, 255
    HIV/AIDS prevention and, 255
    message development, 237
    models, 235, 237
    skills, 226, 244
Communication devices, 195–197, 200
Communication disorders in people with AIDS
    cognitive-linguistic function, 191, 194
    communicative function, 190
    message comprehension, 190–191,
        193–194, 198
    message conveyance, 194–196, 200
    patient compliance, 189
    reports, 189
    speech problems, 195, 197
Communication strategies
    of AIDS, 3
    implementation of, 6

planning of, 6
prerequisites to, 6
proactive, 10
(*See also* Strategic HIV/AIDS Prevention
    Communication Campaigns)
Communicative barriers: per HIV/AIDS
    response, 221
    function, 190
Community outreach, 100–101, 181, 217,
    222–225, 241, 247
Condoms, 21, 76, 82, 84, 94, 99, 101, 102,
    105, 107, 120, 124, 127, 132–134,
    154, 176, 219, 220, 222, 225–226, 240
    distribution, 94
    female, 220
Conference, AIDS, 242
Confirmation of a Candidate paradigm,
    163–164
    assessing media coverage, 163
    phases of, 164
Confirmation paradigm, 163–164
Cosmopolitan, 115, 125, 129, 134
*Covering the Plague—AIDS and the American
    Media,* 143

Delaney, Martin, 108
Dannemeyer, William, 146, 181, 182
Dental dams, 101, 102, 129
Discrimination, AIDS
    criminal law, 176
    employment, 176, 179, 206, 220
    health care/benefits, 176, 181, 220
    housing, 176, 179, 181
    insurance, 81, 176, 179, 181, 184, 206
    personal liberties, 176
Disorders: AIDS-related, 191, 194–197
    communication, 189
    dementing, 190, 197–200, 209
    HIV-based, 190
    strategies to deal with persons with varying
        disorders, 192–193, 196–200
Depression, 136
DiPaolo, Joey, 224
Discriminating (sexual) partner choice,
    127–128, 130, 133–135, 219
Disease: historical substrate, 204–205
    prevention, 255–257
    sexually transmitted, 204, 209, 226, 235
    states, 209–210
"Doctors, Liars, and Women" video, 98

Doctor-Patient (*see* Physician-Patient)
Durand, Yannick, 101
Drug treatment programs, 103
Drug manufacturers (*see* pharmaceutical
    manufacturers)

Ebony Magazine, 78, 190
Effective communication, 243
    complexity of, 6, 15
    four areas strategic to, 4
    impact on patient recovery, 4, 189
    of individuals with impaired
        communication ability, 189–200
Emerson College Aids conference, 242
Employers, 177, 242
Epidemics, 204–205 (*See also* AIDS epidemic)
Events, AIDS awareness, 242
Exchange theory (*see* Theory)

Families and AIDS, 56, 218, 224–227
    home care, 56
Fauci, Tony, 106
Federal government funding for HIV/AIDS:
    programs, 256
    research, 107
Federation of Parents Association, 223
Fernandez, Joseph A., 222–225
Fettner, Ann, 105
First Amendment rights: of free speech/free
    press, 184, 185
Food and Drug Administration (FDA), 92, 94,
    144
    policy on drugs for treating AID 92, 105,
        107
Formative research, 23, 25–26
    concept development, 25
    testing and evaluation, 25–26
    (*See also* Consumer orientation)
FRAIDS, 7–8, 71–75, 78, 79, 83–84, 122,
    180
    contributing factors to, 73
    treatment of, 8, 72–73, 80–81

Gay and Lesbian Community Center, 91
Gay Men's Health Crisis, 56, 92
Gay organizations, 92
    leadership crisis, 92
General Program Against AIDS, 178

Gertz, Alison, 130, 134
Global AIDS Program, 178
Gonorrhea, 2
Gould, Robert, 125–126
Grabowski, Henry, 92

Hall, Arsenio, 147, 152, 157
Halston, 151
Harris, Jeffrey, 126
Health care delivery, 57
   concept of illness trajectories, 57
   context of, 57
   criticisms of, 55
   financing issues, 176, 177, 256
   locus of care, 56–57, 62–67
   percent of GNP, 244
   primacy of physician–patient relationship,
     57
   rationing, 178
   triadic model, 55, 57, 68
Health care as negotiation, 5, 59–62
Health communication:
   as academic field, 5
   areas strategic to, 4
   benefits of, 5, 6, 236–237
   care partners, 7 (*See also* Care Partners)
   COAST Model of Health Communication,
     10, 235–237
   complexity of, 6
   compliance
     health care professionals, 98, 236–237,
       244
     patient, 37, 55, 236–237, 244
   components of, 6, 235–236
     to individual health, 6
     to public health, 6
   control theories, 4, 5, 8
   definition of, 3–5
   as negotiation, 37–38, 55, 235–237
   neoAristotlelean approach to, 5
   patient satisfaction, 244
   philosophy of ancient Greece, 4
   as preventive health approach, 6
   role of, 3
   themes of, 2
   triad, 7, 55–68
   view of, 4, 5
Health insurance companies, 91–92
Health Threat Communication, 117–132
Hearst, Norman, 127–129

Helms, Jesse, 97
Hemophilia, 144, 181, 182, 209, 216
Heterosexual:
   confusion, 132
   community, 142
   HIV/AIDS statistics, 121, 123–126, 130,
     132, 221
Heterosexuality, 148
   U.S. cases of, 182
HIV, 2, 103
   incubation period, 75–76
   infection prevention, 76
HIV/AIDS antibody tests, 103
   testing, 77, 79, 141, 176, 182, 206–207,
     209
   universal, of health care professionals,
     176, 182, 207, 209
HIV/AIDS counseling, 244
HIV/AIDS disclosure, 151, 153, 154, 158,
     165, 219–220, 256–257
HIV/AIDS Education Teams, 224–225
HIV/AIDS health care delivery, 57
HIV/AIDS infection statistics, 56, 126, 128,
     129, 131, 142, 147, 175–177, 199,
     209
HIV/AIDS leadership, 91–92, 159, 222–227
HIV/AIDS Prevention Communication
     Campaigns
   (*see* Strategic HIV/AIDS Prevention
     Communication Campaigns)
HIV/AIDS reporting, 76–77
   by CDC, 76
   by physicians, 76–77
   by state law, 76–77
HPA-23, 144
HTLV-III, 2
Home care, 56
   increasing need for, 56
Home health care market, 55
Home Health Services, 56
   care partner involvement, 55–56
   family involvement, 56
   Medicare spending, 55
   Medicaid payments, 55
   outpatient treatment, 62
Homophobia, 79, 105
Homosexuals, males, 131, 221
Hudson, Rock, 142–144, 151, 234
Hulley, Stephen, 127–129
Human immunodeficiency virus
   (*see* HIV)

Human T-cell lymphotropic virus Type III (*see* HTLV-III)

Illegal drug use, 16, 17
  IV drug use, 22, 74, 102–103, 106, 126, 131, 146, 148, 157
  safer drug use, 98, 102–103, 106, 107
Illness
  AIDS-related, 98
  care partners involvement in, 55–68
  chronicity of, 7, 56
  definition of, 4
  management of, 55–68, 210–213
  trajectories, 57, 62
"In the Shadow of Love," 243
Infotainment, 149, 181–182, 187, 216–217
Institute for Immunological Disorders, 91
Insurance
  companies, 91–92
  discrimination, 81, 176, 179, 181, 184, 206
  national health, 178–179
Inter-tect Agency, 81

Jackson, Jesse, 152–153
Jamaica, 178
Jeffries, Leonard, 181–182
Johnson, Earvin (Magic), 114, 142, 147–149, 151–165
  global attention, 151
  media content analysis relating to HIV/AIDS disclosure, 152–164
    spokesperson conversion process, 154, 157–160, 165
Jong, Erica, 122
Journal of American Medical Association, 127, 128
Journalistic practices, 141–142, 256

Kimberly Bergalis Patient and Health Provider Act of 1991, 146
Kinsella, James, 143
Koch, Edward, 94, 100
Koop, C. Everett, 147, 182
Kramer, Larry, 91–92, 96, 98, 107
Krim, Matilda, 123
Kroger, Fred, 242

Leadership, national (AIDS), 247
Lurie, Rachel, 102, 106

Mansell, Peter, 91, 92
Massachusetts Institute of Technology, 126
Masters and Johnson, 126
Media campaigns, 2–3
Media coverage of AIDS, 8, 23, 95, 106, 142–143, 149, 151–166, 175, 177, 183–187
  celebrities, 8–9, 141–149, 165, 184–185, 256
  content analysis of, 9, 141–149, 152–154, (Illus.) 155, (Illus.) 156, 180, 181, 183
  characterization of HIV/AIDS victims, 114, 144, 146, 179–184, 216–217, 256
  criticisms of, 184, 255–257
  editorial policies, 184
  effectiveness of education, 8, 142–144, 146, 165, 177, 181–185, 256
  ethic of, 9, 149, 165–166, 180, 184–185, 235, 243, 256
  fear of media coverage, 95
  magazine coverage, 8, 114, 151
  mass media coverage, 114
  newspaper coverage, 114, 151
    agendas and biases, 164
    editorial policies, 184
  press coverage, 8
    performance, 165
    possible phases, 153
  profit motives, 184, 187
  proposed policy governing media coverage of HIV/AIDS, 186–187, 241
  public's "right to know," 184–185, 256
  radio, 114
  results of, 9
  sensationalization of, 8, 216, 234
  stages of, 8, 147–149
  substantive issues, 143
  target audience of, 152
  television, 114, 143, 144, 147, 151–152, 157, 158, 223–224, 243, 245
  trends, 158
Mediated image, 153, 154, 157, 158, 164, 165
Mediated reality, 152–154, 157, 159–163

Medical residents attitudes regarding AIDS
    patients, 61, 205–206
Medicaid payments, HIV/AIDS, 56
Medical establishment:
    AIDS policy, 206–207
    conservatism, 108
    major teaching and research hospitals, 108
    neglect of HIV prevention, 256
    perceptions, 205–206
    research
        institutes, 108
        priorities, 178
    unethical behavior, 243, 256
Medicare spending, HIV/AIDS, 56
Montefiore Medical Center, 217
Munchausen syndrome, 72

National Academy of Sciences, 75
National Cancer Institute, 18
National Commission on AIDS, 147, 175,
    177, 234
National Institute of Allergies and Infectious
    Diseases, 106
National Institute on Deafness and Other
    Communication Disorders Task Force,
    191
National Research Council, 25
National Security, U.S., 177
National Strategic Research Plan, 191
Needle exchange programs, 103, 107
Needles, 17, 22, 98, 102, 120, 131, 179, 256
Neurosurgery, 209–211
New Museum of Contemporary Art, 93
New York City Adolescent AIDS Program
    (see Adolescent AIDS Program)
New York City Board of Education, 222, 223
    (See also Adolescent AIDS Program)
New York University News Study Group,
    141–142
Nichols, Henry, 216
Nichols, Marie H., 11
Noble, Robert, 132

O'Connor, Catholic Archbishop John Cardinal,
    94

Padian, Nancy, 124–125
Pearl, Monica, 102

Pharmaceutical manufacturers, 92, 105,
    108
Physician
    AIDS knowledge, 98
    attitudes toward people with AIDS,
        205–206
    educational training of, 3, 80, 203, 205,
        244
    preventive measures against AIDS, 203,
        243
    responsibility, 206
    traditional role in patient care,
        203–204
    treatment of persons with AIDS, 98
    trust, loss of, 203
Physician-patient communication
    as genre, 4, 235–237
    education, 203
    gatekeeping, 57–58
    impact on patient recovery, 4,
        236–237
Physician-patient relationship, 37–38, 57
    information exchange, 58
    gatekeeping, 57, 58
    primacy of, 57
POISE, 3
Policymaking, 2, 76, 78, 176–178, 180–187,
    227
President's National Advisory Commission on
    AIDS, 148
Prevention messages, 127
    (See also Campaigns, Strategic Health
        Communication Campaign Model,
        and Strategic HIV/AIDS Prevention
        Communication Campaigns)
Prisoners, 106, 107
Project Inform, 108
Promiscuity, 122, 160
Prostitutes, 106, 107, 128, 209, 216,
    235
Public:
    health strategy, 15, 257
    policy debate, 176
    policy issues, 176
    state laws, 76

Racism, 106
Reagan, Ronald, 126, 144
Risk Evaluation Program (REP), 216
    (See also Adolescent AIDS Program)

Safer drug use, 98, 102–103
Safer sex, 17, 83 98–102
  for women, 100–101, 105, 107, 124
St. Patrick's Cathedral, 94–95, 104
Schwartzkof, Norman, 216
Seligman, Martin, 135–136
Sexual abuse, 220–221
Sexual history disclosure, 128, 146, 148, 160,
  182, 221, 240
  private investigators, 81
Sexual partner selection, 133
Sexual practices, 16, 17, 81–84, 94, 100, 102,
  120–122, 124, 127–131, 134, 148,
  152, 209, 216, 219–221
  high risk, 122, 209
  survival sex, 220–221
Sexual segregation, 176
Shanti Project, 5
Shea Stadium, 96, 99, 100, 104
Skills, communication, 226, 244
  (*See also* Health communication as
    negotiation)
Social activism, 105
Social awareness, 106
Social Marketing Process, 27
  (*See also* Campaign implementation)
Social reform, 8
Souter, David, 104
South Africa, 256
Speech-language pathologists, 190, 197
Staley, Peter, 96–97, 105–106
Strategic Health Communication Campaign
  Model, 6, (illus.) 19
  communication analysis, 18, 23–27
    target audience analysis, 23–24,
      234–235
    segment audience groups, 23–24,
      234–235, 240, 241
    formative research, 23, 25–26
    channel selection, 23–24
  evaluation/reorientation, 18, 29–31
  implementation, 18, 27–29
  predictive value, 21
  prevention messages, 21
  stages of, 18–30
Strategic HIV/AIDS Prevention
  Communication Campaigns, 15, 82,
  243
  and behavioral change, 15–17, 18–19, 22,
    23
  incentives, 22

audience identification, 20
audience/program planner interaction, 20,
  100
campaign objectives, 19–20, 25, 28
conclusions of, 31–32
consumer orientation, 20, 100
cost-effective evaluation, 30
evaluation (*see* Outcome evaluation)
goals of, 15, 19–20
implementation, 27
message strategies, 16–17, 100
monitoring for changes, trends, 20
organizational restraints, 20
outcome evaluation, 30
principles of, 18
process evaluation, 28
recommendations, 30–31
target groups, 16
  adolescent, 10, 16, 17
  highest risk, 16
  interrelated risks, 16
  low risk, 16, 145
  participatory planning, 17, 20
Student programs
  New York City Adolescent AIDS Program,
    10, 217–227
Students, 73–74, 82–83, 94, 131, 176, 179
Suicide, AIDS-related, 224
Surveys, 204, 240
Syphilis, 3
Syringes, 17

Teenage sexuality, 130–131, 133
Theory:
  Behavior theory, 21, 23
    levels of analysis (5) of, 23
    predictive value, 23
    strategic planning value, 23
  Exchange theory, 21
    Costs of, 21, 27
    Benefits of, 21–22
    Product promotion, 21, 28
    Service promotion, 21
Time, 121, 131, 133
Trust, 207, 220–221

U.S. Centers for Disease Control (*see* Centers
  for Disease Control)
U.S. Preventive Task Force, 255

U.S. Public Health Service, 81
University of California, San Francisco
    (UCSF), School of Medicine, AIDS
    Coordination Council Task Force on
    AIDS, 207
University of Southern California Medical
    Center, 211

Village Voice, 92

Wachter, Robert M., 106–107
Wall Street, 100
White, Ryan, 144, 151, 181, 182, 216
Wilson, Hank, 95
Women's Day, 99
Women's Health Action and Mobilization
    (WHAM!), 99
World Health Organization, 178

Zidovudine (AZT), 107, 161, 219
Zimbabwe, 177